Adolescent Medicine: Pharmacotherapeutics in Medical Disorders

Edited by Donald E. Greydanus, Dilip R. Patel, Hatim A. Omar,
Cynthia Feucht and Joav Merrick

Health, Medicine and Human Development

Edited by
Joav Merrick

Health is a key component of human development, growth, and quality of life. The *Health, Medicine and Human Development* book series aims to provide a public forum for book publications from a multidisciplinary group of researchers, practitioners, and clinicians for an international professional forum interested in the broad spectrum of health, medicine, and human development. We welcome research on a wide variety of substantive areas that will promote and impact healthy human development, including prevention, intervention, and care also among people in vulnerable conditions.

Bricker JT, Omar HA, Merrick J, eds.
Adults with Childhood Illnesses: Considerations for Practice.
Berlin: de Gruyter, 2011.
ISBN 978-3-11-025521-8
e-ISBN 978-3-11-025568-3

Derevensky JL, Shek D, Merrick J, eds.
Youth Gambling: The Hidden Addiction.
Berlin: De Gruyter, 2011.
ISBN 978-3-11-025520-1
e-ISBN 978-3-11-025569-0

Greydanus DE, Patel DR, Omar HA, Feucht C, Merrick J, eds.
Adolescent Medicine: Pharmacotherapeutics in General, Mental and Sexual Health
Berlin: De Gruyter, 2012.
ISBN 978-3-11-025522-5
ISBN 978-3-11-025570-6

Adolescent Medicine: Pharmacotherapeutics in Medical Disorders

Edited by
Donald E. Greydanus, Dilip R. Patel, Hatim A. Omar,
Cynthia Feucht and Joav Merrick

DE GRUYTER

Editors

Donald E. Greydanus, MD
Michigan State University
College of Human Medicine
Kalamazoo, MI
United States
Greydanus@kcms.msu.edu

Dilip R. Patel, MD
Michigan State University
College of Human Medicine
Kalamazoo, MI
United States

Hatim A. Omar, MD
Division of Adolescent Medicine
Kentucky Children's Hospital
University of Kentucky, Lexington
United States
haomar2@uky.edu

Cynthia L. Feucht, PHARMD
Ferris State University
School of Pharmacy
Kalamazoo, MI
United States
cynthia.feucht@gmail.com

Joav Merrick, MD, MMedSc, DMSc
National Institute of Child Health and Human
Development
Ministry of Social Affairs
Jerusalem
Israel
jmerrick@zahav.net.il

ISBN 978-3-11-027580-3
e-ISBN 978-3-11-027636-7

Library of Congress Cataloging-in-Publication Data
A CIP catalog record for this book has been applied for at the Library of Congress.

Bibliographic information published by the Deutsche Nationalbibliothek
The Deutsche Nationalbibliothek lists this publication in the Deutsche Nationalbibliografie;
detailed bibliographic data are available in the Internet at http://dnb.dnb.de.

Typesetting: Apex CoVantage
Printing: Hubert & Co. GmbH & Co. KG, Göttingen
Cover image: iStockphoto/Thinkstock

♾ Printed on acid-free paper
Printed in Germany
www.degruyter.com

Dedication

Finis coronat opus

This book is dedicated to Adele Dellenbaugh Hofmann (1926–2001), who was a leading force in the development of adolescent medicine in the twentieth century. This "fifth" is for you, Adele, a woman for all times and for all seasons.

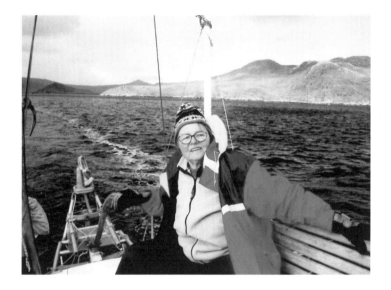

Adele Hofmann was a founder of the Society for Adolescent Medicine and served as its president from 1976 to 1977. The next year she founded the Section on Adolescent Health as a unit within the American Academy of Pediatrics, which now gives an award in her name.

She contended that the passage to adulthood and emancipation meant difficult years for children and parents.

> *"What we're talking about is a decade," she once said, "an age of human growth and development that has tremendously unique things happening emotionally and biologically."*

Over the years she published many articles on the legal rights of minors, teenage behavior and sexuality, and youths with special risks. Together with Donald Graydanus she wrote the authoritative textbook *Adolescent Medicine*, which was first published in 1986 and won an award from the American College of Internal Medicine the year after and went into its third edition in 1997 at McGraw Hill, where it remains in print.

She also wrote *The Hospitalized Adolescent* (1976), which received an American Nurses Association award, and *Consent and Confidentiality in Child and Adolescent Care* (1984).

She was born in Boston, a granddaughter of Frederick Samuel Dellenbaugh, an artist, writer, and explorer. She graduated from Smith College in 1948 and from the University of Rochester Medical School in 1952. She trained at Babies Hospital of Columbia Presbyterian Medical Center and was a National Foundation Fellow in Endocrinology at Presbyterian Hospital. She directed pediatric and adolescent programs at New York University, Bellevue Hospital, St Luke's Hospital, and Beth Israel Hospital, all in New York. After moving to California, she was affiliated with the Children's Hospital of Orange County and the University of California at Irvine.

Contents

    10.3.1 Enzymes and cellular receptors associated with
           lipid metabolism 237
10.4 Familial hypercholesterolemias. 238
10.5 Secondary hyperlipidemia 239
    10.5.1 Management 239
    10.5.2 Anticoagulants. 242
10.6 Syncope. 244
    10.6.1 Management 244
10.7 Cardiac evaluation for ADHD medication 245
10.8 Conclusions 247

11 Pulmonary disorders 249
    John H. Marks

    11.1 Introduction 249
    11.2 Community-acquired pneumonia 249
        11.2.1 Epidemiology. 250
        11.2.2 Diagnosis 250
        11.2.3 Pharmacologic management 251
    11.3 Cystic fibrosis. 252
        11.3.1 Epidemiology. 253
        11.3.2 Differential diagnosis 253
        11.3.3 Pharmacologic management 253
        11.3.4 Management of chronic cystic fibrosis 255
    11.4 Asthma 257
        11.4.1 Epidemiology. 258
        11.4.2 Differential diagnosis 258
        11.4.3 Pharmacological management. 258
    11.5 Conclusions 265

12 Musculoskeletal disorders and sports injuries 269
    Cynthia L. Feucht and Dilip R. Patel

    12.1 Introduction 269
    12.2 Salicylated NSAIDs 270
    12.3 Nonsalicylated NSAIDs 272
        12.3.1 Side effects of nonsalicylated NSAIDs. 272
        12.3.2 Drug interactions 279
        12.3.3 Efficacy of NSAIDs in musculoskeletal injuries 279
    12.4 Use and abuse of analgesics. 286
    12.5 Conclusions 288

13 Concepts of rheumatoid disorders. 293
    Donald E. Greydanus, Mary D. Moore, and Cynthia L. Feucht

    13.1 Introduction 293
        13.1.1 Symptomatology 293
        13.1.2 RD studies. 296

ACKNOWLEDGMENTS

Foreword

It was 50 years ago that adolescent medicine became recognized in the United States as a new field of clinical practice focused on the unique needs of youth transitioning from childhood to adulthood through a decade of complex physical and psychosocial changes (1). In 1960 J. Roswell Gallagher at the Boston Children's Hospital, often considered the founder of the field, published the first textbook, titled *Medical Care of the Adolescent*, that helped to establish recognition for the enthusiastic physicians setting up adolescent clinics and inpatient units primarily in university pediatric departments across the United States (2). As the specialty grew, academic faculty, including now iconic names like Stan Friedman and Elizabeth McAnarney, began publishing a number of excellent comprehensive textbooks on adolescent care.

Adele Hofmann, with the strong contributions of her former fellow Donald E Greydanus, published *Adolescent Medicine* in 1983 (3). It was followed by second and third editions (1989, 1997) with Hofmann and Greydanus as editors, and, in 2006, a fourth edition in her memory edited by Greydanus and renamed *Essential Adolescent Medicine* (4). For those of us privileged to have contributed chapters to these and the many other superb texts on adolescent medicine published over the years and more importantly for those of us using them daily as references in our clinical practice, caring for teens, one constraint has been very clear. Owing to limited space in each chapter, only a minimal discussion can be included about medications and drug therapy. In the twenty-first century, a vast number of pharmacologic agents are becoming available and widely used in adolescents. Major advances in medical treatment have resulted, along with direct marketing of drugs to consumers by the pharmaceutical industry, increased patient expectations of a drug for every symptom, and professional concern about overmedicating youth, making the need for full information about medication management a high priority.

It was also some 50 years ago, in 1961, that Senator Estes Kefauver proposed the legislation that the U.S. Food and Drug Administration (FDA) be given the authority to require that pharmaceutical firms prove their drugs were effective and safe before putting them on the market. Although this safeguard is taken for granted by consumers today, prior to this there was no such requirement. After much debate about whether the government should be given such authority (the Kefauver hearings), the legislation passed. It also resulted in the legally mandated "package insert" intended to provide drug information, although most clinicians find its contents to be minimally useful (5). Internet searches for drug information primarily produce the same package insert text.

Health professionals today are expected to adhere to scientific, evidence-based treatment guidelines, yet we who treat adolescents face several challenges. With the exception of medications for a few specific conditions such as attention deficit disorder, many pharmaceuticals still have not been tested in adolescent populations. The assumption has long been that when adult body weight is reached (typically 110 lb), drug pharmacodynamics become similar and therefore dosages, side effects, risks, and adverse reactions are largely extrapolated from the adult literature. Searching independently for research or treatment reviews that address adolescent patients can be time-consuming and confusing. Hence those of us prescribing medications for teens have had little age-specific "evidence" to rely on.

Relying on the regulatory role of the FDA to ensure safety of pharmacologic choices can also be problematic. As concern about postmarketing adverse drug reactions has increased, the FDA has increased its use of "black box warnings." In November 2004, owing to studies suggesting risk to bone health, the FDA put a black box warning on the very effective long-acting injectable contraceptive Depo-Provera, widely used in teens, and advised limiting its use to 2 years. As a result, thousands of adolescents began stopping Depo-Provera in 2005 (6). During the following 2 years (2006–2007), there was a temporary increase in U.S. teen pregnancy rates after years of steady decline (7). In 2004 the FDA also put a black box warning on the antidepressants known as selective serotonin reuptake inhibitors (SSRIs), advising that their use in children and adolescents could increase risk of suicidal thoughts. Antidepressant prescription rates for teens promptly decreased, but then adolescent suicide rates unexpectedly increased by 18%, again after years of decline (8). These two examples are not presented as cause and effect and many other factors may be related to the associated findings. The key conclusion is that since most of the important health issues of adolescents involve pharmacological treatment, the risks and benefits of such choices must be well understood. That is, a reliable source of detailed information and discussion is urgently needed, especially for clinicians in primary care.

The editors of this book have done a superb job of filling this need. Dr. Donald Greydanus and his talented coeditors have assembled a team of international experts on specific adolescent medical conditions to discuss the state-of-the-art pharmacologic treatment of the principal disorders in their fields. The full range of common conditions is covered and each chapter includes a brief discussion of the definition, epidemiology, and differential diagnosis of the condition. Each then proceeds with a full discussion of the medications used in treatment management. Busy office practitioners will be especially grateful that the information presented is succinct and useful.

This is the first textbook on adolescent medicine focused specifically on the medications used to treat the common clinical diagnoses of this age group. It will quickly become an invaluable reference kept close within reach next to the health professional's favorite adolescent medicine clinical textbook. I am excited to recommend it highly to the many physicians and allied health professionals dedicated to providing excellent primary care for adolescents in a wide range of clinical settings throughout the United States and internationally. This is the long-needed book we have been waiting for; it will maximize our ability to recommend the best treatment plans for our new-millennium adolescent patients.

Roberta K. Beach, MD, MPH, FAAP
Professor Emerita, Pediatrics and Adolescent Medicine
Department of Pediatrics, Division of Adolescent Medicine
University of Colorado School of Medicine
170 Dahlia Street
Denver, CO 80220 USA
Email: DrRKBeach@msn.com

References

1. Alderman EM, Rieder J, Cohen MI. The history of adolescent medicine. Pediatr Res 2003;54(1):137–47.
2. Gallagher JR. Medical Care of the Adolescent. New York: Appleton-Century-Crofts; 1960.
3. Hofmann AD. Adolescent Medicine. Menlo Park, CA: Addison-Wesley; 1983.
4. Greydanus DE, Patel DR, Pratt HD. Essential Adolescent Medicine. New York: McGraw-Hill; 2006.
5. Avorn J. Teaching clinicians about drugs – 50 years later, Whose job is it? N Engl J Med 2011;364(13):1185–7.
6. Omar HA, Kives S. Depot medroxyprogesterone acetate (DMPA, Depo-Provera) in adolescents: What is next after the FDA black box warning. J Pediatr Adolesc Gynecol 2005;18(3):183.
7. Martin JA, Hamilton BE, Sutton PD, and Ventura SJ. Births: Final data for 2008. Natl Vital Statistics Rep 2010;59(1): 1. http://www.cdc.gov/nchs/data/nvsr/nvsr59/nvsr59_01.pdf.
8. Brent D. Antidepressants and suicidal behavior: Cause or cure? Am J Psychiatry 2007; 164:989–91.

Contributors

Orhan K. Atay MD
Director, Department of Pediatric
Gastroenterology
Bronson Methodist Hospital
601 John St., Suite M-351
Kalamazoo, MI 49007
United States
Chapter 5

Roberta K. Beach MD, MPH, FAAP
Professor Emerita, Pediatrics and
Adolescent Medicine
Department of Pediatrics, Division of
Adolescent Medicine
University of Colorado School of Medicine
170 Dahlia Street
United States
DrRKBeach@msn.com
Foreword

Madeline A. Chadehumbe, M.D.
Division of Pediatric Neurology
Michigan State University
Helen DeVos Childrens Hospital
1300 Michigan St
Ste 102
Grand Rapids, MI 49503
United States
Madeline.Chadehumbe@devoschildrens.org
Chapter 4

Arthur N. Feinberg MD
Professor of Pediatrics & Human
Development
Michigan State University College of
Human Medicine
Pediatric Clinic Director
MSU/Kalamazoo Center for Medical Studies
1000 Oakland Drive
Kalamazoo, MI 49008–1284
United States
Feinberg@kcms.msu.edu
Chapter 2

Cynthia L. Feucht, PharmD., BCPS
Adjunct Professor of Pharmacy Practice
Ferris State University, School of Pharmacy
Clinical Pharmacist, Borgess Ambulatory
Care
1701 Gull Road
Kalamazoo, MI 49048
United States
cynthia.feucht@gmail.com
Chapter 8, 12, 13, 14

Renuka Gera, MD
Professor and Associate Chair, Department
of Pediatric Hematology/Oncology
Assistant Dean for the Lansing Campus
Michigan State University, College of
Human Medicine
Principal Investigator, Children's Oncology
Group
B215 Clinical Center, 138 Service Road
East Lansing, MI 48824
United States
Renuka.gera@hc.msu.edu
Chapter 6, 7

**Donald E. Greydanus MD Dr. HC
(ATHENS)**
Professor, Pediatrics & Human
Development
Michigan State University College of
Human Medicine
Pediatrics Program Director
Michigan State University/Kalamazoo
Center for Medical Studies
Kalamazoo, MI 49008–1284
United States
Greydanus@kcms.msu.edu
Chapter 1, 8, 9, 13, 14, 15

Manmohan K. Kamboj M.D
Department of Pediatric Endocrinology
Section of Endocrinology, Metabolism and
Diabetes
Nationwide Children's Hospital
700 Children's Drive (ED425)
Columbus, OH 43205
United States
Manmohan.Kamboj@
Nationwidechildrens.org
Chapter 3

Roshni Kulkarni MD
Professor and Director
Division of Pediatric & Adolescent
Hematology/Oncology
Director (Pediatric), MSU Center for
Bleeding & Clotting Disorders
Distinguished Hematology Consultant-Div.
of Blood Disorders, NCBDDD, CDC
Pediatrics & Human Development
Michigan State University
B220 Clinical Center
East Lansing, MI 48824–1313
United States
Roshni.Kulkarni@hc.msu.edu
Chapter 6

James Loker MD
Bronson Pediatric Cardiolology
Bronson Methodist Hospital
601 John St. Suite M-351
Kalamazoo, Michigan 49007 USA
United States
lokerj@bronsonhg.org
Chapter 10

John H. Marks MD
Associate Professor, Pediatrics & Human
Development
Michigan State University College of
Human Medicine
Division of Pediatric Pulmonology
Pediatrics Program
1000 Oakland Drive
Kalamazoo, MI 49008–1284
United States
Marks@kcms.msu.edu
Chapter 11

Mary D. Moore MD
Director, Pediatric Rheumatology
Michigan State University College of
Human Medicine
Pediatric Residency Training Program
Kalamazoo Center for Medical Studies
Kalamazoo, Michigan, USA
United States
Moore@kcms.msu.edu
Chapter 13

Hatim A. Omar MD
Professor, Pediatrics & Obstetrics/
Gynecology
Director, Adolescent Medicine & Young
Parents Program
University of Kentucky
Kentucky Clinic, J422
Lexington, Kentucky 40536–0284
United States
haomar2@uky.edu

Dilip R. Patel MD
Professor, Pediatrics & Human
Development
Michigan State University College of
Human Medicine
Adolescent and Sports Medicine Director
Pediatrics Program
Michigan State University/Kalamazoo
Center for Medical Studies
1000 Oakland Drive
Kalamazoo, MI 49008–1284
United States
Patel@kcms.msu.edu
Chapter 12

Elna Z. Saah, MD
Assistant Professor, Department of Pediatric
Hematology/Oncology
Michigan State University College of
Human Medicine
B215 Clinical Center, 138 Service Road
East Lansing, MI 48824
United States
elna.saah@ht.msu.edu
Chapter 6, 7

Ajovi B. Scott-Emuakpor, M.D., Ph.D.
Professor, Department of Pediatrics/Human
Development
Director, Pediatric & Adolescent Sickle Cell
Program
Division of Pediatric and Adolescent
Hematology/Oncology
Michigan State University–B220 Clinical
Center
138 Service Road
East Lansing, MI 48824–1313
United States
Scottemu@msu.edu
Chapter 6

Tor A. Shwayder MD
Director, Pediatric Dermatology
Henry Ford Medical Center
3031 Grand Boulevard
Detroit, MI 48202
United States
tshwayd1@hfhs.org
Chapter 2

Olufemi Soyode MD
Division of Pediatric Neurology
Michigan State University
Helen DeVos Childrens Hospital
1300 Michigan St
Ste 102
Grand Rapids, MI 49503
United States
olufemi.soyode@devoschildrens.org
Chapter 4

Ruqiya Shama Tareen MD
Associate Professor, Department of
Psychiatry
Michgian State University College of
Human Medicine
Psychiatry Residency Program
Kalamazoo Center for Medical Studies
1722 Shaffer Road, Suite 3
Kalamazoo, Michigan 49048
United States
Chapter 2

Therdpong Tempark MD
Fellow in Pediatric Dermatology
Henry Ford Medical Center
Dept of Dermatology
3031 Grand Boulevard
Detroit, MI 48202
United States
Chapter 2

Alfonso D. Torres MD
Director, Pediatric Nephrology
Pediatrics Program
Michigan State University/
Kalamazoo Center for Medical Studies
1000 Oakland Drive
Kalamazoo, MI 49008–1284
United States
Torres@kcms.msu.edu
Chapter 15

Abbreviations

1,25 diOHD	1,25-dihydroxy vitamin D
25OHD	25-hydroxy vitamin D
5-HT	5-hydroxytryptamine/serotonin
AAP	American Academy of Pediatrics
ABCs	airway, breathing, and circulation
ABPM	ambulatory BP monitoring
ABVPC	doxorubicin (Adriamycin), bleomycin, vinblastine, prednisone, and cytoxan
ACE	angiotensin converting enzyme
ACEI	angiotensin converting enzyme inhibitor
ACH	anticholinergic
ACTH	adrenocorticotrophic hormone
AD	autosomal dominant
ADH	antidiuretic hormone
ADHD	attention deficit/hyperactivity disorder
AED	antiepileptic drug
AHA	American Heart Association
AIDS	acquired immunodeficiency syndrome
AIH	autoimmune hepatitis
AIHA	autoimmune hemolytic anemia
AKI	acute kidney injury
ALD	adrenoleukodystrophy
ALL	acute lymphoblastic leukemia
ALT	serum glutamic-pyruvic transaminase
AML	acute myelogenous leukemia
AMN	adrenomyeloneuropathy
ANAs	antinuclear antibodies
ANC	absolute neutrophil count
ANCA	antineutrophil cytoplasmic antibody
anti–DNAase B	antideoxyribonuclease B
anti-dsDNA	antibodies to double-stranded DNA
AOR	adjusted odds ratio
Apo B	apolipoprotein B
aPTT	activated partial thromboplastin time
AR	autosomal recessive
ARBs	angiotensin receptor blockers
ARDS	adult respiratory distress syndrome
ARF	acute rheumatic fever
AS	ankylosing spondylitis
ASA	acetylsalicylic acid (aspirin)

ASCO	American Society of Clinical Oncology
ASO	antistreptolysin-O
AST	aspartate transaminase
ATG	antithymocyte globulin
ATP	adenosine triphosphate
ATPase	adenosine triphosphatase
ATRA	all-*trans* retinoic acid
AUC	area under the curve
AVN	avascular necrosis
AVP	arginine vasopressin
BCIE	bullous congenital ichthyosisform erythroderma
BEACOPP	bleomycin, etoposide, doxorubicin (Adriamycin), oncovin, prednisolone, procarbazine
BI	bullous ichthyosis
BJHS	benign joint hypermobility syndrome
BLT	Buschke-Loewenstein tumor
BM	bone marrow
BMI	body mass index
BMT	bone marrow transplant
BP	blood pressure
B-PAP	bilevel positive airway pressure
BSA	body surface area
BUN	blood urea nitrogen
BWS	Beckwith-Wiedemann syndrome
BZD	benzodiazepines
CA	condyloma acuminata
CAD	coronary artery disease
CAH	congenital adrenal hyperplasia
CAKUT	congenital abnormalities of the kidneys and urinary tract
CA-MRSA	community-acquired methicillin-resistant *S. aureus*
CAP	community-acquired pneumonia
CBC	complete blood count
CBZ	carbamazepine
CCP	cyclic citrullinated peptide
CCT	crude coal tar
CD	Crohn's disease
CDC	Centers for Disease Control and Prevention
CETP	cholesterol esterase transfer protein
CF	correction factor
CF	cystic fibrosis
CFRD	CF-related diabetes mellitus
CFTR	cystic fibrosis transmembrane conductance regulator
CFUs	colony forming units
CHr	reticulocyte hemoglobin concentration
CI	confidence interval
CI	contraindicated

CIE	congenital ichthyosiform erythroderma
CINV	chemotherapy-induced nausea and vomiting
CKD	chronic kidney disease
CLM	cutaneous larva migrans
CMN	congenital melanocytic nevi
CMP	complement membrane protein
CMV	cytomegalovirus
CNS	central nervous system
CoA	coenzyme A
COX	cyclooxygenase
COX-1	cyclooxygenase-1
COX-2	cyclooxygenase-2
CPAP	continuous positive airway pressure
CPK	creatine phosphokinase
CPP	central precocious puberty
CPR	cardiopulmonary resuscitation
CPS	complex partial seizure
CR	controlled release
CrCl	creatinine clearance
CREST	Calcinosis, Raynaud's syndrome, Esophageal dysmotility, Sclerodactyly, Telangiectasia
CRH	corticotropin-releasing hormone
CRI	chronic renal insufficiency
CRP	C-reactive protein
CSD	cat-scratch disease
CSII	continuous subcutaneous insulin infusion
CT	computed tomography
CV	cardiovascular
CVC	central venous catheter
CVD	cardiovascular disease
CVL	central venous line
CYP	cytochrome P
D-HUS	diarrhea-negative HUS
D+HUS	diarrhea-positive HUS
DAT	direct antiglobin test
DAX	dosage-sensitive sex reversal, adrenal hypoplasia critical region, on chromosome X, gene 1
DBP	diastolic BP
DCCT	Diabetes Control and Complications Trial
dDAVP	decompressing acetate
DDD	dense deposit disease
DEA	U.S. Drug Enforcement Administration
DEET	N,N-diethyl-meta-toluamide
DEXA	dual-energy x-ray absorptiometry
DHEA	dehydroepiandrosterone
DHEAS	dehydroepiandrosterone sulphate

DI	diabetes insipidus
DIC	disseminated intravascular coagulation
DKA	diabetic ketoacidosis
DLCO	diffusing capacity of the lungs for carbon monoxide
DM	diabetes mellitus
DMARD	disease-modifying antirheumatic drug
DMSA	dimercaptosuccinic acid
DNA	deoxyribonucleic acid
DOMS	delayed-onset muscle soreness
DPCP	diphenylcyclopropenone
DPI	dry-powder inhaler
DR	delayed-release
DSM-IV-TR	*The Diagnostic and Statistical Manual of Mental Disorders, Fourth Edition, Text Revision*
DSPD	delayed sleep phase disorder
DVT	deep vein thrombosis
EBV	Epstein-Barr virus
ECG	electrocardiogram
ECHO	echocardiogram
EEG	electroencephalogram
EHEC	enterohemorrhagic *E. coli*
EHK	epidermolytic hyperkeratosis
EIA	enzyme immunoassay
EIB	exercise-induced bronchospasm
EIMD	exercise-induced muscle damage
ELISA	enzyme-linked immunosorbent assay
ELNT	Euro-Lupus Nephritis Trial
EM	electron microscopic
EM	extensive metabolizer
EoE	eosinophilic esophagitis
EPS	epidermal nevus syndrome
EPS	extrapyramidal
ER	extended release
ERT	enzyme replacement therapy
ESM	ethosuximide
ESR	erythrocyte sedimentation rate
ESRD	end-stage renal disease
ET	epidermolytic toxin
ET	essential tremor
EULAR/PReS	European League against Rheumatism/Pediatric Rheumatology European Society
FAB	French American British
FDA	U.S. Food and Drug Administration
FEPs	free erythrocyte porphyrins
FFAs	free fatty acids
FH	familial hypercholesterolemia

FISH	fluorescent in situ hybridization
free T4	free thyroxine level
FSGS	focal segmental glomerulosclerosis
FSH	follicle stimulating hormone
G6PD	glucose-6-phosphate dehydrogenase
GABA	gamma-amino butyric acid
GABHS	group A beta-hemolytic *Streptococcus*
GBM	glomerular basement membrane
GBP	gabapentin
GBS	group B streptococcal
G-CSF	granulocyte colony-stimulating factor
GER	gastroesophageal reflux
GERD	gastroesophageal reflux disease
GH	growth hormone
GHB	gamma-hydroxybutyrate
GHD	growth hormone deficiency
GI	gastrointestinal
GM-CSF	granulocyte macrophage colony-stimulating factor
GN	glomerulonephritis
GNC	Gram-negative cocci
GnRH	gonadotropin-releasing hormone
GSD I	glycogen storage disease type I
GSD II	glycogen storage disease type II
GTCS	generalized tonic-clonic seizure
H2	histamine-2
HAART	highly active antiretroviral therapy
HbA1c	glycated hemoglobin
HbA2	hemoglobin A2
HBeAG	hepatitis Be antigen
HbF	fetal hemoglobin
HBsAg	hepatitis B surface antigen
HBV	hepatitis B virus
hCG	human chorionic gonadotropin
HCTZ	hydrochlorothiazide
HCV	hepatitis C virus
HD	Hodgkin's disease
HDL	high-density lipoprotein
HFA	hydrofluoroalkane
HFMD	hand, foot, and mouth disease
HIT	heparin-induced thrombocytopenia
HIV	human immunodeficiency virus
HLA	hepatic lipase
HLA	human leukocyte antigen
HMG-CoA	hydroxy-methylglutaryl coenzyme A
HPA	hypothalamic-pituitary-adrenal
HPG	hypothalamo-pituitary-gonadal

HPV	human papillomavirus
HS	hereditary spherocytosis
HSCT	hematopoietic stem cell transplantation
HSP	Henoch-Schönlein purpura
HSV	herpes simplex virus
HUS	hemolytic-uremic syndrome
HZV	herpes zoster virus
IBD	inflammatory bowel disease
IBS	irritable bowel syndrome
IBS-C	IBS constipation-predominant
IBS-D	IBS diarrhea-predominant
IBS-M	mixed or alternating stool pattern
I:C	insulin:carbohydrate
ICP	intracranial pressure
ICS	inhaled corticosteroid
ICU	intensive care unit
IDD	intellectual and developmental disability
IDDM	insulin-dependent diabetes mellitus
IDL	intermediate-density lipoprotein
IE	ifosfamide and etoposide
IEMs	inborn errors of metabolism
IFA	immunofluorescent antibody
IFN	interferon
IGF1	insulin-like growth factor 1
IGFBP3	insulin-like growth factor binding protein 3
ILAE	International League Against Epilepsy
ILVEN	inflammatory linear verrucous epidermal nevus
IM	intramuscular
INR	international normalized ratio
I/O	intake and output
IR	immediate release
ISKDC	International Study of Kidney Disease in Children
ISN/PRS	International Society of Nephrology/Renal Pathology Society
IT	intrathecal
ITP	immune thrombocytopenia
IV	intravenous; intravenously
IVF	intravenous fluids
IVIG	intravenous immunoglobulin
JA	juvenile arthritis
JCA	juvenile chronic arthritis
JHS	joint hypermobility syndrome
JIA	juvenile idiopathic arthritis
JPD	juvenile plantar dermatosis
JRA	juvenile rheumatoid arthritis
KOH	potassium hydroxide

LABA	long-acting beta agonist
LCAD	long-chain acyl CoA dehydrogenase
LCAT	lecithin cholesterol acyl transferase
LCD	liquor carbonis detergent
LDH	lactic dehydrogenase
LDL	low-density lipoprotein
LDLR	LDL receptor
LE	leukocyte esterase
LE	lupus erythematosus
LEV	levetiracetam
LFT	liver function tests
LH	luteinizing hormone
LI	lamellar ichthyosis
LMWH	low-molecular-weight heparin
LN	lichen nitidus
LOX	lipoxygenase
LP	lichen planus
LPL	lipoprotein lipase
LRINEC	Laboratory Risk Indicator for Necrotizing Fascitis
LTG	lamotrigine
LVH	left ventricular hypertrophy
MAC	membrane attack complex
MAOI	monoamine oxidase inhibitor
MAP	high-dose methotrexate, doxorubicin (Adriamycin), and cisplatin
MAS	macrophage activation syndrome
MCAD	medium-chain acyl CoA dehydrogenase
MCD	minimal change disease
MCHC	mean corpuscular hemoglobin concentration
MCV	mean corpuscular volume
MDI	metered-dose inhaler
MDS	myelodysplastic syndrome
MELAS	mitochondrial myopathy, encephalopathy, lactic acidosis, and stroke-like episodes
MLD	metachromatic leukodystrophy
MMF	mycophenolate mofetil
MMI	methimazole
MN	membranous nephropathy
MODY	maturity-onset diabetes of youth
MOSF	multiorgan system failure
MPGN	membranoproliferative glomerulonephritis
MPH	methylphenidate
MPO	myeloperoxidase
MPS	mucopolysaccharidoses
MR	magnetic resonance
MRA	magnetic resonance angiography
MRC	Medical Research Council of Britain

MRD	minimal residual disease
MRI	magnetic resonance imaging
MRSA	methicillin-resistant *S. aureus*
MSUD	maple syrup urine disease
MTHFR	methylenetetrahydrofolate reductase
NADPH	nicotinamide adenine dinucleotide phosphate
NAEPP	U.S. National Asthma Education and Prevention Program
NAFLD	nonalcoholic fatty liver disease
NAPQI	*N*-acetyl-p-benzoquinoneimine
NASH	nonacoholic steatohepatitis
NBCIE	nonbullous congenital ichthyosiform erythroderma
NCEP	National Cholesterol Education Program
NCM	neurocutaneous melanosis
NEP	neutral endopeptidase
NF	necrotizing fasciitis
NFAT	nuclear factor of activated T cells
NHF	National Hemophilia Foundation
NHL	non-Hodgkin's lymphoma
NIDDM	non-insulin-dependent diabetes mellitus
NIH	U.S. National Institutes of Health
NK1	neurokinin-1
NMS	neuroleptic malignant syndrome
NO	nitric oxide
NPD	Nieman-Pick disease
NPH	neutral protamine Hagedorn
NSAIDs	nonsteroidal anti-inflammatory drugs
NTE	not to exceed
OCD	obsessive-compulsive disorder
OH	obstructive hypoventilation
OR	odds ratio
OSAHS	obstructive sleep apnea/hypopnea syndrome
OSAS	obstructive sleep apnea syndrome
OSH	orthostatic hypotension
OSP	outer surface protein
OTC	over-the-counter
OXC	oxcarbazepine
PAN	panarteritis nodosa
PB	phenobarbital
PCH	paroxysmal cold hemoglobinuria
PCOS	polycystic ovarian syndrome
PCP	*Pneumocystis carinii*, now *Pneumocystis jirovecii*
PCR	polymerase chain reaction
PE	phenytoin equivalent
PET	positron-emission tomography
PFT	pulmonary function testing

PH	primary hypertension
PHT	phenytoin
PK	pyruvate kinase
PKU	phenylketonuria
PLA2R	phospholipase A-2 receptor
PLC	pityriasis lichenoides chronica
PLEVA	pityriasis lichenoides et varioliformis acuta
PLMD	periodic limb movement disorder
PM	poor metabolizer
PML	promyelocytic leukemia
PO	oral
POTS	postural orthostatic tachycardia syndrome
PPI	proton pump inhibitor
PPP	peripheral precocious puberty
PR	pityriasis rosea
PSC	primary sclerosing cholangitis
PSGN	poststreptococcal glomerulonephritis
PSRA	poststreptococcal reactive arthritis
PT	prothrombin time
PTS	postthrombotic syndrome
PTU	propylthiouracil
PUVA	psoralen plus ultraviolet A
PWS	Prader-Willi syndrome
RA	rheumatoid arthritis
RAI	radioactive iodine
RARa	retinoic acid receptor a
RAS	renal artery stenosis
RBC	red blood cell
RDs	rheumatoid diseases
RDW	RBC distribution width
REM	rapid eye movement
RF	rheumatoid factor
RFM	rufinamide
rhu GM-CSF	recombinant human granulocyte and macrophage colony-stimulating factor
RLS	restless legs syndrome
RNP	ribonucleoprotein
RSD	reflex sympathetic dystrophy
RSV	respiratory syncytial virus
SABA	short-acting beta agonist
SAM-e	S-adenosylmethionine
SARS	severe acute respiratory syndrome
SBP	systolic BP
SC	subcutaneous; subcutaneously
SCAD	short-chain acyl coenzyme A (CoA) dehydrogenase
SCC	squamous cell carcinoma

SCD	sickle-cell disease
SCD	sudden cardiac death
SCFE	slipped capital femoral epiphysis
Scr	serum creatinine
SDB	sleep-disordered breathing
SEER program	National Cancer Institute's Surveillance Epidemiology and End Result program
SF	steroidogenic factor
SHBG	sex hormone binding globulin
SIADH	syndrome of inappropriate antidiuretic hormone
SJS	Stevens-Johnson syndrome
SLE	systemic lupus erythematosus
SNRI	serotonin-norepinephrine reuptake inhibitor
SPEA	streptococcal pyrogenic exotoxins A
SPF	sun protective factor
SPS	simple partial seizure
SQ	subcutaneously
SSKI	saturated solution of potassium iodide
SSPE	subacute sclerosing panencephalitis
SSRIs	selective serotonin reuptake inhibitors
SSSS	staphylococcal scalded skin syndrome
STD	sexually transmitted disease
sTfRs	soluble transferrin receptors
T1DM	type1 diabetes mellitus
T2DM	type 2 diabetes mellitus
TB	tuberculosis
TCAs	tricyclic antidepressants
TEN	toxic epidermal necrolysis
TENS	transcutaneous electrical nerve stimulation
TGM1	transglutaminase-1
TIBC	total iron-binding capacity
TMP	trimethoprim
TNF	tumor necrosis factor
TNF-α	tumor necrosis factor alpha
TOBI	tobramycin solution for inhalation
TPM	topiramate
TPMT	thiopurine S-methyltransferase
TRPC6	transient receptor potential cation 6 channel
TRPV1	TRP vanilloid
TS	Tourette's syndrome
TS	Turner's syndrome
TSH	thyroid stimulating hormone
TSS	toxic shock syndrome
TTP	thrombotic thrombocytopenic purpura
UARS	upper airway resistance syndrome
UC	ulcerative colitis

UFH	unfractionated heparin
UPPP	uvulopalatopharyngoplasty
URI	upper respiratory infection
UTIs	urinary tract infections
UV	ultraviolet
UVB	ultraviolet B
VCUG	voiding cystourethrogram
VDC	vincristine, doxorubicin, and cyclophosphamide
VDRs	vitamin D receptors
VKA	vitamin K antagonists
VLCAD	very long-chain acyl CoA dehydrogenase
VLCFAs	very long-chain fatty acids
VLDL	very low-density lipoprotein
VP	ventriculoperitoneal
VPA	valproic acid
VTE	venous thromboembolism
VWD	von Willebrand disease
VWF	von Willebrand factor
VWF: Ag	von Willebrand factor: antigen
VWF: RCo	von Willebrand factor: ristocetin cofactor
WBC	white blood count
WD	Wilson's disease
ZNS	zonisamide

1 Introduction – Pharmacotherapeutics in medical disorders

Donald E. Greydanus and Joav Merrick

> If you would understand anything, observe its beginning and its development.
>
> Aristotle (384–322 BC)

The search for optimal medications to support health has mostly likely been present since hominids emerged out of primate evolution over 250,000 years ago. The appearance of *Homo sapiens* as the surviving hominid species over 60,000 years ago heightened this quest (1). One concept that was learned early in human civilization is that medications can be harmful as well as potentially beneficial. Witness the Genesis 3:6 account of Adam and Eve and their demise from eating the "forbidden" fruit.

Folklore and anecdotal information dominated human knowledge for more than 50,000 years, until the work of the Chinese emperor Shen-Nung (2737 BC), who became a meticulous, official, and erudite classifier of medicinal herbs (2). One of the classic paintings of this ruler, who was called the Red Emperor, shows him holding *Ephedra* (ma huang) leaves, confirming the idea that our first medications derived from herbals.

Anecdotal evidence gained over thousands of years of the Chinese and Indian civilizations still remains essentially lost in Western civilization, which slowly developed its own ideas of the best medications for physical and mental health. One of the earliest sources of a Western pharmacopoeia was Egypt, whose early scholars produced the Ebers Papyrus (1550 BC), a classic scroll with 110 pages containing 700 formulas of vegetable, mineral, and animal origin (3).

The ancient Greek civilization began to develop principles of science, although this did not benefit the search for pharmacologic agents until much later in the history of Western civilization. Athletes of the ancient Olympics (776 BC–AD 393) consumed various products in efforts to acquire optimal health and sports performance; these products included figs, mushrooms, strychnine, and others. Whereas progress in some branches of science and philosophy was impressive in ancient Greece, discoveries in the use of medicines to cure human maladies was slow. Consider the lament of Aristotle, one of the most famous and brilliant Greek philosophers, about the state of medicine in ancient Greece: "the physician does not cure man, except in an incidental sense" (4). Indeed, clinical pharmacology had a long way to go!

A major reason for the slow progress of science in this regard was the reliance of human beings for thousands of years on conflicting dogmas based on a complex mix of divination, prophecy, magic, and religion. This was the reaction of humans to a mystifying, cruel, and often violent world. Hippocrates of Cos (460–377 BC), the founder of Western medicine, began to turn this page with his Hippocratic corpus and his now classic dicta to "First do no harm" and also to observe the patient closely.

Diseases were often enmeshed with attempts to understand magic and religion. Epilepsy and mental illness, for example, were blamed on demonic possession and the treatment was exorcism, not pharmacologic prescriptions. Claudius Galen (AD 130–210), the famous Greek physician and surgeon caring for the upper class of ancient Rome and its superstar gladiators, linked many diseases (including epilepsy and mental illness) with masturbation in adolescents and young adults. His concern with hebetic sexuality lingers with us even in the twenty-first century:

> Watch carefully over this young man, leave him alone neither day nor night; at least sleep in his chamber. When he has contracted this fatal habit (i.e., masturbation), the most fatal to which a young man can be subject, he will carry its painful effects to the tomb – his mind and body will always be enervated. (5)

The fall of the Roman Empire in the fifth century of the Common Era led to a dramatic decline in scientific information as humans turned ever most desperately to magic, mysticism, and religion to deal with a violent and unforgiving environment. There were some bright spots that supported a continuing flame of knowledge, such as the Persian physician Rhazes (Muhammad ibn Zakariya Razi, AD 865–925), whose book on disorders of children took the first serious look at this age group.

The West very gradually arose from it sycophantic and saturnine slumber. For example, a book that was released in the late eleventh century dealt with medical disorders of children; called *De Mylierum Passionibus*, it was written by Trotula Platearius of Salerno, Italy. The development of the Renaissance (fourteenth–seventeenth centuries in Europe) led to an explosion of medical knowledge in the areas of anatomy, physiology, surgery, and others (as well as in philosophy, art, and language). Thomas Phaer (1510–1560), an English lawyer and physician, published the first book (*The Boke of Chyldren*) that made a real distinction between the phases of childhood and adulthood.

As each century passed, more progress in understanding the causes of diseases occurred, allowing for improvements in their management. Epidemics of major infections ravaged Europe, such as the Black Plague (due to *Yersinia pestis*), which led to the death of one third of Europe's population in the mid-fourteenth century. Dr. Edward Jenner (1749–1823) was a general physician in England whose landmark observations and experimentation with cowpox in the latter part of the eighteenth century led to the development of the smallpox vaccine and eventually the tremendous triumphs of vaccinology in the twentieth and twenty-first centuries (6).

The term *biology* was launched in the early nineteenth century and initiated the attempts to separate out the etiology of diseases from ancient and persistent philosophical theories (1). Old theories of anatomy were challenged by Andreas Vesalius (1514–1564) in Italy with his classic *De Humani Corporis*. Concepts of blood circulation were given a modern interpretation by William Harvey of England, based on earlier work such as that of the Arabic physician Ibn al-Nafic (1242), the father of circulatory physiology. The theories of Hippocrates and Galen were finally challenged amid a stunning upsurge of intellectual curiosity and inquiry. An American pathologist Dr. John Scudder of Ohio, wrote a pediatric textbook challenging the notion that treatment of adults would suffice for children. He noted: "There are sufficient differences in the action of remedies upon the adult and child, to demand a careful study of the subject" (i.e., the child) (7).

The seeds of pharmacology were sown by the previously mentioned Red Emperor, Shen-Nung and Egyptian Ebers Papyrus. Pedanius Dioscorides (AD 40–90) was a surgeon and botanist in Rome whose travels around the Roman Empire led to his classic work on herbal and medicinal products, *De Materia Medica* (*Regarding Medical*

Matters) (8,9). This pharmacopeia influenced medical treatment for over a millennium. The Persian physician and chemist Avicenna (Ibn Sina) (AD 980–1037) wrote a medical textbook called *The Canon of Medicine*, which became a standard of pharmacologic regimens for the next six centuries.

After thousands of years of observations, the modern era of clinical pharmacology can be traced to the English physician William Withering (1741–1799); he was also a chemist and botanist who discovered digitalis (foxglove) and carefully wrote about both its benefits for heart failure and its toxic effects. The first department of pharmacology was developed by Rudolf Buchheim (1820–1879) at the University of Giessen, Germany, in 1847.

The advancing progress of the seventeenth and eighteenth centuries led to an explosion of new knowledge in various fields of science in the twentieth century. Work in clinical pharmacology culminated in new drugs for medicine and psychiatry in children, adolescents, and adults. Though Hippocrates recommended willow-leaf tea (containing salicylates) for relief of pain and fever, it was not until 1897 that chemists Felix Hoffmann and Arthur Eichengrün identified acetylsalicylic acid, which was then marketed in 1899 as Aspirin (10). Canadian surgeon Frederick Banting and medical student Charles Best identified insulin in 1922, which became the drug prolonging the lives of countless numbers of people with diabetes mellitus in the twentieth and twenty-first centuries (11). Sir Alexander Fleming, a Scottish biologist and pharmacologist, identified penicillin from mold (*Penicillum notatum*) in 1928, stimulating the further development of antibiotics.

Pharmacology had arrived after thousands of years of observation with more and more drugs identified as being beneficial. Psychiatrist Charles Bradley published his landmark study in 1937 observing the benefit of a stimulant called Benzedrine (racemic mixture of dextroamphetamine and levoamphetamine) on 30 children with various mental health conditions including what would later be called attention deficit hyperactivity disorder (ADHD) (12). In the same year researchers Molitich and Eccles published one of the first placebo-controlled research studies on the benefits of Benzedrine in 93 youths labeled as juvenile delinquents (13).

Edward Kendall was an American chemist at the Mayo Clinic (Rochester, Minnesota, USA) who, along with the help of others such as physician Philip Hench, identified cortisone in 1949 (14). Chlorpromazine was introduced in 1950 as one of the first antipsychotic medications, which have now evolved into second- and third-generation antipsychotics (15,16). The Argentine child psychiatrist M. Knobel identified the stimulant methylphenidate as beneficial for children with ADHD, which was then called hyperkinesis with organicity (17). In the 1950s the famous sex educator Margaret Sanger, researcher Gregory Pincus, and physician John Rock became protagonists of the incredible story that led to the development of Enovid, which became an FDA-approved drug for menstrual disorders in 1957 and an FDA-approved oral contraceptive in 1960 (18).

Angiotensin converting enzyme (ACE) inhibitors were introduced in 1956 based on the work of Leonard Skegg, and ibuprofen was introduced in 1969 based on the work of chemist John Nicholson and pharmacologist Stewart Adams of Nottingham, England (19).

Research has continued and each decade has produced more and more drugs for the benefit of medical and mental health (20). However, pharmacologic trials are increasingly directed more by the pharmaceutical industry than by independent researchers, raising concerns over the validity and neutrality of such research (16,21,22). It must be remembered that each drug has side effects and the risk/benefit profile must be carefully identified in a neutral and unbiased manner for the well-being of the patient (23). It is important to note that the word *pharmacology* comes from the Greek word *pharmakon*, with the dual meaning of "poison" in classic Greek and "drugs" in modern Greek. Some drugs can be poison; therefore clinicians must monitor both positive and negative aspects of drug administration very carefully and obsessively. Plants can be wondrous, as noted with willow leaves (salicylates) or foxglove (*Digitalis purpurea*), but also deceptively dangerous, as seen with *Canabis sativa* (marijuana) or *Erythroxylon coca* (cocaine).

Pharmacologic management of human disease is clearly part of the twenty-first-century medical armamentarium. This book is dedicated to this concept, seeking to discuss the pharmacologic or pharmacotherapeutic approach to a specific group of people, the adolescent. Interest in this population has developed over the past half-century, as carefully chronicled by Professor Dr. Robin Beach and Professor Dr. George Chrousos in their forewords to this book. Other approaches are acknowledged in the first part of this book, but the emphasis is on the use of drugs or medications to relieve disease in this important part of humanity, the adolescent. Adolescents of this second decade of the twenty-first century and those adolescents soon to come will determine the future of our planet and life into the twenty-second century. Pharmacology will remain an ever-growing part of clinicians' efforts to improve their patients' mental and medical health. DEG thanks his fellow-editors in the development of this book and the editors thank the many experts who gave up some of their valuable time in preparing their chapters.

> The young physician starts life with 20 drugs for each disease, and the old physician ends life with one drug for 20 diseases.
>
> Sir William Osler, MD (1849–1919)

References

1. Magner LN. A history of the life sciences, 3rd ed. New York, NY: Marcel Dekker; 2002.
2. Greydanus DE, Patel DR. Sports doping in athletes. Pediatr Clin North Am 2010;57(3): 729–50.
3. Scholl R. Der Papyrus Ebers. Die grösste Buchrolle zur Heilkunde Altägyptens (Schriften aus der Universitätsbibliothek 7), Leipzig, Germany: University of Leipzig, 2002.
4. Wheelwright P. Aristotle. New York: Odyssey Press, 1951: 68.
5. Greydanus DE, Geller B. Masturbation: Historical perspective. NY State Med 1980;80: 1892-6.
6. Koppaka R. Ten great public health achievements – United States, 2001–2010. MMWR 2011;60(19): 619–23.
7. Scudder NJM. The eclectic practice of diseases of children. Cincinnati: American Publishing Co., 1869: 19.
8. Brater DC, Daly WJ. Clinical pharmacology in the Middle Ages: Principles that presage the 21st century. Clin Pharmacol Ther 2000; 67(5): 447–50.
9. Vallance P, Smart TG. The future of pharmacology. Br J Pharmacol 2006;147(Suppl 1): S304–S307.
10. Griffiths R. The discovery of aspirin. Am Philatelist 2003;34: 701–7.

11. Hughes E. Breakthrough: The discovery of insulin and the making of a medical miracle. New York: St. Martin Press; 2010.
12. Bradley C. The behavior of children receiving Benzedrine. Am J Psychiatry 1937;94: 577–85.
13. Molitch M, Eccles AK. The effect of Benzedrine sulfate on the intelligence scores of children. Am J Psychiatry 1937;94: 577–85.
14. Woodward RB, Sondheimer F, Taub D. The total synthesis of cortisone. J Am Chem Soc 1951;73: 4057.
15. Greydanus DE, Patel DR, Feucht D. Preface: Pediatric and adolescent psychopharmacology: The past, the present, and the future. Pediatr Clin North Am 2011;58(1): xv–xxiv.
16. López-Munoz F, Alamo C, Cuenca E, Shen WW, Clervoy P, Rubio G. History and discover and clinical introduction of chlorpromazine. Ann Clin Psychiatry 2005;17(3): 113–35.
17. Knobel M, Wolman M, Mason A. Hyperkinesis and organicity in children. Arch Gen Psychiatry 1959;1(3): 310–21.
18. Bynum WF. The western medical tradition. Cambridge, England: Cambridge University Press, 2006.
19. Moore N. Forty years of ibuprofen use. Int J Clin Pract 2003; 135: 28–31.
20. Greydanus DE, Calles Jr JL, Patel DR. Pediatric and adolescent psychopharmacology. Cambridge, England: Cambridge University Press, 2008.
21. Greydanus DE, Patel DR. The role of pharmaceutical influence in education and research: The clinician's response. Asian J Paediatr Pract 2006;9: 35–41.
22. Kölch M, Ludolph AG, Plener PL, Fangerau H, Vitiello B, Fegert JM. Safeguarding children's rights in psychopharmacological research: Ethical and legal issues. Curr Pharm Des 2010; 16(22): 2398–406.
23. Ventegodt S, Greydanus DE, Merrick J. Alternative medicine does not exist, biomedicine does not exist, there is only evidence-based medicine. Int J Adolesc Med 2011;23(3): 7–10.

2 Dermatology

Arthur N. Feinberg, Tor A. Shwayder, Ruqiya Shama Tareen, and Therdpong Tempark

2.1 Introduction

Dermatologic conditions are a very important part of adolescent medicine and can have considerable influence on an adolescent's medical as well as psychological health. The goals of this chapter are to discuss the more common skin conditions encountered in adolescents in the day-to-day practice of a primary care physician. We present a brief summary of etiology and pathogenesis of the conditions followed by a discussion of standard case management, including newer developments where pertinent. The chapter is divided into six main sections:

- Skin infections and infestations (bacterial, viral, fungal, and parasitic)
- Dermatitis (nonallergic, allergic, and idiopathic)
- Hypersensitivity reactions (urticaria, erythema multiforme and drug eruptions)
- Miscellaneous skin conditions (acne, nevi, papulosquamous disorders)
- Dermatologic manifestations of systemic disorders (pruritus without rash, inflammatory bowel disease)
- Collagen vascular disorders, and endocrine disorders
- Disorders of the hair and nails

2.2 Skin Infections and Infestations

2.2.1 Bacterial infections

Bacterial infections of the skin are summarized clinically in ▶Tab. 2.1 (1,2,3,4,5,6).

Impetigo

A common skin infection, impetigo affects about 2.8 percent of children under 4 years and 1.6 percent of those 5 to 15 years of age. Certain conditions that compromise the immune system can lead to impetigo, including, burns, diabetes mellitus, B-cell immunodeficiency states, and so on. Infection has a predilection for the face, especially around the mouth and nose area. Typical lesions can be bullous or nonbullous as well as have a mixed presentation occurring within the same area. Previously group A beta-hemolytic *Streptococcus* (GABHS) was thought to be the main causative agent, especially of the nonbullous form, but current literature suggests *Staphylococcus aureus* as the predominant etiology in both forms of impetigo.

Contact dermatitis presents with tiny vesicles on erythematous skin, but they are very itchy and usually occur on exposed areas with a history of contact with a sensitizing agent. Small clear fluid-filled vesicles of herpes simplex infection are more common on the lips and perioral area and can be quite painful. Varicella vesicles easily

Tab. 2.1: Characteristics of common bacterial infections.

Skin layers/ Structures	Disease	Common sites	Predominant organism	Secondary organism
Epidermis	Impetigo	Face	*Staphylococcus aureus*	*Streptococcus pyogenes* (GABHS)*
	Superficial folliculitis	Face, scalp	*S. aureus*	
	Furunculosis	Face, scalp, axillae	*S. aureus*	
	Staphylococcal scalded skin syndrome		*S. aureus* phage group II	
	Scarlatina	Face and scalp; can involve whole body	*S. pyogenes* (GABHS)	
Epidermis/ subepidermis	Toxic shock syndrome	Whole body	*S. aureus*	
	Ecthyma	Legs, buttocks	*Pseudomonas aeruginosa*	Many gram-negative and some gram-positive organism
Dermis	Carbuncle	Back, thighs	*S. aureus*	
	Erysipelas	Face	*S. pyogenes* (GABHS)	
	Deep folliculitis	Scalp	*S. aureus*	
	Folliculitis decalvans	Scalp		
Dermis and upper subcutaneous tissues	Cellulitis	Legs	*S. aureus*	*S. pyogenes* (GABHS)
Deeper dermis, subcutaneous tissues, and fascia	Necrotizing fasciitis Type I: mixed aerobic & anaerobic infection	Legs and arms Less commonly: trunk, perineum, buttocks, head, & neck	Facultative streptococci, staphylococci, enterococci Gram-negative bacilli, such as *Escherichia coliKlebsiella, Pseudomonas, EnterobacterProteus,* and anaerobes, such as *Peptostreptococcus, Bacteroides,* and *Clostridium* spp.	

(Continued)

Tab. 2.1: Characteristics of common bacterial infections. (*Continued*)

Skin layers/ Structures	Disease	Common sites	Predominant organism	Secondary organism
	Necrotizing fasciitis Type II: monomicrobial		*S. pyogenes* (GABHS)	*Streptococcus agalactiae* and *Streptococcuspneumoniae* *Vibrio vulnificus* *Clostridium* *S. aureus Aeromonas* spp.

*Group A beta-hemolytic *Streptococcus*.

rupture and encrust like impetigo but involve the whole body and occur in crops with lesions of different stages present in same area. Ecthyma is usually a solitary ulcerative lesion surrounded by tiny vesicles; it leaves a scar, unlike impetigo, which seldom does. Pemphigus foliaceus is a rare disease usually involving the face in a butterfly-like fashion; it also presents with vesicles and occasional bullae on an erythematous base.

Bullous impetigo

Accounting for 70 percent of cases, this starts as innocuous reddish papules that coalesce and form small bullae; these easily rupture, forming erosions covered with the typical honey-colored thick crust.

Nonbullous impetigo

This less common form presents with expanding honey-colored crusts, leaving a raw erosive area.

Secondary impetigo

Secondary infection of minor cuts, insect bites, and excessive scratching of eczematous scabies and other pruritic lesions, especially in diabetic or immunocompromised children, can result in impetigenous lesions, usually of the nonbullous type.

Management

Prevention of the spread of infection is important, although topical disinfectants are not indicated. The first line of treatment for small lesions confined to one or two areas is a topical antibiotic like mupirocin, bacitracin, or fusidic acid. Topical antibiotics are not only superior to placebo but mupirocin and bacitracin have been found to be superior to oral erythromycin. Amoxicillin/clavulanate (125/30 mg per mL) three times daily, cephalexin 30 mg/kg per day in two divided doses, erythromycin 40 mg/kg per day in two to four divided doses, and dicloxacillin 90 mg/kg in two to four divided doses per day for 7 to 10 days have all resulted in satisfactory outcomes.

Cellulitis

Cellulitis is rapidly spreading infection of the skin and subcutaneous tissues that results from the introduction of an infecting organism through a minor cut, prick, or any break in the skin. Any part of the body can be involved but cellulitis typically occurs on the lower extremities. In young children, however, involvement of the face is common. The diffuse, rapidly progressive lesion with no clear margins presents with typical signs of acute inflammation (i.e., warm and tender to the touch and shiny red in appearance because of swelling). Immunocompromised hosts are susceptible to cellulitis and its complications. *S. aureus, S. pyogenes*, and *Enterococcus* species are common offenders. Rarely, infection with *Haemophilus influenzae*, especially in infants, and with *Clostridium difficile* can occur. Cellulitis can present with signs of systemic infection such as fever, malaise, pain, lymphangiitis, and lymphadenitis.

Periorbital (preseptal) and orbital (postseptal) cellulitis

These are mostly unilateral conditions often due to a spread of infection from the adjacent inflamed sinuses (7). Local skin infection may also be the initiating factor. Infections can be recurrent and often present during the winter months in young children, with the average age of presentation being 6.8 years; there is a 2:1 male preponderance. The most common agents involved are *S. aureus, S. epidermidis,* and *S. pyogenes*. Orbital cellulitis constitutes an emergency, as it can lead to serious complications such as cavernous sinus thrombosis, meningitis, permanent loss of vision, and diplopia.

Management

Prompt recognition and initiation of antibiotics is required for quick resolution and prevention of complications. Penicillins, cephalosporins, amoxicillin/clavulanate, and macrolides are all effective in uncomplicated cases. Adolescents with diabetes and/or immunocompromised status may require hospitalization and intravenous administration of second- or third-generation cephalosporins with or without aminoglycosides. Attempts to isolate the organism are indicated if empiric treatment fails bring any signs of improvement. Orbital cellulitis should be treated as an emergency; hospitalization and intravenous antibiotics are necessary, as well as consultation with ophthalmology and otorhinolaryngology.

Erysipelas

This localized infection of the skin and subcutaneous tissues is caused by group A beta-hemolytic *Streptococcus*; it usually affects the face and extremities. Unlike cellulitis, lesions are sharply demarcated and may present with a prodrome of fever, chills, nausea, vomiting, and arthralgia. Erisypelas responds well to oral antibiotics but sometimes intravenous antibiotics are indicated. Other well-localized lesions with defined margins – such as a drug reaction or contact dermatitis – may pose a diagnostic challenge, but targeted questioning may delineate the history of exposure.

Folliculitis

An infection of hair follicle, folliculitis is divided into types based on the depth of hair follicle involved, infecting agent, and area involved.

Superficial folliculitis

This is the most common form, which can affect any area of the body with hair follicles, mostly areas with poor hygiene and maceration. *S. aureus* is the usual causative organism. Small pustules with hair in center generally resolve without treatment and with no scarring. Chronic recurring infection responds to topical antibiotics such as mupirocin 2 percent, clindamycin, or erythromycin.

Deep folliculitis

Less commonly infection reaches to the base of follicle, resulting in painful papules and pustules and eventual healing with scarring. Treatment with oral antibiotics targeting *S. aureus* is indicated.

Gram-negative folliculitis

This is common in adolescents with acne vulgaris who are being treated with a long-term antibiotic regimen, giving gram-negative bacteria such as *Klebsiella, Enterobacter,* and *Proteus* an opportunity to overpopulate and infect the hair follicles. Usually the folliculitis affects the areas where acne is predominant, such as the face and chest.

Hot-tub folliculitis

Erythematous itchy papules or pustules overlying large areas of the trunk, extremities and other areas usually present after few hours to as much as 3 days after exposure to a hot tub, whirlpool, or swimming pool that had not been chlorinated properly or in which the pH was suboptimal. Outbreaks have been reported with the use of community pools, whirlpools, and water slides. In cases of severe infection, fever, malaise, sore throat, and lymphadenopathy may occur. Lesions are self-limiting over a few days. Drying can be hastened by 1 percent acetic acid soaks.

Furunculosis

A perifollicular erythematous abscess due to *S. aureus*, furunculosis commonly affects intertriginous areas but can also occur on the scalp and at other sites where hair follicles are abundant. When they occur inside the auditory canal or nasal cavity, furuncles can be very painful. Nasal carriage can be the primary source of infection. Hyperhidrosis can predispose to furunculosis, and maintaining good hygiene of intertriginous areas may be the key to preventing autoinoculation and recurrence. Community-acquired methicillin-resistant *S. aureus* (CA-MRSA) is becoming a more frequent cause of furunculosis. Children with immunocompromised status (e.g., human immunodeficiency virus [HIV] or inherited immune deficiencies) are susceptible to treatment-resistant and recurrent furunculosis.

Carbuncle

These are collections of multiple inflamed furuncles in a small area. Favored sites for carbuncles are where the dermis is thick, such as the thighs, back of the neck, and trunk. A carbuncle is a large erythematous, painful, indurated mass located deep within subcutaneous tissue. Multiple small furuncles comprised by a carbuncle connect to each other via subcutaneous tracts and ultimately drain pus to the surface.

Management

Solitary furuncles of less then 5 cm in diameter respond well to excision and drainage only. In cases where multiple or larger lesions are present or where systemic signs of inflammation are evident, an oral antibiotic like minocycline or doxycycline (in children 8 years of age and older) at 100 mg every 12 hours is indicated. Clindamycin can be used in cases of MRSA furunculosis at a dose of 2 to 8 mg/kg per dose every 6 to 8 hours. In patients with MRSA furunculosis leading to systemic infection, hospitalization and a course of intravenous antibiotics (e.g., vancomycin) is necessary.

Incision and drainage is the treatment of choice for carbuncles. Surgical consultation may be indicated for large carbuncles so as to excise and drain the abscesses and clean some of the tracts. Deep-seated carbuncles are hard and fixed, feeling like a malignant tumor on palpation. If they perforate, they cause deep lesions that heal with scarring. Oral antistaphylococcal antibiotics are indicated only in cases of systemic involvement or when concomitant cellulitis is present.

Scarletina

Also known as scarlet fever, scarlatina is a presentation of acute systemic *S. pyogenes* infection. It is given this name owing to its distinctive reddish, punctate, sandpapery skin rash and mucous membrane involvement. A patient will have high fever, sore throat, vomiting, and listlessness. The rash appears on the second day and starts on the upper trunk; it soon becomes generalized, sparing the perioral area and leaving a pale ring around the mouth. It soon concentrates in the axillae and groin. Mucous membranes also have a bright red hue with petechial lesions on the palate. The tongue becomes smooth and red ("strawberry tongue"). Laboratory studies reveal leukocytosis and an elevated antistreptolysin O titer. A swab culture will confirm the hemolytic *Streptococcus*. Empiric treatment with penicillin should be started as soon as possible to avoid the nonsuppurative complication of rheumatic fever.

Staphylococcal scalded skin syndrome (SSSS) and toxic shock syndrome (TSS)

SSSS is predominantly a disease of younger children; 98 percent of patients are under 6 years of age and 62 percent are under 2 years of age. Inoculation the of skin is usually via bloodstream seeding from a distant infection in the pharynx, conjunctiva, or middle ear. The pathogenesis of SSSS is *S. aureus*, which produces an epidermolytic toxin (ET), mostly group phage II, causing lysis of the epidermis at the granular layer. Cleavage of the epidermis results in a positive Nikolsky sign, producing bullae that easily burst with minor pressure. Systemic signs of infection like high fever usually appear first, followed in 24 to 48 hours by an orange-red macular rash resembling scarlatina with a sandpaper-like quality to the touch. The skin becomes extremely tender and peels away easily, leaving large denuded areas. The rash starts from the scalp and face and descends downward, with axillae and groins being commonly affected. It is important to consider other epidermolytic conditions in the differential diagnosis, such as toxic epidermal necrolysis, erythroderma, and drug eruptions.

TSS

Staphylococcal TSS was first elucidated as a severe complication associated with the use of tampons during the menstrual period. At present about 50 percent of cases are menstrual-related and 50 percent are nonmenstrual, specifically postsurgical or post-infectious. The pathogenesis is due to the TSST 1 toxin, which accounts for 90 percent or more of menstrual cases. Staphylococcal enterotoxins are more prevalent in non-menstrual cases. It presents with a flu-like prodrome then progressing to high fever and hypotension. The dermatologic manifestations are diffuse erythema involving the palms and soles. In nonmenstrual cases the erythema may be more concentrated at the site of surgery or infection. The patient may progress to shock, adult respiratory distress syndrome (ARDS), and multiorgan system failure (MOSF). The diagnosis is clinical, as bacterial cultures are reliably positive in only in 5 percent of cases.

Streptococcal TSS is due to increased virulence related to its M protein as well as the presence of streptococcal pyrogenic exotoxins A (SPEA). It occurs as a complication of delivery, surgery, viral infection such as varicella, or the use of nonsteroidal anti-inflammatory drugs (NSAIDs). It presents with a prodromal flu-like picture and then proceeds to a diffuse erythema (10% of the time scarletinaform). Unlike staphylococcal infection, it is followed by ecchymosis and sloughing, appearing more like necrotizing fasciitis. Complications include sepsis, ARDS, and MOSF.

Management

Blood culture may be negative in TSSS but one should attempt to obtain culture and sensitivity to ensure the correctly targeted antibiotic treatment. Local treatment with a potassium permagnate 1:9000 bath of the skin may provide some comfort, although excessive use may cause dryness and further dehydration. The mainstay of treatment remain the penicillinase-resistant systemic antibiotics (e.g., naficillin, flucoxacillin, and methicillin), which, in severe cases, can be given by the intravenous route. Ree-pithelialization of the skin usually occurs quickly and without scarring. Despite the severity of the rash, the prognosis of uncomplicated SSSS is favorable, with a mortality rate of less than 5 percent.

The antibiotics of choice for staphylococcal TSS are clindamycin 600 mg IV every 8 hours and vancomycin, 30 mg/kg per day in two divided doses. Intensive care support is critical in cases of shock. For streptococcal TSS, studies have shown that *S. pyogenes* does not respond well to penicillin, though susceptible, primarily because of the status of the host. Therefore empiric antibiotics should include clinda-mycin 900 mg IV every 8 hours and imipenem 500 g IV every 6 hours for 14 days. Antibiotics may need to continue until no additional surgical debridement is needed or there are no systemic signs.

Necrotizing fasciitis

A life-threatening infection invading all layers of skin and going beyond subcutaneous tissues including fat and superficial layer of fascia, necrotizing fasciitis (NF) affects younger children and neonates, especially if they have another infection like pharyngitis, chickenpox, or infection of the respiratory or urinary tract (8). Children with lowered immunity and other debilitating conditions like diabetes, trauma, or surgery are more susceptible. Two types of NF are known based on the organism involved. Type I NF is caused by multiple organisms both aerobic and anaerobic. Type II NF is caused mostly by a single agent, usually *S. pyogenes*, but other organisms are also known to be responsible for it (▶Tab. 2.1). Infection is rapid and presents with severe systemic signs of infection. The skin becomes erythematous, followed by the development of severe edema and hemorrhagic bullae. The patient complains of severe unrelenting pain, which, once the nerve endings are damaged, can be replaced by numbness in the affected area. Crepitus in subcutaneous tissue signifies infection with a gas-producing organism like *Clostridium* or *Enterobacter*.

Management

Prompt recognition of NF and isolation of the organism is the key to recovery. A scoring system – known as the Laboratory Risk Indicator for Necrotizing Fascitis (LRINEC) – has been used to facilitate the early diagnosis of NF. It includes the basic laboratory screens, total WBC, hemoglobin, sodium, glucose, serum creatinine, and C-reactive protein. A cutoff score of 6 is used to alert the clinician to the possibility of NF. Tissue oxygen saturation of less then 70 percent has been used to identify NF in the lower extremities in adults. In about 13 percent of cases, subcutaneous gas can be detected by radiography. Computed tomography (CT) is superior to plain radiographs as it can also detect early soft tissue changes like fat stranding, fascial thickening, and dissection along the fascial plains. Magnetic resonance imaging (MRI) has also been shown to be highly sensitive in diagnosing NF. Recently ultrasound has been used more frequently and has shown some efficacy.

A multidimensional approach to these patients is the key to resolution of NF, including surgical and infectious disease consultation, sterile precautions, hydration, and nutritional status. Emergency surgical exploration and debridement is the key component of treatment; multiple debridements may be necessary. Hyperbaric oxygen and intravenous immunoglobulins with varying degrees of evidence for support have been used as adjunctive treatments to hasten the healing process. Empiric treatment with broad-spectrum antibiotics with coverage for MRSA as well as *S.pyogenes* should be started as soon as possible and changed to a more specific regimen once results of culture and sensitivity are available. Refer to the treatment of streptococcal TSS above for antibiotic selection.

Ecthyma gangrenosum

This is a relatively rare infection resulting from occlusive vasculitis usually associated with *Pseudomonas* septicemia. It affects mainly patients who are immunocompromised. Victims of burns have a high rate of *Pseudomonas* septicemia. It usually affects the buttocks and anogenital area but can occur anywhere. It presents as a small innocuous macule, which becomes purulent and develops into a thick-walled hemorrhagic bullous lesion that ultimately becomes a gangrenous ulcer. The pathognomonic feature is a grayish-black eschar surrounded by an erythematous ring. A localized form at the site of infection is also reported; it is more common in immune deficient hosts, especially children with hematologic cancers. Non-*Pseudomonas* ecthyma gangrenosum has also been reported. Differentiation between ecthyma gangrenosum and pyoderma gangrenosum on clinical grounds can be difficult. Histopathologic features and the absence of septicemia in pyoderma can distinguish between two almost identical gangrenous ulcers. In rare cases pyoderma can be complicated by superimposed ecthyma gangrenosum.

Management

Blood cultures and the culture of aspirate from a lesion can confirm *P. aeuroginosa*. Biopsy and histopathology may be necessary at times. Localized smaller lesions can be treated with topical silver sulfadiazine. For larger lesions with *Pseudomonas*, systemic antibiotics such as the beta-lactam penicillins – including piperacillin-tazobactam, ceftazidime, cefepime, imipenem – or the aminoglycosides gentamicin or tobramycin will be efficacious.

Cat-scratch disease (CSD)

CSD, a common infection acquired by playing with kittens and stray cats, is caused by the gram-negative bacillus *Bartonella henselae* (9). It is more commonly seen in humid climates and especially during autumn and winter. The initial scratch is followed by the development of a reddish papule within next 1 to 2 weeks, which later becomes larger and firmer, with the development of high-grade fever in about 30 percent of patients. Regional adenopathy occurs most commonly in lymph nodes draining the arms and legs, especially in the axillae, groins, and epitrochlear areas. The head and neck region is involved in up to 49 percent of cases. Lymphadenopathy may persist for weeks, and CSD is the most common cause of chronic lymphadenopathy in young children. The lesions heal completely within about 2 weeks with symptomatic treatments including warm soaks, analgesics, and antipyretics. Skin lesions can be confused with pyogenic granuloma, Kaposi's sarcoma, and epithelioid hemangioma. Other diseases with lymphadenopathy – including tuberculous adenitis, infectious mononucleosis, tularemia, and tumors – can cause a diagnostic dilemma, especially in patients (about 10%) where a typical CSD skin lesion was not present or noted.

Management

An immunofluorescent antibody (IFA) test or the enzyme immunoassay (EIA) test can be used to confirm the diagnosis when in doubt. DNA polymerase chain reaction (PCR) assays are less commonly used but are highly sensitive. The atypical presentation of Parinaud oculoglandular syndrome – with high fever, regional lymphadenopathy and ocular involvement – is seen in about 5 percent of patients. Encephalopathy and severe systemic disease occur in about 2.5 percent of cases. Treatment is generally not necessary in typical CSD, but in immunocompromised patients or patients with severe systemic infection treatment with antibiotics may be effective. Macrolide antibiotics are most commonly used, such as azithromycin at doses of 10 mg/kg per day for 2 to 5 days or rifampin 20 mg/kg per day in divided doses for 2 to 3 weeks. Children over 12 years of age can be treated with ciprofloxacin 20 to 30 mg/kg per day for 2 to 3 weeks or trimethoprim/sulfamethoxazole (8/50 mg/kg per day) for 7 to 10 days. In severely ill patients with systemic involvement, gentamicin 5mg/kg per day IM or IV every 8 hours is efficacious.

Treponemal infections

Syphilis, due to *Treponema pallidum*, has an incubation period of 9 to 90 days (average of 3 weeks). Supportive laboratory data are reviewed (see chapter 18 in Greydanus DE, Patel DR, Omar HA, Feucht C, Merrick J: Adolescent Medicine – Pharmacotherapeutics in General, Mental and Sexual Health, de Gruyter, Berlin, 2012) (10). The spirochete gains access via mucosal abrasions during sexual activity with the induction of a local immune response and secondary hematogenous spread. The dermatologic manifestation of primary syphilis is classic chancre, a well-defined painless erythematous ulcer with a firm (rubbery) base; there is often associated inguinal adenopathy, unilateral or bilateral, nontender and nonsuppurative.

Secondry syphilis appears 6 weeks to 6 months after disappearance of the chancre and can present with a wide variety of findings in its role as "the great imitator," with fever, malaise, headache, arthralgia, generalized lymphadenopathy, hepatosplenomegaly, rhinitis, sore throat, alopecia (moth-eaten, patchy), and a polymorphic rash usually involving the palms and soles. The rash may be macular, papular, maculopapular, morbilliform, and, on occasion, pustular, papulosquamous, annular, or nodular. Skin manifestations of secondary syphilis will resolve spontaneously over 2 or more weeks if not treated, but lack of treatment would leave the patient at risk for further manifestations of syphilis.

Warts due to syphilis, known as condylomata lata, are moist warty papules seen in moist areas of the body such as the perineum and intertriginous areas. A mucous patch, usually a red papule, is another manifestation of syphilis appearing in the mouth, tongue, and genital areas.

Management

Primary, secondary, and early latent stages of syphilis are treated with benzathine penicillin G (2.4 million units IM) in one dose; late latent and tertiary syphilis are treated with a similar dose for 3 weeks. Penicillin-allergic patients may be desensitized. Alternative antibiotic treatment includes tetracycline 500 mg orally four times daily for 14 days or doxycycline 100 mg orally twice daily for 14 days.

Lyme borreliosis (Lyme disease)

This is an infection transmitted by the deer tick *Ixodes damini*, which introduces the spirochete *Borrelia burgdorferi* (11,12,13). Lyme disease is the most common vector-borne disease in United States, with about 15,000 cases being reported annually. Initially confined to the wooded New England states, it is now considered endemic in 15 states. The hallmark lesion is erythema migrans, which develops in about 75percent to 80 percent of patients at the site of tick bite in days to weeks. It can occur over any part of the body and typically leaves a central pale region that slowly expands. Low-grade fever, malaise, arthralgia, myalgia, regional adenopathy and headache are common and, in the absence of a definitive erythema migrans, are difficult to distinguish from a common flu-like illness.

Atypical and chronic cutaneous manifestations can occur in a subset of patients, including acrodermatitis chronica atrophicans usually affecting extensor surfaces of extremities and present as an indurated, hyperpigmented plaque. Systemic involvement can present in various forms, including, in about 15 percent of patients, lymphocytic meningitis with signs of meningeal irritation, encephalitis, and cranial nerve involvement. Facial nerve palsy in young children living in endemic areas is common in up to 34 percent to 65 percent, depending on different studies from different geographic locations. Other systemic manifestations include hepatosplenomegaly, chronic fatigue, migratory pain, and cardiac and joint involvement.

Management

Prevention of tick bite should be emphasized to patients living or traveling in endemic areas; they should avoid heavily wooded areas, not sit on the ground, wear proper clothing, and apply n,n-diethyl-meta-toluamide (DEET) sparingly. Permethrin can also be sprayed on clothing. Prophylactic antibiotics to prevent Lyme disease after a tick bite are not recommended, as up to 70 percent to 80 percent of deer ticks are not infective. Purified recombinant outer surface protein(OSP) vaccine has been approved for use in children 15 years of age and up, with 49 percent efficacy in the first year and ultimately 76 percent efficacy in preventing Lyme disease. Serologic testing is not useful in endemic areas as there is up to a 30 percent chance of false results. Indirect florescent antibody and enzyme linked immunosobent assay (ELISA) tests are available.

Patients may test negative in the early phase of infection, with results later becoming more sensitive and specific. Recommended treatment for early Lyme disease in children presenting with Bell's palsy, mild carditis, and arthritis is based on age. In children below 9 years of age, penicillin or ampicillin 25 to 50 mg/kg per day in divided doses for a total dose of about 1 to 2 g/day is effective, while children older than 9 years can be treated with tetracycline 250 mg four times a day or doxycycline 100 mg twice daily. In complicated late Lyme disease where persistent arthritis, severe carditis, meningitis, or encephalitis is present, ceftriaxone 75 to 100 mg/kg per day or penicillin G 300,000 U/kg per day is recommended.

2.2.2 Viral infections

Viral exanthems are summarized briefly in ▶Tab. 2.2 (14).

Measles (rubeola)

This has been much a less common infection since the advent of a vaccination regimen in 1963, although in the late 1980s to early 1990s a resurgence of measles occurred in the United States mainly because of a decline in levels of antibodies and vaccination administration in certain populations. There have been other isolated outbreaks, as in

Tab. 2.2: Viral Exanthems of Childhood.

Exanthem	Virus	Incubation	Hallmark
Measles	Paramyxovirus	10–12 days	Koplik's spots
Rubella	Togaviridae/rubivirus	14–21 days	Cephalocaudal progression of rash
Erythema infectiosum	Parvovirus B19	4–15 days	Slapped cheek, lacy reticular rash on extremities
Roseola infantum	Human herpesviruses 6 and 7	5–15 days	Rosy pink rash
Chickenpox	Varicella zoster	10–21 days	Polymorphous lesions in crops
Hand-foot-mouth	Coxsackie A16, etc.	3–7 days	Painful palmer, plantar, & buccal vesicles
Mollusum contagiosum	Molluscipox virus		Pearly umbilicated dome-shaped papules
Verucca vulgaris (warts)	Human papillomavirus		Dome-shaped/filiform/cauliflower/flat lesions

San Diego, California, in 2008, where there was a single case involving a nonvaccinated child who had returned from a trip abroad and then exposed 839 people. Measles is highly contagious, is acquired by droplet infection, and starts with high fever, sore throat, rhinorrhea, conjunctivitis, photophobia, cough, and malaise. Simultaneous involvement of mucous membranes also occurs, with the appearance of tiny grayish-white lesions on the buccal mucosa known as Koplik's spots.

A maculopapular rash appears 3 to 4 days after the prodrome, starting usually on the forehead and behind the ears and then spreading to involve the face, trunk, and limbs. When the rash is fully erupted, fever subsides and resolution of the rash is usually rapid, without scarring. Complications that can occur during the acute phase of infection include superimposed bacterial infection leading to otitis media, gastroenteritis, pneumonia, and rarely encephalitis. A serious dematologic complication of is the appearance of purpura secondary to thrombocytopenia ("black measles"). Persistence of virus within the central nervous system for months to years after initial infection can give rise to a post-infectious form of encephalitis known as subacute sclerosing panencephalitis (SSPE), which can occur in 1 of 100,000 patients.

Management

Supportive treatment includes rest, hydration, balanced nutrition, and protection from direct sunlight. Symptomatic treatment with antipyretics and cough suppression is helpful. In secondary bacterial infection, culture and sensitivity testing and targeted antibiotic therapy are indicated. Hospitalization is needed in patients with encephalitis, in whom corticosteroid treatment is appropriate.

Varicella (chickenpox)

This is highly contagious and quickly spread by direct contact and droplet infection. After an incubation period of 1 to 2 weeks, the disease starts with flu-like symptoms, fever, sore throat, and headaches. After 2 to 3 days of prodrome, a rash first appears on the trunk and spreads laterally. The mildly pruritic rash comes in crops starting as erythematous macules, which evolve into vesicles (like "dewdrops on a petal"), and then into pustules. This eventually gives rise to a polymorphous rash with lesions in different stages of evolution and healing. Lesions rupture and become encrusted before completely healing. Usually there is no scarring or pigmentary change, though this may occur if pruritus is more severe than usual. Varicella usually runs a benign course, but there may be rare secondary infections of the lesions with group A *Streptococcus* or *S. aureus*. More serious complications such as necrotizing fasciitis, meningitis, encephalitis, transverse myelitis, or Guillain-Barré syndrome can occur.

Management

Supportive and symptomatic treatment is all that is needed in cases of an uncomplicated varicella infection. Aspirin should be avoided because of the possibility of inducing Reye's syndrome. Antibiotic treatment will be indicated in secondary bacterial infections. Varicella vaccine became available in the United States in 1995 with the indication for routine vaccination for healthy children at 12 to 18 months of age or for older children who have not yet had a varicella infection. Varicella vaccine is considered effective in up to 85 percent of cases, but it appears that protection against varicella declines 1 year postvaccination. Children vaccinated at less than 14 months are more susceptible to breakthrough infection. Secondary infections are treated with appropriate antibiotics for group A *Streptococcus* and *Staphylococcus*, as discussed previously.

Rubella (German measles)

When acquired postnatally, this is a benign self-limiting disease which begins 2 to 3 weeks after exposure and presents with a prodromal phase comprising mild fever, sore throat, eye pain, headache, and lymphadenopathy of the head and neck. In next 1 to 5 days a maculopapular rash appears on the face, which then progresses to involve the rest of the body. The rash begins to clear by day 3 without leaving any marks. Postpubertal girls are susceptible to persistent arthritis and arthralgia for several weeks. Encephalitis and thrombocytopenic purpura are rare complications.

Erythema infectiosum (fifth disease)

This disease, due to parvovirus B19 infection, is usually seen in 4- to 10-year-old children, but it can also occur in adolescents, with outbreaks occurring in late spring and fall. Following a prodromal phase with low-grade fever, sore throat, headache, myalgia, and arthralgia, a confluent erythematous maculopapular rash appears bilaterally on the cheeks in a butterfly pattern, sparing the nasal bridge and giving the "slapped cheeks" appearance. Mucous membrane involvement is evident, with reddish punctate lesions on the buccal mucosa. The rash then spreads to the trunk and the extensor surfaces of the limbs, where it persists for about 5 to 9 days, leaving behind a lacy or reticular pattern that fades over time. Exposure to an irritant like sunlight within next few weeks to months may cause recurrence of the rash. Transmission of acute infection from mother to fetus results in failure of erythropoiesis, causing the development of hy-drops fetalis in 10 percent. Aplastic anemia is seen in patients who are susceptible owing to underlying hemoglobinopathies or hemopoietic defects.

Hand-foot-and-mouth disease (HFMD)

Infections with these enteroviruses (group A and B coxsackieviruses) are highly conta-gious and spread by the oral-fecal route, with an epidemic occurring in the United States about every 3 years. A brief prodromal phase of 12 to 36 hours presents with abdominal pain, anorexia, a burning sensation in the mouth, malaise, and low-grade fever, followed by the development of painful erosive lesions on the hard palate and buccal mucosa. A painful vesicular rash appears on the hands and feet, more pro-nounced on the hands, especially on the palms and along the sides of the fingers. Symp-tomatic treatment including attention to nutrition is all that is needed, as painful oral lesions lead to avoidance of food.

Molluscum contagiosum

This common infection of school-aged children, due mainly to poxvirus 1, is highly contagious in close quarters, especially with community facilities such as shared bath-tubs, swimming pools, and so on. Typical dome-shaped skin-colored papules are 2 to 8 mm in size and can occur as single or multiple lesions, which then become umbili-cated and turn pearly white. Common sites are the face, hands, trunk, and genitalia. Secondary bacterial infections can occur, especially in the large papules, which can reach up to multiple centimeters in size.

Management

Topical application of cantharidin (as 0.7% Cantharone) is safe when applied sparingly and effective especially in localized lesions. Other less common therapies include the use of the immunomodulatory agent tacrolimus, which, although effective, may predis-pose to herpetic infection. Cryotherapy with liquid nitrogen application on each lesion for 6 to 10 seconds is effective and may have to be repeated in 3 weeks. Imiquimod has also shown some efficacy, but evidence is limited. Excision and curettage and electro-dessication can be employed when lesions are few and localized. Oral cimetidine may shown some efficacy, especially when molluscum is associated with atopic dermatitis. As this condition is benign and self-limited (albeit over 6 to 12 months), watchful waiting is also appropriate in relatively mild cases.

Verruca vulgaris (viral warts)

This human papillomavirus (HPV) infection is very common, affecting up to 10 percent of children. The most common group affected is between 12 and 16 years of age, and the virus is transmitted by direct person-to-person contact and autoinoculation. Sun exposure can increase susceptibility to warts. Common warts are well-circumscribed small papular lesions with a keratinized surface most commonly seen on the hands, arms, and legs, especially on the knees and elbows. Filiform warts have frond-like projections usually found in the perioral area and on the lips. Flat-topped smooth warts occur on sun-exposed areas such as the face, neck, and backs of the hands. Planter and palmar warts are more commonly surrounded by an outer keratinized ring. Anogenital warts are cauliflower-like soft lesions known as condyloma acuminata.

Management

Warts are self-limiting in 30 percent cases within 3 months; 78 percent involute in 2 years. Warts in children have a higher rate of spontaneous resolution. Keratolytic agents like salicylic acid 10 percent to 25 percent applied topically is effective in 67 percent of hand warts and 84 percent of plantar warts within 12 weeks. Cryotherapy has a cure rate of 31 percent to 52 percent depending on the intensity of treatment. Pain and blister formation at the site of treatment have been reported. Only one study has reported use of topical immunotherapy with dinitrochlorobenzene; it involved 40 children and resulted in an 80 percent cure rate. Imiquimod, an immune modifier, has shown some efficacy in anogenital warts in adults but no data are available in children and adolescents. Intralesional bleomycin has also shown efficacy up to 82 percent to 94 percent, but the number of subjects studied was small. Mosaic warts are much more resistant to treatment.

HIV/AIDS

The acute exanthem of HIV infection is an erythematous morbilliform rash on the trunk and extremities that manifests itself after a 2- to 4-week incubation period with a prodrome of fever, lymphadenopathy, and night sweats (15). The rash resolves within 5 to 7 days.

Noninfectious skin lesions

Sweet's syndrome – a manifestation of underlying systemic disease characterized by painful violaceous indurated plaques with neutrophilic infiltrate of the dermis – has been reported in children with HIV/AIDS. Eosinophilic folliculitis is an altered immune response to the common skin antigens and is seen in advanced HIV infection, especially when CD4 lymphocyte counts decrease to less than 200 cells per cubic millimeter. Also, acute urticaria can become chronic urticaria with angioedema and give rise to indurated lesions with a peau d'orange appearance. Many common skin diseases, such as atopic and seborrheic dermatitis, become more extensive and difficult to treat in patients with HIV/AIDS. Psoriasis, although not more common in this population, can be very problematic.

Trimethoprim/sulfamethoxazole is the most common drug-related cause of such reactions, but other drugs can also caused eruptions, including Stevens-Johnson syndrome and toxic epidermal necrolysis.

Bacterial infections in HIV

Many bacterial skin infections – such as impetigo, folliculitis, furuncles, and so on – have a very aggressive and extensive course in the HIV/AIDS population. Bacillary angiomatosis presents with pinpoint erythematous macular lesions, which may form a larger lesion like pyoderma; this is seen more commonly in HIV/AIDs patients and may be confused with Kaposi's sarcoma. Biopsy may be the only way to distinguish between them. It does respond very well to the macrolide antibiotics, such as doxycycline and erythromycin. The incidence of group B streptococcal (GBS) infection in infants exposed to HIV in utero is late and more severe than that in nonexposed infants.

Viral infections in HIV

Herpes simplex (HSV) and herpes zoster (HZV) infections are very common among HIV/AIDS patients. Both of these infections are much more serious, recurrent, and recalcitrant to therapy than in patients without HIV. HZV infections can be debilitating and can involve multiple dermatomes at one time. Since lesions can be extensive, necrotic and atypical, laboratory testing with Tzanck preparation, biopsy of lesions, or viral culture is necessary. Acyclovir is the treatment of choice. The incidence of HPV infection among HIV/AIDS patients has increased not only owing to increased susceptibility to this infection (due to immunosuppression) but also because of the decreased clearance of established infections and reactivation of latent infections. Condyloma acuminata (CA) is the most common presentation of HPV among HIV/AIDS patients. These lesions tend to be much larger and numerous and may spread to involve extensive areas of the body. Hypopigmented verruciform papules can spread easily in children. Common warts including veruccae vulgaris and veruucae plantaris are 16 percent to 17 percent more common in this population. Mulloscum contagiosum occurs in 20 percent of HIV/AIDS patients; it can become generalized, affecting large area of body and reaching sizes up to 1 cm.

HPV is responsible for several carcinomas in situ or premalignant lesions including a giant CA also known as Buschke-Loewenstein tumor (BLT) and intraepithelial neoplasia of anogenital region, which can progress to become anal, vulvar, or penile carcinoma. Acute cytomegalovirus (CMV) infections are seen in up to 90 percent of HIV/AIDS patients. Skin manifestations of CMV are varied, ranging from vesicular, morbilliform rashes to indurated plaques to ulcerative lesions. These lesions respond well to foscarnet, ganciclovir, or cidofovir. Epstein-Barr virus can cause oral hairy leukoplakia and Burkitt's lymphoma or large cell lymphoma, which can be treated with acyclovir at a dosage of 200 to 400 mg five times a day and with highly active antiretroviral therapy (HAART).

Fungal infections in HIV

The most common fungal infection in HIV patient is candidiasis, which, as oral thrush, may be the only presenting sign of HIV in the early phase. Other areas of involvement include the axillae, groin, vagina, and under other skin folds where maceration is likely. Systemic fungal infections are common in advanced cases of HIV/AIDS – for example, *Cryptococcus neoformans* infection presenting with a pleomorphic rash. *Histoplasma capsulatum* may present with skin lesions in about 17 percent of cases. Spirotrichosis can cause ulcerative papules or nodules along with systemic involvement.

Yeast infections

Superficial candidal infection is most common, affecting the skin and mucous membranes. *Candida albicans* is a budding yeast; it is a commensal organism of the mucous membranes and is found around the skin adjacent to mucous membranes and in the gut and vaginal areas. Carriage in these areas is one other way of acquiring infection. Candidal mucocutaneous infections are common in the very young and old and in debilitated populations. Any condition predisposing to defects in immunity, especially of cellular immunity, can predispose to candidal infections. *Candida* is known to have specific immunomodulatory effect that can also dampen the host's immune response. Diabetes mellitus is often complicated by mucocutaneous candidal infections. Other situations predisposing to candidiasis include the use of antibiotics or corticosteroids, malnutrition, and HIV infection. *Candida* favors the moist, occluded areas of skin, most commonly intertriginous, perineal, and perianal areas, especially in obese patients. Diagnosis can be confirmed by the identification of pseudohyphae in a microscopic potassium hydroxide (KOH) preparation.

Management

Attempts should be made to keep the affected areas well aerated. The use of mild soap and water with gentle cleansing is recommended. Wet wipes without strong additives like fragrances or preservatives are also effective. In recurring infection, using barrier preparations like petrolatum, titanium oxide in paraffin, or zinc oxide cream can provide added protection against infection. Combination preparations of corticosteroid plus antifungal agents should be avoided. In any dermatitis where the diagnosis is in doubt or that is present for more than 72 hours, use of a topical antifungal agent twice daily with continuation for a week after disappearance of the rash is appropriate. Nystatin, ketoconazole, clotrimazole, econazole, miconazole, oxiconazole, and ciclopirox are effective anticandidal agents.

2.2.3 Fungal infections

Fungal infections are summarized in ▶Tab. 2.3 (16,17).

Fungi are saprophytes; they were originally soil keratinophiles that evolved to be able to infect animals and humans. They can be unicellular, like *Candida*, or multicellular, like dermatophytes. *Candida* species can infect both skin and mucous membranes, while dermatophytes can infect only keratinized areas like skin, hair, and nails. Skin infections are localized to the stratum corneum, the superficial layer of skin, and never invade the deeper layers. Dermatophytes, also known as tinea and commonly called ringworm, have a specific predilection for different sites of the body. Dermatophytes are divided in three main groups: trichophytons, epidermophytons, and microspora. They spread by direct contact with soil, infected surfaces, or contact with infected body areas. The types of infections are classified based on the body area affected. Tinea capitis (head) and tinea unguum (nails), as examples, are discussed below.

Tab. 2.3: Clinical aspects of fungal infections.

Clinical presentation	Fungi	Site of infection	Other presentations
Tinea corporis	*Microsporum equinum* *Microsporum fulvum* *Microsporum gypseum* *Trichophyton equinum* *Trichophyton gallinae* *Trichophyton rubrum* *Trichophyton tonsurans*	Anywhere on body except groin, hair, and nails	
Tinea gladiatorum	*Epidermophyton floccosum* *Trichophyton verrucosum* *Trichophyton tonsurans*	Highly contagious Anywhere on body except groin, hair, and nails	
Tinea facie Tinea barbae	*Trichophyton mentagrophytes*	Face and beard area	
Tinea cruris	*Trichophyton rubrum*	Groin, perianal and perineal areas	Tinea corporis, pedis, and manuum
	Epidermophyton floccosum		Tinea corporis and pedis
Tinea pedis	*Trichophyton interdigitale*		Tinea pedis

Tinea corporis

Dermatophyte infections of the body excluding groin area, feet, scalp, facial cheeks, and nails are known as tinea corporis. *Trichophyton rubrum* is the most prevalent organism. Most commonly infection is acquired via direct skin-to-skin contact. After invading the stratum corneum, the organism produces hyphae and grows outward, producing the typical round or annular lesions with erythematous, slightly raised margins surrounding a clear center. The expanding border is scaly and, when scraped, can provide a sample to identify hyphae microscopically.

Tinea gladiatorum

A highly contagious variant of tinea corporis, this is common in populations where physical contact with bare skin occurs. Most cases are reported in wrestlers, but other physical contact sports have been sources of reports of outbreaks of such lesions. The infection is more prevalent in seasons of active competitions and intense training. Skin lesions are unlike typical tinea corporis and may appear as scaly erythematous papules and plaques. Lesions have a predilection for the head, neck, and arms and are seldom seen on the legs. Spread of infection to other athletes is frequent and covering of localized lesion during sports encounters should be practiced. In cases of extensive rash, there should be avoidance of contact sports. Resumption of such activities can occur after treatment for 1 week.

Tinea cruris

Commonly known as "jock itch," this is a superficial fungal infection of inguinal folds and perineal/perianal areas commonly seen in adolescent males and postpubertal females. Moist, nonaerated areas of skin, as between skin folds, can give rise to maceration, which is a perfect breeding ground for dermatophytes such as *Trichophyton rubrumTrichophyton mentagrophytes*, or *Epidermophyton floccosum*. It is more common in the summer months and in children or adolescents who are obese or who wear tight fitting undergarments, especially in young girls who wear nylon pantyhose. In children participating in team sports the cooccurrence of tinea pedis and tinea cruris is common. At times it is difficult to differentiate between other rashes affecting this area, such as erythrasma, a chronic intertriginous infection due to *Corynebacterium minutissimum*, which fluoresces orange under Wood's lamp examination. Other fungal infections, such as candidiasis, can be distinguished by the presence of pinkish-red smooth lesions without a definite border and satellite punctate lesions in adjacent areas. In younger children, especially those wearing diapers, contact dermatitis can present a diagnostic problem, but usually a correlation to the offending agent will be clear. Psoriasis and seborrheic dermatitis are also included in the differential diagnosis.

Tinea pedis

This is a common condition in children and athletes, commonly known as athlete's foot. Sometimes the term *moccasin foot* is used to describe extensive infection where the whole foot is involved in the distribution of a shoe covering the foot. Infection is usually in between toes, where moist skin nurtures dermatophytes, producing itchy, macerated lesions with fissuring and often a foul odor. Common risk factors are use of community shower stalls at schools, swimming pools, sports clubs; the sharing of slippers, socks, and shoes; wearing shoes for long time, especially when not wearing absorbent socks; and walking barefoot on a sandy beach or other moist ground that can harbor fomites. Most common organisms are the same as in tinea cruris (▶Tab. 2.3). Tinea rubrum affects relatively dry area of the foot such as the heels, soles, and sides, producing somewhat thickened pink lesions covered with fine silver scales. The differential diagnosis includes contact and atopic dermatitis, psoriasis, and candidal infection between the toes.

Pityriasis (tinea) versicolor

This superficial fungal infection is caused by *Malassezia*, a different genus, and especially by the species *Malassezia fufur*. It gives rise to typical fine scaly macular lesions mostly affecting the trunk, back, and arms but can also involve other areas, especially in children, where involvement of the face is common. It is more frequent in hot and humid climates and in those who use topical corticosteroids and oil-based skin products. It presents differently according to the skin color of the individual affected, hence the name *versicolor*. In light-colored individuals, typical leaf-like macular lesions are hyperchromic or brownish, while in dark-colored skin the macules are hypochromic. Lesions have a fine white scale on their margins and occur in large numbers. A "Christmas tree" distribution is seen on the back and is pathognomonic of this condition. Lesions are completely asymptomatic and the only reason patients seek help is for cosmetic concerns. Vitiligo can be confused with tinea versicolor, especially in dark-skinned individuals.

Management

Most infections are diagnosed purely on clinical grounds, although a KOH preparation can provide a cheap, quick, and highly sensitive (88%) method of confirming the diagnosis with the office setting. Scrapings of the lesion border are placed on slide with a drop of 10 percent to 20 percent KOH; the typical septate hyphae of dermatophytes are then easy to detect. Wood's light Examination is not as useful in dermatophyte infections other than tinea capitis as *Microsporum* will fluoresce whereas the more common *Trichophyton* will not.

Topical antifungals

These are highly effective in most superficial infections except in tinea capitis and tinea unguium, where systemic antifungal treatment is indicated. Commonly used topical preparations are terbinafine, miconazole, and clotrimazole, which can be applied twice daily for 2 weeks. Butenafine has the advantage of once-daily application for 2 weeks with same effectiveness, but it is more costly. The patient should apply topical medication to about 2 cm of surrounding area past the advancing edge of the infection and should be educated to avoid risk factors predisposing to reinfection.

Combination therapy

Combination preparations including antifungals and corticosteroids are widely used; they are prescribed mostly when the diagnosis is not fully established. There is growing concern that such treatment leads to a partial resolution and quick relapse of infection, resulting in prolonged treatment for months. A common preparation of this kind, clotrimazole/betamethasone, has shown a 45 percent failure and 36 percent relapse rate. Therefore such combinations are not recommended.

2.2.4 Infestations

Head lice

Infestation with *Pediculus humanus capitis* is very common all over the world, with prevalence rates ranging from 2 percent in United Kingdom to 13 percent in Australia and 100 percent in some remote communities of central and South America (18,19). Approximately 6 to12 million people are infested with head lice each year in the United States. It usually affects children between ages of 3 to 12 years, with a higher preponderance for girls and a lower predilection for African Americans. Head-to-head contact is the main source of transmission, but sharing combs, hats, scarves, hair bands, and so on, or sleeping on the bedding of the infested person can also cause transmission. Outbreaks in preschools and elementary schools are common. In the United States treatment costs associated with head lice are estimated to be $1 billion annually. Head lice feed on the host's blood and can cause significant itching, which leads to frequent scratching, which, in turn, may give rise to secondary infections like impetigo. Diagnosis is best established by visualizing the live lice, which at times can be very difficult, as they tend to hide in areas where the hair is thickest, as in the nape of the neck. Use of a louse comb can aid in diagnosis. Diagnosis cannot be established by finding occasional eggs, especially more than ¼ inch from the skull, as these would most likely be dead nits from a previous infestation. Finding many nits within ¼ inch of the scalp can be predictive of active infestation in about one third of cases.

Management

Prevention of spread is the most effective way of controlling the infection. Teaching patients not to share personal items like combs, hairbrushes, hats, and so on, can be effective in limiting spread. Once the diagnosis is established, application of permethrin 1 percent, pyrethrins, or 0.5 percent malathion in children older than 24 months can be effective. Permethrin 1 percent is very effective in the form of a cream rinse when left in the hair for 10 minutes and rinsed. The residue it leaves behind continues to kill nymphs emerging from the eggs. A second application is suggested in 7 to 10 days, preferably on the ninth day. Pyrethrin preparations are derivatives of chrysanthemums and should be avoided in children with allergies to ragweed or chrysanthemums. Alternatively, treatment on the first and seventh day and thereafter between 13 to15 days has been proposed. Efficacy has decreased owing to the development of resistance. Malathion 0.5 percent is an organophosphate; it is applied to dry hair and left for 8 to 12 hours with good ovicidal activity. Repeat application is not necessary unless live lice are detected, in which case reapplication between days 7 and 9 is recommended. Benzyl alcohol 5 percent is approved for use in infants older than 6 months. Lindane 1 percent (gamma benzene hexachloride) shampoo is contraindicated in neonates and is not recommended for children less than 50 kg in weight because of seizure risk. A single oral dose of ivermectin 200 µg/kg has shown 74 percent effectiveness, which increased to 95 percent when the dose was repeated at 10 days. Prophylactic treatment of persons sharing the same bedding is recommended. All clothes, hairbrushes, combs, and linens used 2 days prior to treatment should be washed in hot water (130°F). Floors and furniture can be vacuumed with minimal risk of transmission after 1 to 2 days.

Scabies

Scabies affects people of all social classes and ages, but it is more commonly seen in children and adolescents (20). It is estimated that about 300 million new cases occur worldwide each year. Scabies is caused by the arthropod *Sarcoptes scabiei var. hominis*, which can not only transmit by skin-to-skin contact but also by contact with contaminated material like bedding or clothing, where it can survive for up to 36 hours. Scabies is more common in crowded urban areas. Children are more at risk owing to their propensity to be in close contact with each other. Teenage girls tend to be the group most affected. After an incubation period of 3 to 6 weeks, the female mite burrows into the epidermis, where it lays eggs. The larvae emerge within 2 to 3 days and mature into an adult mites within 15 days, increasing the population of mites and thus the risk of transmission to others. The ensuing rash is highly pruritic because of a hypersensitivity reaction to the mite. Itching is worse during night when the skin is warmer. Scratching may cause excoriations and breaks in skin, leading to secondary infections like impetigo. The initial lesion is a small erythematous papule, which can become a vesicle or pustule. Typical lesions are small linear brownish lesions called burrows, most commonly seen between the finger webs, but they can also be found along the sides of fingers, on the borders of hand, and the flexor aspects of the wrist. Other areas like the elbows, axillae, buttocks, and genitalia can be affected.

Management

Diagnosis is confirmed by clinical examination and by finding typical burrow lesions in between finger webs. Attempt should be made to extract the mites or eggs from these burrows by gentle scraping and examination under light microscope. Failure to isolate mite or eggs does not rule out scabies, and treatment can be started based on clinical judgment. Videodermatoscopy can provide high-resolution magnification of the skin up to 600 times under incidental light; it is a noninvasive and effective diagnostic tool to locate mites and eggs. Other techniquessuch as epiluminescence microscopy and der-matoscopy have also shown diagnostic accuracy. Permethrin 5 percent cream is effec-tive and safe when applied to the whole body including the head and washed off after 8 to 12 hours, with reapplication recommended after 2 weeks. Transient burning and erythema can occur.

Malathion 0.5 percent, an organophosphate, applied to the body and left for 24 hours, is also effective. Lindane 1 percent has now become a second-line treatment owing to concerns with neurotoxicity in cases of accidental ingestion andwith local irri-tation and continued itching. In randomized controlled trials in comparison with top-ical crotamiton, lindane, and oral ivermectin, permethrin has shown superior results. Permethrin was also found to be more effective in relieving itch in comparison with lin-dane and crotamiton. Oral ivermectin is an effective treatment when topical treatment is not effective or disease is severe and widespread. Oral ivermectin is not indicated in children weighing less than 15 kg.

Cutaneous larva migrans (CLM)

CLM is a common infestation acquired during travel. It is caused mostly by the hookworm *Ancylostoma braziliense* and less commonly by *Ancylostoma caninum*. Hookworms are most commonly found in the tropical and subtropical countries of Southeast Asia, South and Central America, and the southern United States. *A. braziliense* and related hookworms are also common in Australia, the Caribbean region, and in some parts of Europe. The adult hookworm lives in the intestines of cats and dogs; ova are shed via feces in the soil, where the larvae are hatched and survive for several weeks. The most common risk factor for CLM infestation is walking barefoot on a beach, but any contact between uncovered skin and contaminated soil or sand can cause the transmis-sion. Upon becoming attached to bare skin, the larvae secrete hyaluronidase to gain entry into the superficial layers of skin. After an incubation period of up to 6 days, the typical erythematous serpiginous lesion known as creeping eruption or creeping dermatitis develops.

Vesicles and bullae also develop along the larvae's migration track, along with local edema. Intense pruritus may also give rise to excoriation and secondary infection. Since humans are incidental hosts, once the larvae cannot penetrate deep enough to gain entry into deeper tissue, their journey comes to a natural end with death of the larvae. The lesion resolves completely within 8 weeks but in rare cases may persist for longer. On rare occasion systemic invasion can lead to the development of Loffler's syndrome, characterized by a transient pulmonary infiltrate, eosinophilia, and hepatomegaly.

Management

Diagnosis can be established clinically with a temporal relationship to a visit to an endemic area and finding the typical creeping eruption, about 3 mm wide, which grows in length by few millimeters to few centimeters daily. No specific serologic markers or specific diagnostic tests are available for the diagnosis of CLM. Eosinophilia can be present in about 20 percent of cases. Ivermectin is well tolerated and very effective when used as a single dose of 200 µg/kg, with a cure rate of 94 percent. In cases of treatment failure, the same dose can be repeated in 7 days to ensure complete eradication. The rash and pruritus may take few days to resolve. Albendazole for children 6 years of age and older at 15 mg/kg per day in divided doses with a maximal daily dose of 800 mg/day for 3 days is also effective. In younger children topical albendazole 10 percent ointment applied twice daily for 10 days can be effective.

2.3 Dermatitis

2.3.1 Nonallergic dermatitis

Irritant dermatitis

The most common irritant dermatitis occurs in infants in diapers secondary to contact with urine and feces. In children and adolescents, caustics such as acids, alkali, or hydrocarbons are the etiologic agents and usually cause an acute irritating reaction.

Management of irritant dermatitis consists mainly of identifying the offending agent and ridding the patient of it.

Dry-skin dermatitis

This is generally due to excessive drying of the skin with agents such as soaps, alcohols, lotions, or low humidity. It may occur in patterns, an example of which is "lip-smacking" dermatitis, presenting as dry erythematous irritation around the lips. Another example of dry-skin dermatitis is juvenile plantar dermatosis (JPD, or "sweaty sock syndrome"), presenting initially as erythema of the larger toes and subsequent peeling of the weight-bearing aspects of the plantar foot surface. It is often mistaken for tinea pedis ("athlete's foot"), which occurs initially at the smaller toes and later over the dorsum of the foot.

The goal of management of dry-skin dermatitis is to provide sufficient water to the skin plus a means of keeping it there, usually through the liberal use of lubricants. The use of water-in-oil emulsions will also serve this purpose.

Seborrheic dermatitis

Seborrheic dermatitis is due to the overproduction of sebum from sebaceous glands; it appears as a greasy accumulation of scales (21). The lesions are diffuse in infants, seen more over the face and scalp ("cradle cap") as well as in the flexural areas. In adolescents, seborrhea is seen mainly in the scalp (dandruff), nasolabial folds, postauricular area, and chest. It may be confused with fungal lesions, eczema, contact dermatitis, or psoriasis. The etiology of this condition is unknown, although association with the yeast *Pityrosporum* species has been demonstrated. It remains unclear whether this yeast is causal or acts as an agent in the inflammatory process.

Treatment consists of low-potency topical steroids. Keratolytics (salicylic acid), inhibitors of epithelialization (selenium sulfide), and antifungal shampoos (ketoconazole) may be applied locally but should be used judiciously around the face as they can be irritating to the eyes.

2.3.2 Allergic dermatitides

Atopic dermatitis

Atopic dermatitis is a hereditary condition associated with other allergic hypersensitivity reactions such as asthma and/or allergic rhinitis (22,23). Often the respiratory problems are seasonal. In smaller children the rash is more diffuse, but by early childhood and adolescence it appears primarily in the flexural creases and the dorsum of the hands. The skin is often dry. The initial lesion may be erythematous papules or, in the case of darker-skinned individuals, it may be a follicular hyperkeratosis ("chicken-skin") appearance. The skin is invariably pruritic, which then sets off the classic "itch-scratch-itch" cycle. The lesions then may start weeping, becoming excoriated, fissured and eventually lichenified. There also may be postinflammatory hypo- or hyperpigmentation in the affected areas.

There may be physical findings associated with allergy, such as Dennie lines under the eyes or the "allergic salute," consisting of horizontal creases on the bridge of the nose. There may be peripheral eosinophilia or elevated serum IgE levels. Lesions may flare up because of overheating, overdrying, sweating, or other contact allergens. Also, secondary bacterial infection or herpetic infection (eczema herpeticum, Kaposi's varicelliform eruption) may worsen the appearance considerably.

The etiology of atopic dermatitis remains elusive. Although there have been associations with other conditions causing dry skin, such as icthyosis; with food intakeor the presence of house dust mites; or with immunodeficiency as in Wiskott-Aldrich syndrome, there are no studies that convincingly demonstrate a cause-effect link.

The management of atopic dermatitis is long-term and is often fraught with relapses and much frustration on the part of both patients and physicians. If there is a family history of atopy, the patient may be more familiar with the necessary course of treatment, but it is nonetheless important for the clinician to stress the chronicity as well as the frequency of flare-ups.

Management of atopic dermatitis

Following are the four main goals to therapy.

Dryness of skin

Emollients soften the surface of the skin, allowing for the exposure of extra water-binding sites. Examples of this are alpha-hydroxy acids, lactic acid, salicylic acid, and urea, which remove excess scales from the skin. Lubricants aid in the retention of water either by attracting water to the skin or containing vehicles that prevent water from escaping the skin (occlusion). Petrolatum is a commonly used vehicle to aid in the retention of heat and moisture, but it can feel greasy to the patient, with consequent low compliance to therapy. Substances such as cetyl or stearyl alcohol when added to petrolatum will feel more comfortable to the patient as well as increase the ability of the petrolatum to take up water.

   Creams and lotions are oil-in-water emulsions and are effective in less-severe cases. They are more cosmetically pleasing to the patient and are more easily removable. Ointments contain more water-insoluble components, which do have maximal occlusive properties. Because ointments can be disagreeable to the patient, emulsifiers added to them may increase compliance, although they may diminish water retention. Gels are primarily useful to facilitate the penetration of other topical medications. Because they have an alcohol base, they can sting when applied.

Pruritus

Management of prutitus consists of oral sedating antihistamines used primarily at night to prevent scratching and subsequent excoriation. Examples of such medications are hydroxyzine 1 mg/kg per dose at bedtime or cetirizine 2.5 mg in patients under age 6 and 5 mg in those over age 6 at bedtime.

Inflammation

The mainstay of the anti-inflammatory management of atopic dermatitis is the use of topical steroids. The main issues for treatment revolve about the choice of the medication and the means by which it is applied. As the treatment of atopic dermatitis is multi-pronged, it is important to combine skin moisturization with the use of topical steroids and, flexibly, with the ultimate goal of diminishing the potency of the steroids and hopefully their use altogether until the next relapse. The art of management of atopic dermatitis lies in the juxtaposition of different modes of treatment. The choice of a steroid should begin with one of low potency, such as hydrocortisone 2.5 percent or desonide 0.05 percent. If not effective, midpotency steroids such as fluocinolone acetonide 0.025 percent or triamcinolone 0.1 percent may be of help. Less frequently, high-potency steroids such as betamethasone dipropionate cream 0.05 percent may be necessary. It is important to recognize the consequences of overuse of topical steroids, such as skin atrophy and striae, particularly in areas such as the face and genital area. ▶Tab. 2.4 lists topical steroid medications with their potencies.

   Prior to resorting to high-potency topical steroid therapy, often moist occlusive dressings will be effective; that is, the application of damp cotton gauze followed by dry cotton gauze over a moderate-potency steroid. This may be difficult in an adolescent who would

Tab. 2.4: Topical steroids in the treatment of atopic dermatitis.

	Generic name	Brand name
Class I	Clobetasol proprionate	Temovate 0.05%
	Betamethasone dipropionate	Diprolene 0.05% cream or ointment
Class II	Betamethasone diproprionate	Diprosone 0.05% ointment
	Mometasone furoate	Elocon 0.1% ointment
	Halcinonide	Halog 0.1%
	Flucinonide	Lidex 0.05%
	Desoximetasone	Topicort 0.25% cream, 0.05% gel
Class III	Triamcinolone acetonide	Aristocort A 0.1% ointment
	Betamethasone dipropionate	Diprosone 0.05% cream
	Betamethasone valerate	Valisone 0.1% ointment
Class IV	Triamcinolone acetonide	Aristocort 0.1% ointment
	Flurandrenolide	Cordran 0.05% ointment
	Mometasone furorate	Elocon 0.1% cream, lotion
	Triamcinolone acetonide	Kenalog 0.1% cream or ointment
	Fluocinolone	Synalar 0.025% ointment
	Desoximetasone	Topicort LP 0.05% cream
Class V	Flurandrenolide	Cordran 0.05% cream
	Triamcinolone acetonide	Kenalog 0.1% lotion, 0.025% ointment
	Fluocinolone	Synalar 0.025% cream
	Tridesilon	Desonide 0.05% ointment
	Betamethasone	Valisone 0.1% cream or lotion
	Hydrocortisone valerate	Westcort 0.2% cream or lotion
Class VI	Triamcinolone acetonide Flumetasone pivalate	Aristocort 0.01% cream, Kenalog 0.25% cream or ointment
	Tridesilon	Locorten 0.03% cream
		Desonide 0.05% cream
Class VII	Hydrocortisone	Hytone 1% or 2.5% lotion cream or ointment

Adapted from Custer JW, Rau RE, eds. The Harriet Lane Handbook, 18th ed. St. Louis: Mosby/ Elsevier; 2009.

be embarrassed to be seen with such dressings during the day, so they may be employed at home and during sleep. If is often necessary to encourage parents to maintain this treatment continuously. Patient and parental education is of foremost importance to maintain the treatment plan, even in the face of many failures and frustrations along the way.

Treatment failure with these measures may necessitate referral to a dermatologist. Some primary care physicians may try coal tar applications to restore normal keratinization or immunosuppressive agents such as tacrolimus or pimecrolimus. Coal tar preparations stain and have an unpleasant odor, often a barrier to compliance, and immunosuppressive agents may be irritating to the skin.

Complications (secondary infection)

Treating secondary bacterial infections is of paramount importance. The most common infecting agents are *S. aureus, S. pyogenes*, and herpes simplex. Appropriate antibiotic therapy, local or systemic, is necessary to treat these complications.

Contact dermatitis

Contact dermatitis occurs after incomplete antigens, called haptens, penetrate the epidermis, are carried to lymph nodes where they are presented to T lymphocytes, which then migrate back to the skin. Depending on the strength of the antigen (e. g., poison ivy, or urushiol) , it may take a week to process, or considerably longer for weaker allergens such as nickel. Upon a second exposure to the antigen, the inflammatory reaction occurs with the T lymphocytes releasing inflammatory mediators that cause acute erythematous, often vesicular, pruritic dermatitis.

The hallmark of diagnosis is recognition of the distribution and pattern of the dermatitis. Typically it occurs only at the area of contact. Often a streaky appearance is the clue when the patient has brushed against the allergen in a wooded area. If the lesions due to contact with poison ivy or poison oak appear to be diffuse, the patient has probably spread the oil with his or her hands at the time of initial contact. Often the shape of the lesion is helpful. If it is close to perfectly round, it may be secondary to a metallic contact, such as clothing snaps. The location may also be helpful, as when nickel in earrings cause lesions about the earlobes. Allergens in leather or rubber may cause sensitization of the feet and toes. Perfumes, soaps, and makeup will cause dermatitis in the regions to which they are applied.

Treatment consists of local applications of low-potency corticosteroids and antihistamines to lessen the pruritic component. Generally symptoms last for 3 to 4 weeks with or without treatment.

2.3.3 Idiopathic dermatitides

Dyshidrotic eczema

This condition has been erroneously considered to be secondary to dysfunction of the eccrine (sweat) glands. However, histopathology demonstrates normal sweat glands. Because there is a clinical association with atopy and contact irritants, a single etiology remains elusive. Dyshidrotic eczema presents with highly pruritic vesicles starting at the lateral aspects of the digits; it eventually progresses to fissuring and cracking of the palms and soles. Treatment is similar to that for atopic eczema, usually with low-potency corticosteroid ointments and, if necessary, moist applications followed by covered dry dressings.

Keratosis pilaris

This common condition presents as follicular plugs of the stratum corneum and appears most often on the extensor aspects of the upper and lower extremities and buttocks. It may also appear on the facial cheeks in younger children, especially during colder and dryer months. The lesions feel rough and dry and may be either flesh-colored or erythematous. Associations with atopy and icthyosis have been reported, but this condition often occurs independently. It may be chronic and responds to moisturizers (urea) and keratolytics (lactic acid or retinoic acid).

Nummular eczema

This condition may be associated with atopic eczema, but it may also occur independently. It is characterized by coin-like lesions, can be intensely pruritic, and is treated similarly as atopic eczema. The duration of treatment is considerably longer than that of atopic dermatitis.

2.4 Hypersensivity

2.4.1 Urticaria

Acute urticaria

This condition is short-lived and most often a consequence of infection (24). Bacterial etiologies include streptococci whereas viral ones include Epstein-Barr virus, hepatitis, and others. Urticaria may be allergic in nature, with elevated IgE levels and histamine mediation of the skin reaction, although only 3 percent to 5 percent of cases have been reported with this etiology confirmed. Allergic agents include hymenoptera, scorpion, and jellyfish stings; drug reactions; and food allergies, particularly to peanuts, tree nuts, eggs, shellfish, berries, and tomatoes. Scombroid fish with high amounts of histamine may cause this reaction. Urticaria may be a manifestation of systemic diseases, discussed in the following section. The hallmark lesion of urticaria is the wheal and flare, which is very pruritic. It is transitory in nature but with several relapses and remissions over a few days.

The course is generally benign and self-limited; however, there may be associated angioedema with swelling particularly of the hands and feet. During more severe local reactions, there may be blistering with weeping clear fluid, often mistaken for bacterial cellulitis. Over time, urticarial lesions may appear dusky and be mistaken for ecchymoses. One must always be mindful of a more severe generalized reaction with upper airway obstruction due to oropharyngeal swelling (anaphylaxis).

Several conditions may be confused with urticaria, such as hereditary angiodedma (C1 esterase inhibitor deficiency), erythema multiforme (target lesions), vasculitis, urticaria pigmentosa (mastocytosis), and viral exanthems.

Chronic urticaria

This condition is defined by symptoms lasting for more than 4 to 6 weeks. About 15 percent of them are the physical urticarias, which are secondary to heat, exercise, cold, or pressure (25). Cold urticarias may be hereditary or of immunogenic origin. Severe anaphylactic reactions have been reported in patients with this condition jumping into cold water. Pressure and some cold urticarias are histamine-mediated, but others may be mediated through cholinergic nerves.

Management of urticaria

Acute urticaria that is not severe is best treated with antihistamines. Sedating antihistamines such as hydroxyzine 1 to 2 mg/kg per day and diphenhydramine 5 mg/kg per day are more effective than nonsedating antihistamines. In more severe cases, adrenergic medications may be necessary to manage angioedema. In severe cases of anaphylaxis, airway maintenance is the first priority. Epinephrine given subcutaneously, 0.01 mL/kg of a 1:1000 solution, acts rapidly in this situation. Albuterol inhalers may be used, as well as oral pseudoephedrine, but these may cause significant adrenergic side effects.

Patients should be counseled that the course may last up to 6 weeks. If longer, then further studies are necessary to identify the type of chronic urticaria. Simple placement of ice on a patient's skin for several minutes will produce the wheal and flare. Similarly heat and exercise or pressure will reproduce urticaria. Cold agglutinins and cryoglobulins may be identified. Further studies to look for an infectious or autoimmune etiology may be necessary.

2.4.2 Erythema multiforme

This condition presents as fixed erythematous lesions varying in size and shape without prodrome. They follow an outbreak of herpes labialis in about 50 percent of cases. The lesions last for several weeks and progress to the classic "target" or "iris" lesions, occurring most commonly over extensor surfaces in an acral distribution. They may turn dusky or become encrusted over time. Oral involvement occurs rarely and is not extensive. There are few systemic symptoms and the condition is self-limiting. Subsequent herpes labialis infections will induce recurrences. Although formerly connected with Stevens-Johnson syndrome (SJS, discussed further on under "Life-threatening eruptions"), erythema multiforme is now considered a separate entity. One should no longer use the terms *erythema multiforme minor* and *erythema multiforme major*. Treatment is expectant and occasional use of antihistamines may relieve rare instances of pruritus.

2.4.3 Drug eruptions

The most common drug eruptions are morbiliform (measles-like), urticarial, and fixed. Others include pustular, phototoxic, scarlatineform, bullous, and lichenoid (26,27,28).

Morbilliform eruptions

These rashes are diffuse and maculopapular; they appear about 1 to 3 weeks after institution of the medication. They are the most common and account for up to 50 percent of drug eruptions. There may or may not be pruritus. The rash usually involves the trunk and extremities and may ultimately become confluent. The most common offending agents are antibiotics, anticonvulsants, antifungals, and NSAIDs. It is paramount to elicit a drug history in all patients with rashes. It is also important to consider that the primary illness may be the cause of the rash (strep, EB virus). Amoxicillin may elicit a morbilliform rash in a patient with EB viral infection 50 percent of the time.

Urticarial drug eruptions

These IgE-mediated reactions are the second most common drug eruptions, accounting for about 25 percent of them. They present as a wheal and flare from hours to days after exposure and may be associated with angioedema, although rarely anaphylaxis. The intravenous or intramuscular route is more likely to cause anaphylaxis than oral dosing. Drugs most commonly associated with this condition are NSAIDs and antibiotics (penicillins, cephalosporins, and sulfonamides). Note that cefaclor produces a reaction resembling serum sickness.

Fixed drug eruptions

These present as erythematous lesions of varying size, appearing at first urticarial but then becoming well demarcated and eventually hyperpigmented. The main offending drugs are antibiotics (trimethoprim, sulfonamides, tetracyclines, and ciprofloxacin), anticonvulsants (barbiturates, carbamazepine) and oral contraceptives. They clear slowly over months and recur with reintroduction of the offending agent.

Less common drug eruptions

Less common drug eruptions include vasculitis, erythema nodosum, photosensitivity, lichenoid reactions, and bullous eruptions. Offending agents for vasculitis include anticonvulsants, NSAIDS, antibiotics (penicillins, sulfonamides, and macrolides), gold, diuretics, and cimetidine. Erythema nodosum is associated with oral contraceptives, NSAIDs, sulfonamides, and opiates. Photosensitivity reactions may be phototoxic owing to direct damage due to sunlight, altering the drug. They occur in sun-exposed areas and are often quite painful, resembling severe sunburn. The more common offending agents are antibiotics, particularly tetracycline, sulfa drugs, griseofulvin, NSAIDs, diuretics (furosemide, thiazides), psoralens, and coal tar derivatives. The other photosensitivity reaction is a true allergy presenting as severe urticaria in sun-exposed areas. Ultraviolet light acts directly on the drug, altering it to an allergenic form. The most common offending agents are perfumes, para-amino benzoic acid, phenothiazines, and sulfonamides. Lichenoid reactions occur months after exposure to drugs such as diuretics, beta blockers, and phenothiazines, and their violaceous plaques are often mistaken for rashes associated with collagen vascular disorders.

Life-threatening eruptions

Stevens-Johnson syndrome (SJS) and toxic epidermal necrolysis (TEN) were once considered part of the spectrum of erythema multiforme but are now separated from that condition (29). It is difficult to distinguish SJS from TEN clinically and pathologically (separation at the dermal-epidermal junction); therefore some consider the two conditions a continuum, with TEN being a more severe form. Some experts have defined SJS as epidermal detachment of less than 10 percent of body surface area, TEN as more than 30 percent. They present with a 1- to 2-week prodrome consisting of fever, headache, malaise, vomiting, and/or diarrhea. Skin involvement consists of blisters progressing to bullae with epidermal necrosis. There is mucosal involvement, frequently occurring 1 to 2 days before the cutaneous lesions in at least two sites. Especially involved are the mouth and eyes, with crusty hemorrhagic lesions, but involvement may extend to the lower gastrointestinal tract, kidneys, liver, heart, and genitourinary tract in more severe instances. Skin and mucosal lesions often result in severe scarring, contracture, and dyschromia, and there may be permanent damage to the nails.

Triggers are most commonly antibiotics (sulfonamides, penicillins), anticonvulsants, and NSAIDs. In rare instances herpes simplex and mycoplasmal pneumonia have been implicated. There is evidence that there may be a genetic predisposition for these conditions. One study confirmed evidence of a gene, *HLA-B1502*, associated with SJS in a Han Chinese population after intake of carbamazepine. Outcomes can be poor, with a mortality rate of up to 30 percent reported.

Management of drug eruptions

The hallmark of management of drug reactions is prompt discontinuation of the offending agent. If there is any concern about anaphylaxis, the airway must be maintained and subcutaneous epinephrine 1:1000, 0.01 mL/kg up to 0.5 mL, should be administered immediately with intravenous fluids. Systemic steroids may also be of benefit. In the event of anaphylaxis, the patient should carry information of this allergy usually as a wristband. In addition, it is paramount to document all allergies on the patient's medical record.

Most other reactions (urticarial, fixed, or lichenoid) are not life-threatening and may take several weeks to months to subside. Medication is generally not necessary, although antihistamines may be of benefit for pruritus in urticarial reactions.

Treatment of SJS and TEN is challenging. The conditions manifest themselves clinically as burns and appropriate fluid replacement is necessary. As with burns, the lesions must be kept clean and debrided with serial cultures and appropriate antibiotic therapy as warranted. The use of corticosteroids and intravenous immunoglobulin is controversial. It is important to obtain dermatologic and ophthalmologic consultation to prevent or treat keratitis, iritis, and scarring. Oral and airway hygiene is important, as is support with total parenteral nutrition.

2.5 Miscellaneous Skin Conditions

2.5.1 Acne vulgaris

Acne vulgaris is one of the most common skin problems in primary care and dermatology offices (30,31). It usually begins at the onset of puberty. Genetic susceptibility influences the development of acne and relates to severity.

The pathogenesis of acne involves multiple factors, including abnormal keratinization, hormone and sebum production (androgen stimulation), bacterial colonization (*Propionibacterium acnes*), and host immune response with inflammation.

The obstruction of a pilosebaceous unit on the face, a follicular plug, is a microcomedone caused by an excessive amount of sebum from desquamated epithelial cells in the follicular wall. Adrenal and gonadal androgens during the adolescent period affect sebum production. Microcomedones subsequently change to comedones in blackhead (open head) and whitehead (closed head) forms. *P. acnes*, a gram-positive anaerobic bacterium, colonizes at pilosebaceous follicles. This bacterium hydrolyzes triglycerides to free fatty acids (FFAs) and produces proinflammatory mediators and chemotactic factors that are the causes of inflammation. This results in papules, pustules, and nodulocystic acne. The severity of acne correlates with stage of sexual maturity and rate of sebum production.

The proposed trigger factors of acne are stress (activation of androgen hormone), mechanical factors, topical products (obstruction pilosebaceous unit), and medications (anabolic steroids, progestins, isoniazid, phenytoin, vitamin B12).

The presentation of acne is variable and includes comedones, papules, pustules, cysts, nodules, scarring, and dyspigmentation at the face, neck, chest, and back area.

Management of acne

Topical therapy

• Benzoyl peroxide

The mechanisms of action are antimicrobial, comedolytic, and anti-inflammatory. These actions are useful in mild inflammatory and/or comedonal acne.

There are varieties of concentration (2.5%–10%) and preparation (gel, wash, foam, cream). Benzoyl peroxide also comes in combination with other medications (topical antibacterial, vitamin A). This agent is usually used as a thin coat (pea-sized) to all acne-prone areas once to twice daily.

The common side effects are stinging, drying, redness, peeling of the skin, and bleaching of colored clothes.

• Topical antibiotics

The mechanisms of action are reduction of bacteria on the skin surface and within follicles and anti-inflammatory effects. The most common topical medications are clindamycin and erythromycin. Less commonly used are metronidazole and sulfonamide (sulfacetamide).

These medications are appropriately used in mild to moderate acne as well as mixed inflammatory and comedonal acne, usually once to twice daily.

Recent data show topical antibacterial resistance of *P. acnes* to erythromycin or clindamycin. Multiple drugs resistance is also reported. Recommendations for topical antibiotics are short-term use and avoidance of concomitant oral and topical therapy with the same medication. The combination use of topical antibiotics with topical benzoyl peroxide or topical retinoid decreases the risk of resistance. Antibiotics used in the treatment of acne are summarized in ▶Tab. 2.5.

• Retinoids

The mechanisms of action are normalization of keratinization as well as comedolytic and anti-inflammatory effects. There are varieties of concentration from 0.01 percent to 0.1 percent and various preparations: gel, microgel, cream form, vitamin A, and adapalene. One may combine retinoids with other products, such as benzoyl peroxide and tazarotene. The combination of many products enhances therapeutic efficacy.

These agents are usually used as thin coats (pea-sized) applied once nightly on the dry face because of the effects of skin irritation and sun sensitivity. Postinflammatory hypo- or hyperpigmentation may occur in darker-skinned individuals. To prevent these effects, begin with a lower-strength preparation. The evidence of teratogenicity from topical retinoid use is inconclusive (pregnancy category C classification, no controlled studies in women; risk to the fetus cannot be ruled out).

Tab. 2.5: Oral antibiotics for treatment of acne.

Drug	Dose/ Frequency	Age	Side effects	Remarks
Tetracycline cap (250, 500 mg)	250–500 mg twice daily	Age >9 years	Dental staining GI upset, esophageal irritation Photosensitivity	Administer on an empty stomach Avoid taking with antacid, dairy products Take with a large glass of water
Doxycycline cap (50, 100 mg)	50–100 mg twice daily	Age >9 years	Less dental staining than Tetracycline GI upset Photosensitivity/ photo-onycholysis	Avoid taking with dairy products
Minocycline cap (50 and 100 mg)	50–100 mg Twice daily	Age >9 years	Dental staining (less) GI upset, hepatitis Blue-gray skin pigmentation Drug induced lupus Headache, vertigo (vestibular disturbance) Serum sickness like reaction	Administer on an empty stomach Avoid taking with dairy products
Erythromycin tab (250 and 500 mg)	250–500 mg twice daily	Any age	GI upset	Administer one hour after intake of food
Trimethroprim/ sulfamethoxazole tab (80/400 and 160/800 mg)	80/400, 160/800 mg Once/twice daily	Any age	Drug hypersensitivity reaction Bone marrow suppression GI upset, hepatitis Renal toxicity	Avoid in Glucose-6-Phosphate Dehydrogenase Deficiency Use as second-line drug
Cephalexin tab (250, 500 mg)	250–500 mg twice daily	Any age	GI upset	Use as second-line drug

- Azelaic acid

This medication is produced from the yeast *Pityrosporum ovale*. The mechanisms of action are minimal both in antibacterial and anticomedonal effect. Azelaic acid may be an alternative treatment for mild inflammatory and comedonal acne. The dominant beneficial effect is the ability to ameliorate hyperpigmented lesions.

The available form is a 20 percent cream. The side effects are pruritus, burning, and erythema.

- Dapsone

This medication has Food and Drug Administration (FDA) approval for the treatment of acne. The available form is a 5 percent gel. The supportive evidence of efficacy is lesion reduction in number and improvement of acne severity.

Systemic therapy

- Oral antibiotics

Oral antibiotics are used in cases of moderate to severe inflammatory acne. The mechanisms of action are decrease *P. acnes*, resulting in decreased inflammation from the reduction of neutrophil chemotaxis and proinflammatory cytokines. Oral antibiotics are generally used to control the acne for several months, with improvement in 4 to 8 weeks after initiation.

The most commonly used twice-daily antibiotics are tetracycline, doxycycline, minocycline, and erythromycin. ▶Tab. 2.5 summarizes the antibiotic treatment of acne.

- Isotretinoin

Isotretinoin is *cis*-retinoic acid, a derivative of vitamin A, usually used in recalcitrant acne with severe and nodulocystic lesions. The mechanism of action is to eradicate all types of acne pathogenesis.

This medication is usually started at a dosage of 0.5 to 1 mg/kg per day up to 2 mg/kg per day. A cumulative dose of 100 to 150 mg/kg is associated with successful treatment. The dosage and duration of therapy depends on individual response, and a repeated course maybe necessary.

The potential side effects are dry skin and mucosa, alopecia, pseudotumor cerebri (especially when taken with oral antibiotics), abnormal lipid profiles and liver function tests, exacerbation of inflammatory bowel disease, and teratogenic effects (pregnancy category X classification).

Female patients must be tested to make sure that they are not pregnant before beginning isotretinoin and be supervised to have at least two methods of contraception during the course of treatment. Signature of a consent form with risks and benefits is required before initiation of treatment.

Hormonal therapy

Hormonal therapy is an optional treatment in female patients especially in hyperandrogenic acne (hirsutism, androgenetic alopecia, menstrual irregularity, polycystic ovarian syndrome). The mechanisms of action are reduction of active free testosterone and ovarian androgen production.

Oral contraceptive pills, norgestimate, and ethinyl estradiol are approved by the FDA to treat acne vulgaris.

Spironolactone, an antiandrogenic agonist, is also an optional treatment in females. The side effects are breast soreness, menstrual irregularities, hyperkalemia, and fatigue.

2.5.2 Nevi

Melanocytic nevi

The melanocytic nevus is a common skin disorder that may be congenital or acquired (32). The acquired form may be due to internal factors (genetic, race, skin type, hormone, and pregnancy) or external factors (sun exposure, cutaneous surgery, systemic immunosuppression, medications).

Melanocytic nevi result from the benign proliferation of melanocytes leading to accumulation of nevus cells (nevocyte) in layers of the skin. This condition is divided into junctional nevi (nevocytes in the dermoepidermal junction), compound nevi (nevocytes in the junction and dermis), and intradermal nevi (nevocytes limited to the dermis).The risk of transformation from melanocytic nevus to malignant melanoma is extremely low.

Congenital melanocytic nevi (CMN)

These lesions usually present at birth or in the first year of life. CMN is most commonly classified based on the diameter into three groups:

- Small (less than 1.5 cm in diameter)
- Medium (1.5–19.9 cm in diameter)
- Large/giant (greater than 20 cm in diameter)

Giant melanocytic nevi in the neonatal period are considered when the size is larger than the baby's palm (about 6 cm). CMN usually are brown-colored macules, papules, or patches on any part of the body. Giant melanocytic nevi tend to have color, size and texture variation and become hairy with increasing age. The posterior trunk is the most common location of giant melanocytic nevi.

CMN of all sizes carry an increased risk of malignant melanoma, especially giant melanocytic nevi. The higher malignancy risk of the giant melanocytic nevus is associated with large diameter, increasing of satellite lesions, and location on the back. Malignancy risk rates range between 2 percent and 4 percent for giant congenital nevi. The malignancy risk for small congenital nevi is unknown but is probably less than 1 percent.

Neurocutaneous melanosis (NCM) is due to proliferation of intracerebral melanocytes, which may result in seizure, malignant melanoma of the central nervous system, increased intracranial pressure, and spinal cord compression. NCM is mostly found in giant melanocytic nevi with satellite lesions.

The treatment of giant melanocytic nevi is complicated and controversial. The vast majority are simply followed with biopsy or removal only when worrisome lesions arise. Factors in management include location, size, neurocutaneous melanosis, cosmetic result, risk of malignant melanoma, and anesthetic issues. A multidisciplinary approach with the patients and families should be provided.

Spitz nevus

The presentation of a Spitz nevus is a well-circumscribed reddish-brown dome-shaped papules or nodule, mostly as a solitary lesion. Spitz nevi are predominant in the pediatric population and most commonly occur on the face, neck and lower extremities.

They are usually acquired proliferations of melanocytes with histopathologic features that sometime overlap with melanoma.

The differential diagnosis consists of atypical melanocytic nevus, melanoma, pyogenic granuloma, and early-stage juvenile xanthogranuloma.

Although the potential risk of malignant transformation is minimal, there is no definite consensus on the management of Spitz nevi. Surgical excision to confirm the diagnosis and risk of malignancy is the usual approach. Care should be taken to remove the entire lesion on the first biopsy, as examination of the deep component is essential for a correct diagnosis.

Halo nevus (Sutton's nevus)

This presents as a halo or hypopigmented macule surrounding a pigmented nevus. The halo is usually symmetrical and with a regular in border differing from the irregular halo of melanoma. The most common location of halo nevi is on the back. Half of the patients have multiple lesions.

The pathogenesis of this disorder is unknown. It has been proposed to be an immune-mediated attack on the nevus cells in the lesion. Autoimmune conditions such as vitiligo and thyroiditis are rarely found together with halo nevi.

The treatment of halo nevi is observational. Excision is unnecessary when the central lesion appears benign.

Nevus spilus (speckled lentiginous nevus)

The initial lesion may reveal a large brown patch in the first few years of life; this gradually develops the secondary variably darker lesion of superimposed small pigmented macules and/or papules. It is typically solitary. The trunk and extremities are the most common locations. The lesion varies in size.

The characteristic presentation is multiple dark brown to black macules superimposed on the larger brown patch.

Nevus spilus should be monitored because of the potential risk of malignant transformation.

Becker's nevus

Becker's nevi are acquired. The clinical presentation is a unilateral slightly thickened irregular border of brownish hyperpigmented plaque usually found at the chest wall, upper trunk, and shoulder of adolescent males. Hypertrichosis is a common concomitant finding.

Thepathogenesis of this condition is unclear. Increased androgen receptors in the lesion are presumed to relate to hypertrichosis in these nevi. Becker's nevi are associated with smooth muscle hamartomas that affect arrector pili muscle contractions.

Hyperpigmented patches and hypertrichosis tend to persist for life. Laser therapy is not recommended in most cases because of the unpleasant results.

Epidermal nevus

The epidermal nevus is a hamartoma of the top layer of skin. It presents as localized flesh-colored to brownish verrucous surface of papules or plaques, single to linear in configuration, sometimes along Blaschko's lines.

The differential diagnosis includes lichen striatus and linear lichen planus. Skin biopsy is helpful to distinguish these conditions.

Treatment of epidermal nevi includes surgical procedures (excision, liquid nitrogen, cryotherapy, dermabrasion, laser ablation) and topical treatment (tretinoin, podophyllin, keratolytic agents).

Cutaneous findings of epidermal nevus are concomitant with an array of extracutaneous abnormalities/systemic complications such as limb defect/deformity, seizures, developmental delay, macrocephaly, eye abnormalities, skeletal abnormalities (kyphosis, scoliosis). This is known as epidermal nevus syndrome (EPS).

The inflammation of linear epidermal nevus is termed inflammatory linear verrucous epidermal nevus (ILVEN). This condition is a chronic and inflammatory cause of epidermal nevus variants. The symptoms are characteristically extreme pruritus and recurrent inflammation. Treatment of ILVEN is very difficult. Choices include topical or intralesional corticosteroid, topical retinoid, topical calcineurin inhibitor, topical vitamin D derivatives, CO2 laser, and surgical excision. Responses are often poor.

2.5.3 Papulosquamous disorders

Primary forms of ichthyosis (nonsyndrome ichthyosis)

We discuss congenital forms of icthyosis mainly because they persist into childhood and adolescence and require treatment (33,34,35,36).

Ichthyosis vulgaris

Ichthyosis vulgaris is the most common form of ichthyosis, which is frequently associated with atopic dermatitis. The other minor criteria of atopic dermatitis include xerosis, hyperlinearity of palm-sole, and keratosis pilaris. This condition transmitted as an autosomal dominant trait. The examination of parents' skin may be helpful in diagnosis.

The presentation reveals white to gray scales on the extensor surface of the extremities, particularly the lower legs. The flexor surface and groin are always spared. The scale is small and white to gray, like a fish scale; it is worse in dry weather.

The diagnosis is clinical. Skin biopsy may be done only in cases of uncertainty. The treatments include hydration, then topical emollient and/or keratolytic agents such as urea and lactic acid.

Recessive X-linked ichthyosis

The mode of transmission of this condition is X-linked recessive. The affected patients are males. Females are mostly carriers. The pathogenesis is a defect of the gene encoding the enzyme steroid sulfatase. The onset of this condition is usually in first few months of life. It presents as generalized large dark brownish scales accentuated on the lateral side of neck, preauricular area, abdomen, back, and feet but sparing the palms, soles, central face, and flexural areas.

Corneal opacity is usually found in affected adult males. Because of contiguous gene syndromes, hypogonadism and/or cryptochidism is sometimes present. The treatments include topical emollient and/or keratolytic agents such as urea and lactic acid.

Bullous congenital ichthyosiform erythroderma (BCIE)/Epidermolytic hyperkeratosis (EHK)/Bullous ichthyosis (BI)

The clinical presentation of BCIE is extremely variable. The classic presentation is superficial bullae, broad sheets of desquamation, and generalized erythroderma in the first few days of life. The skin and bullous disease will change to hyperkeratosis in the next first few months.

The characteristic findings are thick, hyperpigmented verrucous scales on the flexural surfaces, intertriginous areas of the body, and on dorsal surfaces of the hands and feet. Palms, soles, and scalp are frequently involved. Unpleasant odor is very common owing to fermented bacteria, yeast, and fungi in the hyperkeratotic skin.

The pathogenesis is a mutation of the keratin gene, leading to abnormal keratin protein. Thickening skin is believed to be a compensatory mechanism for skin protection.

Emollients are the proper management. Mechanical trauma and prolonged use of keratolytic agents should be avoided because of increased skin fragility. A mild antibacterial cleanser (e.g., chlorhexidine) or a bleach bath is beneficial to decrease bacterial fermentation. Oral vitamin A derivatives (isotretinoin, aciretin, etc.) help slough the scale.

Lamellar ichthyosis (LI)

This severe condition is transmitted as an autosomal recessive trait. The pathogenesis is a TGM1 gene mutation resulting in a defective transglutaminase-1 enzyme, which leads to desquamation of the top skin layer.

The diagnosis is based on clinical findings of large plate-like scales, ectropion, eclabium, and scarring alopecia. Ectropion is eversion of the eyelid, which exposes the palpebral conjunctiva and induces keratitis and madarosis. Eclabium is eversion of the lips. The patient usually presents at birth with a collodion membrane. There are generalized large quadrangular dark brown thick scales at the face, trunk, and flexor surfaces of the extremities. The classic scales are centrally attached with raised borders. Palms and soles are frequently involved with a varying degree of keratoderma and fissuring. Scarring alopecia particularly at the hairline is a common finding. The thickened skin also causes the obstruction of sweat ducts, resulting in heat intolerance.

Treatments include topical emollients and/or potent keratolytic agents. Oral retinoids (e.g., acitretin) may be helpful in severe cases. Ectropion should be corrected to prevent long-term visual complications.

Congenital ichthyosiform erythroderma (CIE)/Nonbullous congenital ichthyosiform erythroderma (NBCIE)

CIE is transmitted as an autosomal recessive trait. The pathogenesis is mutation of the TGM1 gene, the same as in lamellar ichthyosis.

The patient initially presents with a collodion membrane at birth. After this is shed, the skin turns red (erythroderma) and develops fine white powdery scales on the face, scalp, and trunk. Hyperkeratosis of the palms and soles with deep fissures is common. Ectropion and scarring alopecia may occur to variety of degrees.

The treatments include topical emollients and/or keratolytic agents such as urea, salicylic acid, alpha hydroxyl acid, propylene glycol, or a combination.

Harlequin ichthyosis

Harlequin ichthyosis is the most severe form of congenital ichthyosis, with a high morbidity and mortality. This condition is transmitted as an autosomal recessive trait. Most of these patients are born prematurely and suffer complications of prematurity (e.g., respiratory distress, sepsis, hypothermia).

The clinical picture is characterized by hard, thickened, armor-like skin with brownish fissures leading to polygonal or triangular plaques. Rigidity of the skin results in facial deformity, ectropion, eclabium, everted O-shaped lip ("fish mouth" deformity). There is limited flexion of the hands and feet. Constriction of the chest wall often results in respiratory and feeding problems.

The treatment of harlequin fetus is controversial. The high mortality rate is due to severe infection, poor feeding, and electrolyte imbalance. The treatment for survivors is systemic retinoid (acitretin), which may improve ectropion, eclabium, and accelerate shedding of skin. Risks and benefits of long-term use of this medication should be discussed before starting treatment. Supportive treatment with emollients may be used as adjunctive therapy.

Lichens

Lichen nitidus (LN)

This condition is most commonly seen in children of preschool and school age. The exact pathogenesis is unknown. The characteristic findings are minute sharply demarcated flesh-colored flat-topped papules arrange in groups that may circumscribe the trunk, genitalia, abdomen, and forearm. Koebner's phenomenon (lesions developing at the site of trauma) can be found in many patients. The condition is seen on the glans penis.

The differential diagnoses include papular eczema, flat warts, keratosis pilaris, micropapular lichen planus, and follicular psoriasis. The characteristic histopathologic features are used to confirm diagnosis in uncertain cases.

The natural course of this condition varies from weeks to months and it clears spontaneously. Supportive treatment with oral antihistamines and topical corticosteroids may be helpful.

Lichen planus (LP)

Lichen planus is a common disorder usually found in all age groups. The exact pathogensis is unknown.The characteristic findings are small flat-topped pruritic polygonal purplish papules ("the four P's"). The distribution is usually seen in the flexural surfaces of the lower legs as well as the ankles, wrist, genitalia, lower back, face, and mucous membranes or along Blaschko's lines. Papules may develop at the site of trauma (Koebner's phenomenon).

The polymorphic variants of lichen planus in pediatric patients consist of bullous LP, actinic LP, annular LP, atrophic LP, hypertrophic LP, linear LP, ulcerative LP, LP pemphigoid, LP lupus erythematosus, and lichen planopilaris. Linear LP is the most common variant in pediatric patients. Follicular LP on the scalp (Lichen planopilaris) can lead to scarring alopecia.

Mucous membranes of the mouth may demonstrate a characteristic reticulated, delicate white line or annular-linear lacy reticulated pattern called Wickham's striae. The buccal mucosa, lip, and tongue are the most commonly affected areas.

Nail involvement is uncommon in pediatric patients with lichen planus but may present with pitting, lusterless nails with a thinning nail plate, longitudinal ridging, and 20-nail-dystrophy.

The differential diagnosis depends on the variants presenting and includes lichen striatus, lichen nitidus, lichen simplex chronicus, lichenoid drug eruption, and papular granuloma annulare.

The diagnosis of LP relies on the characteristic pattern of lesions. The typical histopathologic features from skin biopsy are helpful to confirm the diagnosis.

The treatment of choice of LP is moderate to potent topical corticosteroids and antihistamines. In cases of extensive or recalcitrant symptoms, systemic corticosteroid injection (triamcinolone acetonide 5–10 mg/mL per dose or 1 mg/kg per dose) is effective. Other treatments include topical tacrolimus, oral dapsone, psoralen plus ultraviolet A (PUVA) or ultraviolet B (UVB) light therapy, oral retinoid, cyclosporine, and thalidomide.

Pityriasis lichenoides

Pityriasis lichenoides is an inflammatory papulosquamous skin disorder with characteristic clinical and histopathologic features. This condition has been divided into two forms including the acute form: pityriasis lichenoides et varioliformis acuta (PLEVA, Mucha-Habermann disease) and the chronic form, pityriasis lichenoides chronica (PLC).

The exact pathogenesis of pityriasis lichenoides is unknown. Recent data reveal an abnormal response to an antigenic stimulus provided by unidentified infectious agents, possibly viral. Pityriasis lichenoides is primarily a cutaneous T-cell lymphoproliferative disorder. Nevertheless, the progression of pityriasis lichenoides to cutaneous T-cell lymphoma in children has been rarely reported.

PLEVA is a polymorphous papulosquamous eruption. It presents as asymptomatic or pruritic symmetrical erythematous macules and papules that coalesce in crops and turn to vesicular, necrotic, and purpuric lesions. Lesions are most common on the trunk, proximal thighs, and upper arms. The natural course of disorder usually runs over several weeks to months.

The differential diagnosis is chickenpox, insect bite reaction, leukocytoclastic vasculitis, and vesicular pityriasis rosea.

PLC is a chronic form of pityriasis lichenoides. The course of PLC is variable from months to years. The skin lesions reveal scaling papules and plaques that usually resolve with postinflammatory hypopigmentation or less commonly with hyperpigmentation.

The differential diagnosis is pityriasis rosea, secondary syphilis, and guttate psoriasis.

Histopathology from skin biopsy may be helpful in cases of uncertain clinical diagnosis.

Patients and families should be reassured of the self-limited natural course of this condition. There is no specific treatment. Optional treatments include oral erythromycin, topical corticosteroid, and phototherapy. Topical corticosteroid or oral antihistamine may decrease the pruritus. Oral erythromycin, 30 to 50 mg/kg per day for 1 to 2 months, is partially effective in some cases. Ultraviolet light therapy may be helpful in cases not responding to oral erythromycin. Spontaneous recovery usually occurs in several months to years.

Pityriasis rosea (PR)

Pityriasis rosea is an acute, benign self-limited papulosquamous disorder. The exact etiology of this condition is unknown. There may be a viral like prodrome and/or history of preceding upper respiratory tract infection in some cases.

The clinical manifestation is initially a single isolated lesion defined as a "herald patch." The most common site of the herald patch is on the trunk, upper arm, neck, or thigh. The lesion is characterized by a sharply demarcated oval shape with surrounding fine white scale ("collar sign") usually seen 1 to 2 weeks prior to the appearance of other lesions. Only about 50 percent of cases begin with a herald patch.

The secondary lesions reveal generalized erythematous patches, papules with fine white scale bilaterally and symmetrically discrete to the line of skin cleavage, in a "Christmas tree pattern" on the upper arm, neck, back, trunk, and upper thigh. The white scales reveal a "collarette of scale" surrounding the lesion, characteristic of pityriasis rosea. Each individual lesion is football-shaped with a raised red border, trailing scale, and darker flat interior.

The duration of secondary lesions may be days to weeks. Spontaneous recovery usually occurs within 6 to 12 weeks but may be prolonged over a period of 6 months. There may be residual postinflammatory hypo- or hyperpigmentation.

The diagnosis is based upon the history, distribution pattern, and the characteristics of the lesions. Histopathology of pityriasis rosea is not diagnostic because of the similarity with subacute or chronic dermatitis.

Patients and families should be reassured of the self-limited natural course of this condition. The treatment is supportive with topical or systemic antipruritic medications. Optional treatments include oral erythromycin, topical corticosteroid, and UVB light therapy. Mild to moderate corticosteroid may temporarily reduce pruritus in some patients. Oral erythromycin (dosage 25–40 mg/kg per day over 2 weeks) may shorten the course of disorder. UVB light therapy over 5 to 10 days can significantly improve the eruption and reduce the degree of pruritus as well as hasten the resolution.

Psoriasis

Psoriasis is an immune-mediated papulosquamous disorder (34). Its pathophysiology is postulated to be a combination of genetic predisposition, environmental factors, and innate and acquired immune system problems resulting in hyperproliferation and abnormal differentiation of keratinocytes.

The characteristic lesions of psoriasis are erythematous plaques with well-defined borders and papules with grayish or silvery scales. The papules may coalesce to large plaques, usually seen in a symmetrical pattern on the scalp, extensor surfaces of elbows and knees, and the lumbosacral and anogenital areas.

The term *inverse psoriasis* may be used in a variant of flexural surface involvement of the axillae, groin, perineum, central chest, and umbilical region.

The "Auspitz sign" is a characteristic phenomenon that results from removal of the white scale leading to fine punctuate bleeding points. Koebner's phenomenon may develop at sites of trauma.

Facial psoriasis especially in the periorbital area is more common in children than in adults. This often presents with small round psoriatic plaques in the upper inner eyelid area.

The scalp is one of the most common sites of psoriatic involvement. The presentation is a well-defined white scale on an erythematous base resulting in a variable degree of temporary hair loss. The distribution involves the scalp, eyebrows, pre- or postauricular area, and beyond the hairline. The term *tinea amiantacia* or *pityriasis amiantacia* is used for the generalized white scale pattern.

The most common manifestation of nail change in psoriasis is pitting. The others are discoloration of the nail ("oil drops"), onycholysis, and subungual hyperkeratosis.

Extracutaneous involvement of psoriasis may include psoriatic arthritis and symmetrical anterior uveitis in adult patients, rarely in children.

There are variable patterns of presentation.

Guttate psoriasis

This is usually the first manifestation of psoriasis in children and young adults. The lesion is characterized by drop-like (guttate) round/oval lesions and white scale in a symmetrical distribution on the trunk and proximal aspects of the extremities. Group A streptococcal infection is the most common trigger of this condition. The reason for this sequence of events is unknown.

Pustular psoriasis

This is the most severe variant of childhood psoriasis. An explosion of generalized sterile pustules on the erythematous skin with previous plaque psoriasis or on normal skin characterizes the lesion.

The overlying pustules may be discrete or may rapidly coalesce to a large plaque as a "lake of pus" before drying over 3 to 4 days with desquamation. The repetitive explosions of pustules consequently develop over several weeks.

The trigger factors are withdrawal of systemic corticosteroids, use of a potent topical corticosteroid, and/or respiratory tract infection.

Pustular psoriasis palmaris et plantaris is a chronic eruption, usually symmetrical, on both palms and soles. The lesions are characterized by deep-seated sterile pustules with white scales on top of a bright erythematous base. They finally turn to dark yellow or brown scales in several days. The crop of pustular lesions is often recurrent and sometimes associated with secondary bacterial infection due to *S. aureus*.

The diagnosis of psoriasis depends on the characteristic clinical findings. Histopathology from skin biopsy is used for confirmation.

The natural course of psoriasis is unpredictable but prolonged and chronic. The trigger factors that may aggravate psoriasis are traumatization (Koebner's phenomenon), medications (lithium, antimalarials, beta blockers, withdrawal of systemic corticosteroids) and infection (especially streptococcal).

Management of psoriasis

Topical therapy

- Topical corticosteroids are the most commonly used in treating children. The options depend on the site of lesion, body surface area, and duration of treatment. Risks of side effects should be considered and minimized by monitoring the amount of usage, potency, proper site, and intermittent rotational or combination therapy. The combination of topical corticosteroids with other medications (e.g., topical calcipotriene) is beneficial in older children.
- Calcipotriene is an analogue of vitamin D3, usually combined with topical corticosteroid to facilitate the onset of action. This medication is one of the effective treatments for mild to moderate plaque-type psoriasis in children and adults. The most common side effect is lesional or perilesional irritation, especially on the face and in skin folds.
- Tars are anti-inflammatory and antiproliferative. There are many forms of tar preparations, such as 1 percent to 10 percent crude coal tar (CCT), 5 percent to 10 percent liquor carbonis detergent (LCD), and topical corticosteroid and salicylic acid combinations. The concentration of medications is appropriately selected to age and lesion sites. Tar shampoo is used as monotherapy for scalp psoriasis or in combination with other topical therapy.
- Tacrolimus ointment is a calcineurin inhibitor effective in the facial and neck area and in intertriginous psoriasis (psoriasis inversus).
- Anthralin 0.1 percent to 1 percent cream and ointment is primarily effective in the treatment of chronic plaque-type psoriasis. Short-contact therapy is initially applied for 5 minutes and gradually increased over time as tolerated before being rinsed off. The most common side effects are irritant contact dermatitis and perilesional staining.

Phototherapy

Natural sunlight is beneficial in psoriatic patients. Phototherapy is the most frequently used optional treatment in children with moderate to severe psoriasis who are recalcitrant to topical therapy.

Narrow-band UVB (312 nm) is currently the most effective treatment of psoriasis. Administration three times per week is usually required until clearance occurs. The side effects of UVB therapy include skin darkening and burning.

Systemic therapy

- Antibiotics are used to eradicate streptococci, which are one of the trigger factors of guttate or plaque-type psoriasis. This medication should be prescribed only in case of a positive throat culture, although the culture may also be positive in the carrier stage.
- Methotrexate is started orally at 2.5 mg up to 15 to 20 mg/wk based on ideal body weight (dosage 0.3–0.5 mg/kgper week). The most common side effects are nausea, headache, and fatigue. The most common serious side effect is bone marrow suppression. Supplementary folic acid 1 to 5 mg/day diminishes the risk of mucosal

ulceration and macrocytic anemia. Complete blood count and liver function tests should be monitored for patients on this medication.

- Retinoids (acitretin: dosage 0.5–0.75 mg/kg per day) is often used in combination with topical treatment and UVB therapy. The most common side effect is dryness of skin and mucosa. Other complications are hypertriglyceridemia, teratogenic effects, premature epiphyseal closure, and hyperostosis. Complete blood count, liver function test, and lipid profile should be monitored during administration of the medication.
- Cyclosporine is effective in pediatric plaque-type psoriasis at a dose of 3 to 3.5 mg/kg per day. The supportive data in childhood psoriasis are limited to a small case series. The side effects are hypertension, immunosuppression, and renal and hepatic toxicity.
- Biological agents: Etanercept has been systematically studied in a small number of pediatric patients with plaque-type psoriasis. Infliximab has only case reports of effective treatment in childhood psoriasis.

2.6 Dermatologic manifestations of systematic disorders

The goal of this section is to demonstrate dermatologic manifestations of other conditions. This will enable the clinician to ameliorate dermatologic conditions by approaching the primary cause, often in conjunction with specialty consultation. We select disorders not uncommon in adolescents.

2.6.1 Pruritus without rash

Pruritus can be a manifestation of several conditions. There may often be no physical findings until the areas become excoriated. While malignancies such as Hodgkin and non-Hodgkin's lymphoma are associated with pruritus, relatively few patients with prutitus without skin findings actually have a malignancy. Other malignancies will be associated with abnormal dermatologic findings, which may be prutitic. Examples of such are mycosis fungoides associated with leukemia and carcinoid associated with histamine flush. Renal failure patients, especially at the time of dialysis, will complain of pruritus. Cholestasis will frequently cause itching, especially in the palms and soles, primarily due to deposition of bile salts in the skin. Specific hepatic causes include primary biliary cirrhosis, sclerosing cholangitis, pregnancy, and hepatitis. Endocrine causes include hyperthyroidism and diabetes mellitus. Other conditions common in adolescence associated with pruritus include iron deficiency anemia and occasionally allergies. In patients with immunodeficiencies such as HIV, pruritus may be a complication of the primary condition (eosinophilic folliculitis in HIV), or due to a secondary infection or infestation such as scabies.

2.6.2 Inflammatory bowel disease (IBD)

The primary skin manifestations of IBD consist of mouth ulcerations and perianal fissures and fistulae, more common in Crohn's disease (37) (see chapter 5).

2.6.3 Erythema nodosum

This is the most common skin manifestation of IBD, slightly more common in Crohn's disease than in ulcerative colitis. The lesions are tender red or violaceous subcutaneous nodules most commonly on the pretibial area. They often become more manifest during exacerbations.

2.6.4 Pyoderma gangrenosum

This occurs in about 5 percent of patients with ulcerative colitis and 2 percent of patients with Crohn's disease. The lesions present initially as a red papules and progress to central necrosis with subsequent ulceration.

2.6.5 Less common skin manifestations

Other lesions associated with IBD include psoriasis, epidermolysis bullosa, Sweet's syndrome (neutrophilic infiltrates, also seen in myelogenous leukemia), and primary granulomas (metastatic Crohn's disease).

2.6.6 Management

This consists of treating the primary condition and inducing remission. This should be done in conjunction with specialty consultation from a gastroenterologist for appropriate management of corticosteroid dosages, or, in more severe cases, immunomodulators (azathioprine or 6-mercaptopurine), calcineurin inhibitors (cyclosporine), and monoclonal antibodies (infliximab). Sometimes surgical intervention in IBD will allow for remission of skin manifestations.

Regarding the specific conditions mentioned above, erythema nodosum usually responds well to corticosteroid therapy. Pyoderma gangrenosum may also respond to interlesional steroids, local chromoglycate, oral Dapsone, hyperbaric oxygen, and granulocytopheresis. Sweet's syndrome is particularly sensitive to corticosteroids.

2.7 Collagen Vascular Disease

These conditions are not uncommon in adolescents and identification of dermatologic manifestations is paramount to proper diagnosis and management.

2.7.1 Lupus erythematosus (LE)

Lesions may manifest as vesicles, bullae, or ulcerations of the nasal or oral mucosa as well as the integument (38). Skin lesions may progress to atrophy or scarring. Typical lesions also consist of the malar "butterfly rash"; generalized maculopapular rashes; dermatitis, frequently sun-sensitive; and vasculitis (periungual erythema, Livedo reticularis, telangiectasia, and Raynaud's phenomenon). Dermatitis often results in postinflammatory hypo- or hyperpigmentation (see chapters 13 and 15).

Discoid lesions may be present in 25 percent of patients with clinical SLE or they may be its sole manifestation. They are erythematous plaques often on the face, neck, and trunk. They often heal with scarring, atrophy, telangiectasias, or hyper- and hypopigmentation. Lupus panniculitis, hypertrophic LE and lupus tumidus (photosensitive pink plaques or nodules) may also be a sole manifestation.

Systemic LE (SLE) may have hair and nail manifestations including alopecia, scarring and nonscarring and pitting, ridging, and onycholysis of the nails.

2.7.2 Dermatomyositis

Classic skin manifestations include the heliotrope rash (red-purple eyelids, telangiectasia of eyelid capillaries, periorbital edema, and malar and facial erythema), Gottron's papules (red papulosquamous lesions over knuckles and sometimes extensor surfaces), nail capillary dilatation, and tortuosity and skin ulcers. Calcinosis may occur not only in the skin but also in muscle and fascial planes.

2.7.3 Juvenile idiopathic arthritis (JIA)

The rash associated with JIA is salmon-pink in color; it is fleeting and becomes more prominent with heat, both external and with fever. Skin trauma may bring out the rash (Koebner's phenomenon).

2.7.4 Management

The goal of management of skin and mucous membrane lesions in LE is to prevent scarring and atrophy. An important aspect of dermatologic management in LE is preventative. Patients with photosensitivity should avoid excessive sun exposure, use sunscreens, and select light bulbs for their homes that do not emit UV light. Patients should avoid triggers of Raynaud's phenomenon such as smoking, cold, vasoconstrictors, and caffeine.

Skin lesions in LE that are isolated often respond to topical therapy. Topical steroids are often effective, starting with low-potency medications, although it may be necessary to advance to fluorinated corticosteroids for deeper lesions. However, it is important not to overuse these medications, as atrophy, striae, and telangectasia may be complications. Topical immunosuppressants such as tacrolimus are presently under investigation and may be effective.

If systemic medications are necessary, antimalarial drugs such as chloroquine and quinacrine can be used. It may take 6 to 12 months to see improvement. Ocular pathology is a serious side effect of these medications and the prescribing physician should always be mindful of this. Systemic corticosteroids and immunosuppressive agents may be helpful for bullous lesions but generally are not necessary.

2.8 Endocrinologic Disorders

2.8.1 Thyroid disorders

Patients with hypo- or hyperthyroidism will present with pruritus, sometimes idiopathic, sometimes due to dry skin (see chapter 3). In hyperthyoridism the skin is thin and diaphoretic; in hypothyroidism, it may be cool, pale, and myxedematous. There may be a yellowish hue due to carotenemia in hypothyroidism. Patients with thyroid disease have an increased incidence of vitiligo, especially patients with autoimmune conditions. Hair may be thickened in hypothyroidism and thinned in hyperthyroidism.

2.8.2 Diabetes mellitus

Pruritus in diabetics may be secondary to neuropathy but also may be a consequence of fungal and yeast infections. Antifungals are the treatment of choice.

2.8.3 Adrenal disorders

In patients with adrenal insufficiency, the skin is hyperpigmented, especially in the palmar creases and areas exposed to trauma or sunlight. Pigmentation may be exaggerated in areas that are normally darker. Mucous membranes may display spots of pigmentation. Vitiligo may be present in patients with primary immune disorders.

The dermatologic manifestations of Cushing's disease are primarily skin atrophy, bruisability, and striae. Hyperpigmentation due to overproduction of adrenocorticotrophic hormone (ACTH) may also occur.

2.8.4 Management

Treatment of skin manifestations of endocrinologic conditions is contingent upon management of the primary disorder and should always be done in consultation with an endocrinologist.

2.9 Hair and Nails

2.9.1 Alopecia areata

The sudden onset of localized alopecia is characterized by sharply demarcated round or oval patches of hair loss.

The pathogenesis of alopecia areata is proposed to be a combination of genetic susceptibility, relating to the inner root sheath, and faint association with autoimmune diseases (39). The classic autoimmune disorders include thyroid diseases (Hashimoto's thyroiditis), vitiligo, LE, rheumatoid arthritis, pernicious anemia, and myasthenia gravis. The association with these diseases is not clear and testing for them is directed by family history.

The skin is smooth almost totally devoid of hair with or without scale. The areas of hair loss may be single or numerous. The rim of alopecia reveals the pathognomonic sign of "exclamation hair." The inflammatory process of hair is located at the attenuated hair bulb, resulting in easily loosening. The initial hair loss may reveal an irregular border, area of involvement, length of lost hair, and duration of loss.

The typical pattern of hair loss along the bilateral parietotemporal to posterior occiput is called the ophiasis pattern, usually indicating a poor prognosis. The progressive terminal scalp hair loss including the eyelashes and eyebrows is called alopecia totalis, and the total complete loss of body hair is alopecia universalis. This progression is more common in children than in adults.

One of the differential diagnoses is trichotillomania. Trichotillomania typically presents with an irregular border of hair loss of bizarre shape and with variation in the length of unplucked hair.

The diagnosis is clinical. Histopathology from skin biopsy may helpful in cases of uncertain history and atypical presentation. Nail changes may be found, especially a finely pitted nail in either a horizontal or vertical pattern.

There is variability of the natural course of disease and treatment. Poor prognostic factors are autoimmune diseases, family history of alopecia areata, vitiligo, thyroid diseases, young age of onset, extensive hair loss, ophiasis pattern, Down's syndrome, and nail dystrophy.

2.9.2 Management of alopecia areata

- Topical corticosteroid is the most common therapy for alopecia areata in children (40). Mid- to high-potency preparations are usually prescribed with monitoring of side effects. Regrowth of hair should be assessed 6 to 14 weeks after starting treatment. Intradermal corticosteroid injection is mostly used in older children and in cases of failure of topical treatment. A concentration of triamcinolone acetonide varying from 2.5 to 5 mg/mL is administered as multiple intradermal injections of 0.1 to 0.3 mL per site approximately 1 cm apart and repeated every 4 to 6 weeks.
- Oral prednisolone at a dosage of 0.5 to 1 mg/kg per day for 4 weeks or until the hair loss stops is used in selected difficult cases, but a high relapse rate often occurs after dosage reduction.
- Topical minoxidil may stimulate follicular DNA synthesis with proliferation, differentiation of follicular keratinocytes, and reregulation of hair physiology. The concentrations of minoxidil are 2 percent to 5 percent; it may be applied twice daily. Hair growth is usually seen after 2 months of treatment. The uncommon side effects are allergic contact dermatitis, hypertrichosis, and local irritation.
- Topical immunotherapy (contact sensitizers) has been used in chronic and extensive alopecia areata. These agents will sensitize contacted skin, inducing erythema, scaling, and pruritus. T-suppressor cells are generated in the contacted area, which may result in a nonspecific inhibitory effect on the autoimmune reaction in hair follicles and in regrowth of the hair.
- Diphenylcyclopropenone (DPCP) is the most commonly used topical sensitizer in children. The efficacy of DPCP in alopecia areata ranges from 48 percent to 85 percent. The side effects of DPCP include eczematous reaction; itching; edema of face, scalp and cervical area; and postauricular lymphadenopathy.
- Dithranol (Antralin) 0.25 percent to 1 percent cream is initially used as short-contact therapy with gradually increasing contact time as tolerated prior to rinsing. The side effects of this medication are scalp irritation, folliculitis, and staining of the skin and clothes. It can be used in combination with twice-daily topical corticosteroid therapy.
- PUVA. The presumed mechanism of action of PUVA is a photoimmunologic effect by inhibition of the local immunologic attack on hair follicle. The response rates and high relapse rates vary with the dose. There is a known incidence of induced skin cancers with oral PUVA treatment.

2.9.3 Telogen effluvium

The characteristic pattern is diffuse thinning of the scalp hair. There are several anecdotal trigger factors including emotional stress, high fever, systemic illness, severe infection, surgery, nutritional deficiency, thyroid abnormalities, and systemic lupus erythematosus. Medications (albendazole, amphetamine, retinoids, beta blockers, anticonvulsants, angiotensin converting enzyme [ACE] inhibitors) also affect this condition. These factors may interrupt the normal cyclic pattern of the anagen phase and result in early telogen phase. Telogen phase with an increasedf hair count of 25 percent or more is significantly abnormal.

The diagnosis of telogen effluvium is supported by a prior history of illness or stress for 6 weeks to 4 months and the percentage of telogen hairs in the scalp biopsy of more than 12 percent to 15 percent of terminal follicles.

In cases of telogen effluvium without evidence of historical trigger factors, a complete blood count, serum iron/ferritin, and thyroid function tests are useful screening tests.

The treatment of telogen effluvium is supportive. Spontaneous regrowth of the hair may appear in several months unless the trigger is repeated. Regrowth of the hair is usually complete within 6 months.

2.9.4 Androgenic alopecia

Androgenic alopecia (male-pattern baldness) with a genetic predisposition is the most common cause of hair loss in adults. Androgen hormones gradually transform large scalp hair follicles to smaller follicles and turn anagen phase to telogen phase in a faster than normal cycle.

Androgenic alopecia can occur in either gender but males are affected more severely than females. The male pattern reveals the symmetrical frontoparietal recession of the hairline and/or vertex thinning, whereas the female pattern is relatively unaffected at the hairline but seen the vertex and/or as diffuse thinning. Some cases begin during adolescence.

The diagnosis is based on the pattern of scalp hair loss. Hair plucking of frontal area reveals the increased ratio of telogen to anagen phase, but it is usually unnecessary to do this to make the diagnosis.

Topical treatment with 2.5 percent minoxidil solution is used to stimulate follicular proliferation, dermal papillary vascularization, increased anagen duration, and enlargement of miniaturized follicles. This solution should be routinely applied to maintain hair growth. It works well on vertex and frontal scalp thinning. Topical minoxidil may cause telogen effluvium to occur 2 to 8 weeks after initial treatment owing to the releasing of telogen hair as anagen promotion begins. Irritation, erythema, and hypertrichosis are the common side effects of minoxidil.

Oral finasteride is a specific type II 5-alpha reductase inhibitor resulting in reduction of levels of dihydrotestosterone both in serum and scalp skin. F-nasteride 1 mg/day is effective treatment in men older than 18 years of age. A response to this medication may occur as early as 3 months. Medication should be continued for at least 24 months before reevaluation. The side effect is sexual dysfunction in 4.2 percent of patients.

Spironolactone, an aldosterone antagonist; 50 to 200 mg/day is the optional treatment of androgenetic alopecia in women. Breast soreness and menstrual irregularities are side effects of this medication.

2.9.5 Trichotillomania

Trichotillomania is classified as an impulse-control disorder. The scalp is the most common area of involvement but the eyebrows and eyelashes may be involved as well.

This condition usually occurs in adolescents or older children, predominantly in females. The characteristic hair pattern is bizarre in configuration, having irregular borders and frequent distribution to the side of patient's handedness, with varying length and/or broken hair from traction. The affected areas are commonly found at the frontal, frontotemporal, and vertex areas of the scalp.

Direct evidence from observation of hair plucking and indirect evidence of broken groups of hairs in the patient's room are helpful to confirm diagnosis.

The management of trichotillomania is difficult. The patients should be reassured the cause of disease is stress and that stress reduction will improve the condition. Supportive treatment such as a mild shampoo or a mild topical scalp lotion (hydrocortisone) may be useful to relieve pruritus and irritation. The mainstay of treatment is psychiatric intervention and behavior therapy.

2.9.6 Traction alopecia

Traction alopecia is traumatic hair loss secondary to tensile force on the scalp hair. It presents as oval or linear areas of hair loss along the margin of the hairline depending on type of traction or trauma. This condition is common in females who pull braids, adolescents with ponytails, or those who use barrettes and hair rollers.

Hair will regrow in a few months after stopping traction. However, scarring and little regrowth may occur because of follicular destruction.

2.9.7 Hirsutism and hypertrichosis

Hirsutism is excessive hair growth in women and girls due to androgens. This may appear at the upper lip, neck, anterior chest wall, breast, abdomen, upper inner thigh, and legs. Often it is genetic, with one or both parents being hirsuite.

Hypertrichosis is excessive hair growth in males and females of nonandrogen etiology without evidence of masculinization or menstrual abnormality. The excessive hair growth may occur both in generalized and localized patterns.

The ideal treatment is correction of the cause of these conditions. The simplest methods to eradicate the excessive hair are cutting with razors, scissors, or shaving. Side effects include pseudofolliculitis and irritation. Epilation includes plucking, threading and waxing. Plucking and wax epilation are usually painful and induce folliculitis, pseudofolliculitis, and postinflammatory hyperpigmentation.

Chemical depilatory agents, 2 percent to 10 percent thioglycolates, mercaptans, and sulfide may be effective but cause irritation, have an unpleasant odor, and systemic absorption may occur in extensive areas of usage.

Electrolysis permanently damages hair follicles but is difficult to use in younger children. The side effects include erythema, edema, pain, and postinflammatory dyspigmentation.

Laser hair removal includes the ruby laser (694 nm), the alexandrite laser (755 nm), the diode laser (800–810 nm), and Nd:YAG laser (1064 nm).

Systemic medication to control hirsutism should be used under the supervision of an endocrinologist or gynecologist.

2.9.8 Hair changes with systemic disease

Anagen effluvium

The effects of systemic treatment of radiation and chemotherapy may result in this condition. Hair loss may be prominent at the frontal, vertex, and parietal areas of the scalp or it may be generalized. The severity of generalized hair loss depends on the toxicity of the causative agents.

Several manipulations may minimize hair loss, such as applying ice packs or tourniquets to the scalp for 30 minutes before drug administration.

The medical history, physical examination, and microscopic examination of hair are useful to diagnose this condition.

The ideal treatment is cessation of the causative agents and to wait for hair regrowth.

2.9.9 Infection

Tinea capitis

Tinea capitis is the most common hair infection of childhood (41). The characteristic pattern is localized alopecia and broken hair with scaling. The most common age groups are prepubertal children because the effect of sex hormones in adolescence may change the sebum of scalp to free fatty acid with a protective effect.

There are varieties of dermatophytes that cause tinea capitis, such as *Trichophyton*, *Microsporum*, and *Epidermophyton* species. The predominant species vary according to geographic location. The different pathogens may affect varieties of clinical presentation. *Trichophyton tonsurans* is the major cause of tinea capitis in the United States. Predisposing factors of tinea capitis are large family size, overcrowded living conditions, low socioeconomic status, the postmenstrual period, and an immunocompromised host.

Transmission of these diseases usually occurs by contact with infected spores in shedding scale, hair or fomites from person to person or animal to person.

The classic manifestations vary as patchy alopecia, gray patch, scaling with or without hair loss, follicular pustules/papules, erythema, black dot, kerion, scarring, and favus:

- Gray patch is a noninflammatory type of tinea capitis. The clinical examination reveals the grayish patches of spores covering the hair shaft (ectothrix) and there is usually scaling. *Microsporum* species is the common agent causing this form.
- Black dot presents with small black dots from broken hair shafts with alopecia. The cause of this form is dermatophyte invasion of the medullary hair (endothrix). *T. tonsurans* is the most common etiologic agent.
- Kerion is an inflammatory type of tinea capitis. It presents as a boggy mass, an erythematous plaque with pustules and purulent discharge. Alopecia with loosening hair is

also a significant presentation. Sinus drainage may occur, and kerion is frequently misdiagnosed as a bacterial abscess. This form often results in scarring alopecia from permanent damage to hair follicles.
- Favus is a severe chronic condition. The characteristic pattern is scaly erythematous patches with yellow-red perifollicular papules. Yellow cup-shaped fungal mycelia called scutula are present. This lesion may result in scarring, atrophy, and permanent alopecia.

The differential diagnosis of tinea capitis includes seborrheic dermatitis, psoriasis, alopecia areata, trichotillomania, follicultis, LE, and lichen planopilaris.

A potassium hydroxide preparation of scaling and broken hair confirms the diagnosis. The microscopic examination reveals tiny arthrospores surrounding or within the hair shaft. However, the gold standard of diagnosis is fungal culture.

The treatment of tinea capitis is systemic therapy because of the requirement of penetration of medication to the hair follicles. The drug of choice for tinea capitis is griseofulvin because of its efficacy, safety profile, and cost. The dosage is 20 mg/kg of the ultramicrosize form administered once daily for a month. Problems with liver function are now not thought to be as significant as they once were and thus liver function tests should be obtained only if treatment is going to last more than 1 month.

Topical therapy may be an additional treatment. Shampoo containing selenium sulfide, ketoconazole, or zinc pyrithione used twice daily is adjunctive therapy to eliminate contagious spores of dermatophytes.

Contaminated individual hairbrushes, pillowcases, and hats of infected patients should be cleaned and not shared with others. Symptomatic family members and contacts should be evaluated.

2.9.10 Herpetic whitlow

Herpetic whitlow is the localized form of HSV infection, usually seen in dentists and physicians who have contact with herpetic lesions. Autoinoculation to other sites also may occur. Clinical manifestations are a deep-seated, painful group of vesicles with surrounding erythema. Ipsilateral regional lymphadenopathy may occur.

The differential diagnosis is blistering dactylytis, impetigo, burns, and friction blisters. Viral culture or direct fluorescent antibody testing is helpful to confirm the diagnosis.

The proper treatment is supportive therapy. Spontaneous recovery usually occurs over 3 weeks. However, oral antiviral therapy may relieve pain and speed recovery.

2.9.11 Bacterial

Paronychia

Paronychia is a bacterial infection surrounding the nail. Acute paronychia usually presents as painful erythema with swelling of the proximal and lateral nail fold. The cuticle is sometimes obliterated. The most common pathogen is *S. aureus*. The pathogens in ingrown toenail are usually *Pseudomonas* species and gram-negative organisms.

Chronic paronychia usually manifests as asymptomatic periungual erythema. The most common pathogen is *Candida* species, particularly with repeated and chronic exposure to moisture at work or due to finger sucking.

Systemic candidiasis, acrodermatits enteropathica, multiple carboxylase deficiency, chronic mucocutaneous candidiasis, and immunodeficiency should be considered in cases of multiple involvement of nails in both hands and feet.

The ideal treatment of paronychia is to eradicate the infectious pathogens and keep the finger dry. Either alcohol-propylene glycol vehicle or thymol concentration 4 percent in chloroform is applied to dry the nail fold. Topical clindamycin solution may beneficial in secondary bacterial infection.

2.9.12 Ingrown nail

The distal-lateral edge of the nail curves inward and penetrates the underlying tissue. The causes of this disorder are improper cutting of the nail, tearing of the nail plate, and/or too tightly fitting footwear. There may be a genetic predisposition.

It presents as painful erythema with swelling and may turn to granulation tissue over time. Complications of ingrown nail are paronychia and recurrent dactylitis.

Treatments are use of properly fitting footwear, special trimming, waiting for the nail to grow past the free edge, and control of the infection by compression dressings and topical/systemic antibiotics. Antiseptic soaks such as Hibiclens soap, Dakin's solution, or potassium permanganate may be helpful. Surgical procedure such as partial/total nail avulsion is necessary in painful cases or in frequent recurrence.

2.9.13 Fungal

Onychomycosis/Tinea ungium

The term *onychomycosis* refers to a fungal infection of the nail (42,43,44,). However, *tinea ungium* is a specific term for dermatophyte infection of the nail.

Onychomycosis is more common in adults than children. Toenail onychomycosis is usually associated with tinea pedis. This condition is classified in four patterns of infection site including distal subungual, proximal subungual, lateral subungual, and superficial white onychomycosis.

Distal subungual onychomycosis is the most common form of fungal infection. The separation of the nail plate and nail bed by fungal invasion leads to onycholysis and thickening of the subungual nail.

Proximal subungual onychomycosis is an uncommon presentation in a normal host and is usually seen in HIV or other immunocompromised conditions. The cuticle of proximal nail fold is initially disrupted. Proximal separation of the nail plate and nail bed results in onycholysis, scaling, and discoloration.

Superficial white onychomycosis is a superficial infection of nail plate. The organisms directly invade to the dorsal nail plate. The infected nail plate is fragile and easily removed. *Trichophyton* species is the most common pathogen of the fingernails.

The common findings of onychomycosis are not usually symmetrical and only one to three nails of one hand or foot may be involved. If all of the nails are involved, other diagnoses should be suspected, including psoriatic nail, chronic paronychia, drug-induced onycholysis, trauma, lichen planus, and pachyonychia congenita.

The treatment of onychomycosis is systemic therapy because of poor topical penetration to the nail plate. However, topical therapy (such as Amorolfine, Ciclopirox) is used

Tab. 2.6: Systemic antifungal agents for onychomycosis in children.

Antifungal agents	Dose	Remark
Griseofulvin (tablet)	*Continuous therapy*: 15–20 mg/kg per day	*Continuous* Toenail, 6–12 months Fingernail, 3–6 months
Itraconazole (capsule, oral solution)	*Pulse therapy*: 5 mg/kg per day *Continuous therapy*: 5 mg/kg per day	1 week on, 3 weeks off Toenail, 3 pulses, follow up Fingernail, 2 pulses, follow up *Continuous* Toenail, 12 weeks Fingernail, 6 weeks
Fluconazole (tablet)	*Intermittent therapy*: 3–6 mg/kg per day (one dose/week)	*Intermittent* Toenail, 26 weeks Fingernail, 12 weeks
Terbinafine (tablet)	*Continuous therapy*: <20 kg – 62.5 mg/day 20–40 kg – 125 mg/day >40 kg – 250 mg/day	*Continuous* Toenail, 12 weeks Fingernail, 6 weeks

as adjuctive therapy in some cases. Topical usage is appropriate in superficial white onychomycosis.

Oral griseofulvin is the drug of choice for onychomycosis. Other oral antifungals such as terbinafine (Lamisil), itraconazole (Sporonox), and fluconazole (Diflucan) are increasing in usage with good supportive evidence. ▶Tab. 2.6 lists systemic antifungal agents for onychomycosis.

2.9.14 Onychodystrophy

Pitting nail

This is a common problem in children. Alteration in the proximal matrix results in pitting of the nail plate's surface. The characteristic pattern is a punctuate depression of the nail plate, which may be small, shallow, or large and deep, involving a few or all of the nails. It frequently occurs in normal healthy adolescents. There are many disorders associated with this condition including atopic dermatitis, alopecia areata, psoriasis, and trauma.

Beau's line/Onychomadesis

Beau's line is a transverse groove/furrow of the nail plate resulting from the interruption of nail formation. There are several causes of nail matrix interruption, such as systemic illness, high fever, or systemic maladies such as Kawasaki disease, severe bullous eruption, thyroid disease, radiation therapy, Stevens-Johnson syndrome, and chemotherapy.

The duration of the systemic illness is associated with the distance between the cuticle and the groove.

Onychomadesis is complete separation of the nail plate resulting from arrest of the nail matrix. The causes of Beau's line has also been reported to be the causes of onychomadesis. Trauma to the nail matrix can lead to this deformity.

These conditions are transient phenomena and nails regrow without nail plate scarring.

Trachyonychia (20-nail dystrophy)

Trachyonychia is a deformity of the nail with opaque discoloration, a rough, sandpaper-like surface, and ridging, grooves, or striations. The number of nails involved may be used in lieu of the term *20-nail dystrophy*.

This condition may occur months preceding cutaneous signs of other diseases. Commonly associated disorders are lichen planus, atopic dermatitis, psoriasis, and alopecia areata, but it may occur commonly in a normal healthy adolescent.

The exact cause of this condition is unknown. The natural course varies from 6 months to 16 years. We do not see it in adults, so that it is either self-limiting or progresses to another condition.

An optional treatment is watchful waiting, especially if the primary causative condition clears. Treatment with potent topical corticosteroid at the proximal nail fold may be helpful only in some cases, but reports are anecdotal. Some practitioners use the intralesional corticosteroid triamcinolone 0.5 to 1 mg/kg per month for 3 to 6 months.

2.9.15 Nail changes with systemic and nutritional disorders

Spoon nail/Koilonychia

Koilonychia is a common disorder of the nail plate. Physiologic koilonychia may be found in the great toenail of newborns and young infants. The nail is characterized by a central concavity with turned up distal and lateral margins.

This condition may be a secondary feature of several dermatologic disorders (lichen planus, trachyonychia) and of systemic diseases such as hypothyroidism, hemochromatosis, and iron deficiency anemia.

Clubbing of finger/Acropachy

Clubbing of fingers is one of the presentations of multiple systemic disorders. The most common diseases in adolescent patients include congenital cyanotic heart disease, inflammatory bowel syndrome, chronic hypoxia of pulmonary disease, and endocrinopathy.

Red lunula

This condition can be seen in several systemic diseases such as alopecia areata, lupus erythematosus, psoriasis, dermatomyositis, congestive heart failure, and carbon monoxide poisoning.

Terry's nail

This discoloration is characterized by the pink distal portion and the proximal white portion of the nail. It can be seen in cirrhosis, chronic congestive heart failure, and adult-onset diabetes.

Half-and-half nail/Lindsey's nail

In this condition the proximal nail bed is white and distal half is red, pink, or brown. It is usually seen in renal disease with azotemia.

Yellow nail syndrome

The triad of yellow nail syndrome consists of yellow nail, lymphedema, and respiratory disease. The pathogenesis of this condition is unclear and it is persistent.

This syndrome is associated with severe long-term lymphedema, respiratory distress (especially chronic bronchitis, bronchiectasis, interstitial pneumonitis, and pleural effusion), thyroid disease, lymphoreticular malignancy, rheumatoid arthritis, lupus erythematosus, Hodgkin's lymphoma, and nephrotic syndrome. Treatment with vitamin E and/or a zinc supplement may be helpful.

2.10 Summary

We have discussed common conditions encountered in adolescents during routine practice with particular emphasis on management. Please consult the bibliography below for further details. The chapter contains six tables for quick reference.

References

1. Cole C, Gazewood J. Diagnosis and treatment of impetigo. Am Fam Physician 2007;75: 859–64.
2. Rhody C. Bacterial infections of the skin. Prim Care 2000;27(2):459–73.
3. Stulberg DL, Penrod MA, Blatny RA. Common skin infections. Am Fam Physician 2002;66(1):119–24.
4. King RW, Kulkarni R. Staphylococcal scalded skin syndrome in emergency medicine. Accessed 2011 Jun 15. URL: http://emedicine.medscape.com/article/788199-overview
5. Hogan PA. Pseudomonas folliculitis. Australas J Dermatol 1997; 38(2):93–94.
6. Eneli I, Davies HD. Epidemiology and outcome of necrotizing fasciitis in children: an active surveillance study of the Canadian Paediatric Surveillance Program. J Pediatr 2007;151(1):79–84.
7. Hauser A, Fogarasi S. Periorbital and orbital cellulitis. Pediatr Rev 2010;31(6):242–49.
8. Stoneback JW, Hak DJ. Diagnosis and management of necrotizing fasciitis. Orthopedics 2011;34(3):196.
9. Florin TA, Zaoutis TE, Zaoutis LB. Beyond cat scratch disease: Widening spectrum of Bartonella henselae infection. Pediatrics 2008;121(5):e1413-25.
10. Rawstron SA, Mehta S, Bromberg K. Evaluation of a Treponema pallidum-specific IgM enzyme immunoassay and Treponema pallidum western blot antibody detection in the diagnosis of maternal and congenital syphilis. Sex Transm Dis 2004;31(2):123–26.

11. Steere AC. Lyme disease. N Engl J Med 2001;345(2):115–25.
12. Murray T, Feder HM Jr. Management of tick bites and early Lyme disease: a survey of Connecticut physicians. Pediatrics 2001; 108(6):1367–70.
13. Ilowite NT. Muscle, reticuloendothelial, and late skin manifestations of Lyme disease. Am J Med 1995;98(4A):63S-8.
14. Scott LA, Stone MS. Viral exanthems. Dermatol Online J 2003;9(3):4.
15. Aftergut K, Cockerell CJ. Update on the cutaneous manifestations of HIV infection. Dermatol Clin 1999;17(3):445–71.
16. Andrews MD, Burns M. Common tinea infections in children. Am Fam Physician 2008;77(10):1415–20.
17. Berg D, Erickson P. Fungal skin infections in children. New developments and treatments. Postgrad Med 2001;110(1):83–84, 87–88, 93–94.
18. Centers for Disease Control and Prevention. Accessed 2011 Jun 15. URL: http://www. cdc.gov/parasites/lice/head/diagnosis.html
19. Burkhart CN, Burkhart CG. An assessment of topical and oral prescription and over-the-counter treatments for head lice. J Am Acad Dermatol 1998;38(6 Pt 1):979–82.
20. Chosidow O. Scabies and pediculosis. Lancet 2000;355(9206):819–26.
21. Naldi L, Rebora A. Clinial practice. Seborrheic dermatitis. N Engl J Med 2009;360(4):387.
22. Williams HC. Clinical practice. Atopic dermatitis. N Engl J Med 2005;352(22):2314.
23. Leung DY. Atopic dermatitis: new insights and opportunities for therapeutic intervention. J Allergy Clin Immunol 2000;105(5):860.
24. Sackesen C, Sekerel BE, Orhan F, Kocabas CN, Tuncer A, Adalioglu G. The etiology of different forms of urticaria in childhood. Pediatr Dermatol 2004;21(2):102–8.
25. Kaplan AP. Chronic urticaria and angioedema. N Engl J Med 2002; 346(3):175.
26. Samel AD. Drug eruptions. Up to date. Accessed 2011 Jun 15. URL: http://www.uptodate. com/contents/drug-eruptions
27. Weston WF, Lane AT, Morelli JG. Color Textbook of Pediatric Dermatology, 4th ed. Philadelphia: Mosby, 2007.
28. Cohen BA. Pediatric Dermatology, 3rd ed. Philadelphia: Mosby, 2005.
29. Koh MJA, Tay YK. An update on Stevens-Johnson syndrome and toxic epidermal necrolysis in children. Curr Opin Pediatr 2009; 21:505–10.
30. Antoniou C, Dessinioti C, Stratigos AJ, Katsambas AD. Clinical and therapeutic approach to childhood acne: an update. Pediatr Dermatol 2009;26(4):373–80.
31. Krowchuk DP, Gelmetti C, Lucky AW. Acne. In: Schachner LA, Hansen RC, eds. Pediatric Dermatology, 4th ed. Philadelphia: Mosby, 2011:827–50.
32. Marcoux DA, Duran-McKinster C, Baselga E. Pigmentary abnormalities. In: Schachner LA, Hansen RC, eds. Pediatric Dermatology, 4th ed. Philadelphia: Mosby, 2011:700–46.
33. Paller AS, Mancini AJ. Papulosquamous and related disorders. In: Paller AS, Mancini AJ. Hurwitz Clinical Pediatric Dermatology: A Textbook of Skin Disorders of Childhood and Adolescence, 3rd ed. Philadelphia: Elsevier Saunders; 2005:85–106.
34. Benoit S, Hamm H. Childhood psoriasis. Clin Dermatol 2007;25(6):555–62.
35. Shwayder T. Disorders of keratinization: Diagnosis and management. Am J Clin Dermatol 2004;5(1):17–29.
36. Oji V, Traupe H. Ichthyosis: Clinical manifestations and practical treatment options. Am J Clin Dermatol 2009;10(6):351–64.
37. Peppercorn, MJ. Skin and eye manifestations of inflammatory bowel disease. UpToDate. Accessed 2011 Jun 15. URL: http://www.uptodate.com/contents/skin-and-eye-manifestations-of-inflammatory-bowel-disease
38. Schur PH and Moschella SL. Mucocutaneous manifestations of systemic lupus erythematosus. UpToDate. Accessed 2011 Jun 15. URL: http://www.uptodate.com/contents/mucocutaneous-manifestations-of-systemic-lupus-erythematosus

39. Paller AS, Mancini AJ. Disease of hair and nails. In: Paller AS, Mancini AJ. Hurwitz Clinical Pediatric Dermatology: A Textbook of Skin Disorders of Childhood and Adolescence, 3rd ed. Philadelphia: Elsevier Saunders; 2005:145–83.
40. Alkhalifah A, Alsantali A, Wang E, McElwee KJ, Shapiro J. Alopecia areata update: part II, treatment. J Am Acad Dermatol 2010;62(2):191–202.
41. Kakourou T, Uksal U. Guidelines for the management of tinea capitis in children. Pediatr Dermatol 2010;27(3):226–28.
42. Gupta AK, Skinner AR. Onychomycosis in children: A brief overview with treatment strategies. Pediatr Dermatol 2004;21(1):74–79.
43. Berker D. Childhood nail diseases. Dermatol Clin 2006;24:355–63.
44. Holzberg M. Common nail disorders. Dermatol Clin 2006;24:349–54.

3 Disorders of the endocrine system

Manmohan K. Kamboj

3.1 Introduction

Growth and development are very important considerations in adolescents. Hormone disturbances in any part of the endocrine hormone axis can lead to significant disturbances in growth and pubertal development. Therefore accurate monitoring of growth, maintaining a high index of suspicion for underlying hormone disorders, and timely intervention are all important to minimize these abnormalities and ensure a healthy adolescence. The following discussion focuses on a few of the endocrine concerns important in adolescents (1,2,3,4,5,6,7).

3.2 Thyroid Hormone Disorders

3.2.1 Hypothyroidism (8,9,10,11,12)

Hypothyroidism results from decreased secretion or insufficient availability of thyroid hormone to the body. Hypothyroidism seen in adolescence may be acquired or congenital. Congenital hypothyroidism is present since birth and may be due to thyroid dysgenesis or dyshormonogenesis and requires lifelong thyroid hormone replacement. Acquired hypothyroidism may be due to autoimmune thyroid disorders or to interference with thyroid hormone synthesis by foods, drugs, or medications. Autoimmune hypothyroidism is referred to as Hashimoto's lymphocytic thyroiditis and, as the name implies, is characterized by lymphocytic infiltration and has a genetic predisposition. Iodine deficiency and radiation exposure to the head and neck may also result in hypothyroidism.

The signs and symptoms of hypothyroidism can be very subtle and insidious and may include growth deficits, dry pale skin, coarse brittle hair, bradycardia, cold intolerance, constipation, and meno/metrorrhagia. Findings may include coarsening of facial features, sallow pale skin, hung up deep tendon reflexes, and bradycardia. The thyroid gland is usually enlarged, firm, nontender, cobblestone-like; it may be irregular and nodular. Laboratory investigations reveal low levels of thyroid hormone (T4, free T4, T3, and free T3) and high levels of TSH.

Treatment

The treatment for hypothyroidism essentially is replacement with a synthetic formulation of thyroxine. Levothyroxine, or T4, is the endogenous hormone secreted by the thyroid gland, which is converted to its active metabolitetriiodothyronine, or T3. The doses are titrated by monitoring free T4 and TSH levels with the aim of keeping both of these values within the normal range. The usual dose in adults and older adolescents for the treatment of hypothyroidism is 1.7 mcg/kg per day orally. The pediatric doses vary according to age and comparatively the younger children require a much higher per kilogram dosage than adolescents (see ▶Tab. 3.1).

It is important to be aware of these relative differences in dosage in the different age groups. Overall mild or subclinical hypothyroidism generally may require lower doses. Levothyroxine is available under multiple brand names; the tablets are color-coded and available and multiple strengths, including 25, 50, 75, 88, 100, 112, 125, 137, 150, 175, 200, and 300 mcg. The medication is generally administered once daily about 30 minutes before breakfast. However, more practically, patients are advised to take the dose later in the day if they happen to miss the morning dose. Thyroid function tests including free T4 and TSH should be done about 4 weeks after initiating thyroid hormone replacement and after any changes in medication dose are made. If there is suspicion of underlying adrenal insufficiency, it should be ruled out prior to starting of thyroid hormone replacement. Thyroid hormone replacement is contraindicated in uncorrected adrenal insufficiency.

3.2.2 Hyperthyroidism

Hyperthyroidism results from excessive secretion of thyroid hormone; the most common cause in adolescents is autoimmune hyperthyroidism, also referred to as Graves' disease. It is five to six times more common in adolescent girls than boys and generally has a strong genetic predisposition. Clinical features vary greatly; they may be nonspecific and the onset may be often insidious. There may be weight loss, palpitations, poor exercise tolerance, emotional and psychiatric disturbances, and menstrual irregularities. There may be tachycardia, widened pulse pressure, hypertension, or heart murmur on examination. Ophthalmologic and dermatologic findings are more common in adults than adolescents. Laboratory findings include marked elevation of thyroid hormone levels (T4, free T4, T3, free T3) along with suppression of TSH levels. TSH receptor–stimulating antibodies are usually positive, in addition to positive antithyroperoxidase and antithyroglobulin antibodies.

Treatment

Treatment of hyperthyroidism/Graves' disease maybe a therapeutic challenge (8,9,10, 11,12). Multiple options are available, including medical therapy, surgical therapy,

Tab. 3.1: Dose of thyroid hormone in different age groups.

Age group	Dose of thyroid hormone (mcg/kg per day)
Adults and older adolescents	1.7
Younger adolescents over 12 years of age	2–3
Children between the ages of 6 and 12 years	4–5
Children between the ages of 1 and 5 years	5–6
Children between the ages of 6 and 12 months	6–8
Children between the ages of 3 and 6 months	8–10
Children between the ages of 0 and 3 months	10–15

radioactive iodine therapy. Medications used include two groups of drugs: thionamides including propylthiouracil (PTU), and the methimazole (MMI) group, primarily including Tapazole. The medical therapy is the initial therapy of choice for children and adolescents with hyperthyroidism/Graves' disease employed by most pediatric endocrinologists. ▶Tab. 3.2 lists both of these medical treatment options. Both MMIs and PTU inhibit thyroid hormone formation promptly, but because there is no effect on the release of already formed thyroid hormone, circulating levels of thyroid hormone remain elevated for a few weeks. PTU also has an additional peripheral effect. Both these agents may have significant side effects, primarily including liver disease, blood dyscrasias, fever, urticaria, dermatitis, arthralgias, and neutropenia.

Most of these side effects occur with both agents. Precautions and dose adjustments may be needed for patients who are already on anticoagulants, digoxin, and theophylline and also in patients with renal impairment. Beta blockers may be required in addition to initiation of antithyroid medications to control the catecholaminergic hyperactivity symptoms of hyperthyroidism. These agents offer symptomatic relief to the patient in the interim until thyroid hormone levels can be normalized. Propranolol (Inderal) may be used in these situations.

It must be remembered that these agents are relatively contraindicated in patients with an additional history of asthma or reactive airway disease. Dosages of up to 10 to 40 mg per dose every 6 to 8 hours may be used. Extended-release preparations are now available as well. In acute situations, iodine may be used to acutely block thyroid hormone production, as evident in the Wolff-Chaikoff effect, where thyroid hormone blockade is seen when the thyroid gland is exposed to excessively large doses of iodine. This is a transient phenomenon lasting for 2 to 3 weeks, after which breakthrough occurs and no further thyroid hormone blockade is seen. This is therapeutically used to control hyperthyroidism in the short term. Potassium iodide – in the form of tablets, syrup, saturated solution of potassium iodide (SSKI), and Lugol's iodine (strong iodine solution) – is available with varying concentrations of iodine. The usual dose in children is 50 to 250 mg three times a day orally; in adults it is 50to 500 mg three times a day. The onset of antithyroid effect is usually seen in 1 to 2 days. This treatment is contraindicated in pregnancy. The other major side effects are mentioned in ▶Tab. 3.3.

Tab. 3.2: The two main groups of antithyroid medications.

	PTU	MMI
Dosing	Every 8 hours initially and then may be given twice or thrice a day	Every 8 hours initially and then once or twice a day
Taste and compliance	More metallic taste, poor compliance	Better compliance
Tablet size	50-mg tablets	5- and10-mg tablets
Potency	Less potent	More potent
Dose	5–10 mg/kg per day	0.5–1.0 mg/kg/day
Risk of hepatitis	Higher risk of hepatitis	Comparatively slightly lower risk
Use in pregnancy	Relative preference in pregnancy	Higher teratogenicity (aplasia cutis)

Tab. 3.3: Side effects of antithyroid medications.

Minor adverse reactions – seen in up to 25% of patients
- Elevated liver enzymes
- Leukopenia
- Skin rash
- Granulocytopenia
- Arthritis
- Lymphadenopathy

Major adverse reactions – seen in up to 1% of patients
- Agranulocytosis
- Hepatitis

The second feasible therapeutic option is that of radioactive iodine (RAI) treatment (10,11,12). This is actually the treatment of first choice in adults. Pediatric endocrinologists, however, still hesitate and use this mostly after a trial of medications has failed. The RAI dose usually depends on dosimetry calculations based on thyroid gland size and RAI uptake. The aim of RAI is to achieve complete ablation of the glands, causing postablation hypothyroidism, which then is treated with thyroid hormone replacement. The alternative modality of therapy – especially in younger children, adolescents with very large thyroid glands, those who do not want radioactive iodine therapy, and those in whom medical therapy has failed or shown evidence of side effects – is surgery. Total thyroidectomy is recommended by a surgeon who is well experienced with the procedure. Risks of hemorrhage, vocal cord paralysis, and permanent hypoparathyroidism exist.

3.3 Central Diabetes Insipidus (DI)

Central DI is due to inadequate secretion or release of arginine vasopressin. This may be due to congenital or acquired disorders. The acquired form is more common and may be due to tumors in the hypothalamic/pituitary area, granulomatous diseases, histiocytosis X, septo-optic dysplasia, or Wolfram's syndrome. Patients with DI typically are unable to concentrate their urine, with low urine specific gravity between 1.001 and 1.010 and low urine osmolality of 50 to 300 mosm/kg in face of high plasma osmolality and hypernatremia. Extremely low levels of serum arginine vasopressin (AVP) in situation of hyperosmolality and hypo-osmolar urine strongly suggest DI. A water deprivation test may be useful for further clarification.

Treatment

Adolescents with central diabetes insipidus are treated with vasopressin (13,14). Untreated patients with DI crave cold water. If the thirst mechanism is intact and there is free access to water, individuals can maintain normal plasma osmolality. But this would entail a significant intake of fluid volumes and significant polyuria. Therefore, although it would be possible physiologically, this would be kept up at a great inconvenience and discomfort to the individual.

Vasopressin can be replaced in the form of decompressing acetate, also known as dDAVP. dDAVP is a synthetic vasopressin analogue. It is available in various forms including an injectable preparation, nasal spray, rhinal tube, and oral tablets. It is important to remember that the potencies and concentrations of all these preparations are different.

Synthetic aqueous vasopressin is called pitressin; it may be required in the immediate postoperative period following trauma or surgery in the pituitary and peripituitary area. In these cases most clinicians prefer to use this in the form of a continuous intravenous infusion, the advantage being that the half-life is very short and almost immediate titrations of dose can be made based on the intake and output as well as serum osmolality.

Alternatively, subcutaneous injections may be used. The dose requires titration irrespective of form of administration, which is again dependent on close monitoring of the intake and output (I/O) and serum sodium levels. For nonemergent use, dDAVP may be administered via subcutaneous injections, intranasal administration via rhinal tube or nasal spray, and oral administration with tablets. dDAVP is supplied in the following forms: injectable, with 4 mcg/mL solution; nasal spray, with 10 mcg per dose (5 mL); tablets, 0.1 and 0.2 mg; and rhinal tube solution 0.01 percent, with a rhinal tube that has dose markings.

Administration is generally started at a smaller dose and then titrated upward as needed: With tablets, the starting dose 0.05 mg twice a day. The general dose range is 0.1 to 0.8 mg/day. dDAVP is generally given every 8 to 12 hours. With the nasal spray/rhinal tube the dosage is 0.1–0.4 mL per day or every 8 to 24 hours as needed. The injectable dDAVP at 0.5 to1 mL/day may be administered intravenously or subcutaneously and is generally given twice a day. The relative potency of the different routes of administration differs: the subcutaneous injectable form is most potent, with the intranasal form having 1/10 the potency of the injectable form and the oral form having 1/200 the potency of the injectable form or 1/20 the potency of the nasal form. This is extremely important when changing from one formulation and route of administration to the other.

Contraindications include hyponatremia and moderate to severe renal failure. Adverse effects include headaches, nausea, injection site reactions, abdominal cramping, blood pressure changes, and facial flushing. There may be nasal congestion, rhinitis, or epistaxis with the nasal spray or rhinal tube administration. Close monitoring of intake and output and serum sodium levels in addition to urine and plasma osmolality should be done. It is very important to remember to look at the formulation and route of administration when initiating treatment or changing treatment from one formulation to another. Also, it should be remembered that dDAVP is marketed in a much more concentrated form used in hematology and that this cannot be interchanged with doses used for the treatment of DI.

3.4 Adrenal Gland Disorders

The adrenal cortical disorders are characterized by underproduction (hypoadrenocorticism) or overproduction (hyperadrenocorticism) of adrenal cortical hormones including glucocorticoids, mineralocorticoids, and adrenal androgens (15,16,17,18).

3.4.1 Hypoadrenocorticism

Hypoadrenocorticism may result from multiple causes that may be congenital or acquired; however, even the congenital disorders may present at an older age. Congenital adrenal hyperplasia (CAH) is an important cause of hypoadrenocorticism but is discussed separately. The presentation in these patients may be due to cortisol and/or aldosterone deficiency. Acute adrenal crisis may be life-threatening and may be precipitated by a concurrent illness in a previously undiagnosed patient. Such an episode is characterized by fever, weakness, lethargy, nausea, vomiting, anorexia, hypoglycemia, seizures, hypotension, acidosis, shock, and cardiovascular collapse. Intensive care management is lifesaving.

The clinical presentation, however, may be more chronic and insidious, especially in adolescents, and they may present with muscle weakness, malaise, mental status changes, anorexia, vomiting, weight loss, hypoglycemia, and orthostatic hypotension. Generalized bronze pigmentation of the skin is noted. Additional testing reveals hyponatremia, hyperkalemia, low serum cortisol levels, and high plasma adrenocorticotropic hormone (ACTH) and renin activity. Further testing with an ACTH (cosyntropin) stimulation test reveals poor cortisol reserve. Additional testing including very long chain fatty acids and antiadrenal antibodies is helpful to establish an underlying etiology. Imaging may help visualize adrenal size to look for any tumors, and so on.

Treatment

Acute adrenal insufficiency presentation needs immediate treatment after a critical blood sample for diagnostic laboratory workup is drawn. The treatment includes immediate fluid resuscitation with normal saline and dextrose, which will correct hypoglycemia, hyponatremia, and hypovolemia. Hydrocortisone started immediately at 100 mg/m^2 per day in divided doses every 6 hours. Precipitating factors/illnesses need to be treated appropriately. Once the acute state is treated and for patients who present more insidiously, ongoing treatment consists of physiologic hydrocortisone replacement, which may vary from 8 to 15 mg/m^2 per day in three to four divided doses. Patients with additional salt wasting require mineralocorticoid replacement with fludrocortisone in doses of 0.05 to 0.2 mg/day. Additional salt may be added to the diet as needed to maintain normal serum sodium levels and plasma renin activity. The steroid stress dose coverage is an important concept that patients and families need to understand.

The physiologic dose of hydrocortisone previously noted is insufficient to meet the needs of the body during stress conditions, notably fever, trauma, or any other significant illness. During these times (and as happens in the body normally), the steroid dose must be increased. Based on the degree of stress, dose of hydrocortisone may be increased to two to five times the normal dose of the individual and preferably given every 6 hours. If the patient is unable to take oral medication, injectable hydrocortisone may be administered intramuscularly. The patient and family are educated about the intramuscular administration of hydrocortisone at the time of diagnosis.

Exogenous steroid treatment

Patients on long-term steroid treatment for other medical conditions may exhibit hypothalamic-pituitary-adrenal (HPA) axis suppression at multiple levels. Complete recovery of the HPA axis may take many months. Such a patient should be weaned off the steroids very gradually and carefully. It is important to ensure appropriate stress coverage with exogenous hydrocortisone until there is complete recovery of the adrenal reserve. This may need to be tested for by ACTH stimulation testing.

Congenital adrenal hyperplasia (CAH)

CAH is a congenital autosomal recessive disorder that results from an enzymatic defect in the adrenal steroid pathway. The commonest type of CAH is due to a defect in the 21-hydroxylase enzyme caused by a defect in the CYP21 gene (16,17). This disorder may present in varying forms depending on the degree of enzymatic defect and genetic mutation. Female newborns may present at birth with ambiguous genitalia; the salt-wasting type may present in the first couple of weeks of life with evidence of salt wasting; the simple virilizing form presents with evidence of virilization without salt wasting. The nonclassic form of CAH is more common and usually presents as premature adrenarche in childhood. The newborn screen checks for 17-hydroxyprogesterone level to rule out CAH due to CYP21 gene mutation.

Clinically the 21-hydroxylase deficiency is characterized by low cortisol, hyponatremia, hyperkalemia (for salt wasters), high levels of adrenal androgens, high plasma ACTH, and advanced skeletal age. The treatment for congenital adrenal hyperplasia aims at replacing the glucocorticoids with hydrocortisone. The physiologic requirement of hydrocortisone may vary between 8 and 15 mg/m^2 per day divided into three doses. The patients with salt wasting also requires mineralocorticoid replacement with fludrocortisone and additional salt replacement in early infancy.

These treatment modalities result in normalization of electrolyte abnormalities, hypoglycemia, lowering of ACTH levels, and decreased the adrenal androgens, thus normalizing the HPA axis. This also prevents skeletal age advancement. Patients with CAH also need directives for stress dose coverage for steroids as well as education about intramuscular hydrocortisone replacement, as discussed previously. There are ongoing studies about the use of alternative medications in the form of antiandrogens and aromatase inhibitors, which are believed lower the glucocorticoid requirement.

3.4.2 Hyperadrenocorticism

Hyperfunctioning of the adrenal cortex may result in excessive levels of glucocorticoids, mineralocorticoids, adrenal sex steroids, or a combination of these. Cushing's syndrome may result from an ACTH secreting pituitary tumor stimulating the adrenal gland (Cushing's disease), ectopic corticotropin-releasing hormone (CRH) or ACTH from a nonpituitary tumor, or overactivity of the autonomous adrenal gland. Patient usually presents with a cushingoid appearance.

A similar phenotype may also result from an exogenous steroid intake as well as from exogenous obesity. However unlike exogenous obesity in which children and adolescents have growth acceleration with an advanced bone age; those with Cushing syndrome and exogenous steroid intake present with growth deceleration, short stature, and delayed puberty.

Additional features include generalized muscular weakness, headaches, purplish striae, hypertension, hyperglycemia, and osteoporosis . Laboratory workup reveals loss of normal diurnal variation in cortisol levels and high 24-hour urinary cortisol. Further endocrine testing with a low- and high-dose dexamethasone suppression test, ACTH levels, CRH stimulation test, and pituitary and adrenal gland imaging may be helpful.

Treatment in these patients depends on the underlying cause. Transsphenoidal surgery is utilized to treat Cushing's disease. Adrenalectomy or subtotal adrenalectomy may be indicated in the case of adrenal tumors. After adrenalectomy, these adolescents require adequate adrenal steroid replacement therapies.

3.5 Disorders of Vitamin D, Calcium Metabolism, and Parathyroid Hormone

Vitamin D, calcium, and parathyroid hormone are closely interlinked to maintain calcium homeostasis as well as adequate bone metabolism (19,20,21,22). Most disorders in this category are therefore related to abnormalities at one of these levels. Vitamin D is a prohormone synthesized in the skin or supplied in the diet. Vitamin D deficiency therefore may result from a combination of deficient sun exposure and inadequate dietary intake.

The precursor of vitamin D in the skin is vitamin D3, the animal source–derived dietary vitamin D is D3, and the plant source–derived vitamin D is D2; both of these are metabolized similarly in the body. Vitamin D is hydroxylated in the liver to 25-hydroxy vitamin D (25OHD), which is further metabolized in the kidney by 1-alpha-hydroxylase to 1,25 dihydroxy vitamin D (1,25 diOHD); this is the active form of vitamin D. The molecular effects of vitamin D are mediated via vitamin D receptors (VDRs). 1,25 diOHD is mainly responsible for calcium and phosphorus absorption in the intestine and therefore the primary regulator of bone mineralization.

The main source of vitamin D is from sunshine exposure, vitamin D supplementation in dairy products and cereals, or multivitamin preparations. However, multiple factors including dark skin, sun exposure only at dusk and dawn, cloudy longer winters, insufficient area of skin exposed to sun, northern latitudes, and use of sunscreens can all compromise the amount of vitamin D generated in the skin. A high prevalence of vitamin D deficiency is noted even in otherwise healthy adolescents and even athletes.

The present recommendation for daily vitamin D intake is 400 international units. However, controversy continues regarding adequate serum levels of vitamin D. It is generally accepted that serum levels of less than 30 ng/mL of 25OHD are consistent with vitamin D insufficiency and levels more than that are considered sufficient

3.5.1 Rickets

Rickets results from undermineralization of the cartilaginous epiphysial growth plate and therefore is specific to the growing skeleton and will not be seen once epiphyses have closed; then, instead, osteomalacia is noted. Rickets therefore may be seen in younger adolescents but is a much more common condition in younger children. Rickets may result from multiple causes including nutritional vitamin D deficiency; familial X-linked hypophosphatemia or vitamin D–resistant rickets; vitamin D–dependent rickets due to impairment of 1-alpha-hydroxylase; or hereditary vitamin D resistance.

The treatment of rickets will vary depending on the underlying etiology. First, nutritional rickets is preventable and can be prevented by adequate exposure to sunlight and/or oral supplementation of vitamin D. For nutritional rickets, vitamin D replacement is effective.

Various protocols exist to guide vitamin D replacement. Vitamin D in the form of vitamin D analogues or calciferol is available for this treatment. Vitamin D (2000–4000 IU) can be given in daily doses for 6 to 8 weeks, with improvement noted in the vitamin D levels in serum as well as in radiologic healing of the bony manifestations. "Stoss" therapy has been used, especially in patients with poor compliance and more often in developing countries, when large doses of vitamin D (150,000–300,000 IU) can be administered at one time.

Risks of hypercalcemia exist; therefore the administration of massive doses is not recommended as routine therapy. Patients who have additional concerns with malabsorption may need higher replacement doses of vitamin D, usually in the range of 4,000 to 10,000 IU/day. Some anticonvulsants may interfere with hepatic P450 enzymes, and their long-term use has been associated with rickets and osteomalacia. These children and adolescents may require supplementation with vitamin D all year around. They should have adequate calcium intake ensured as well, either in the diet or with oral supplementation.

In addition, if adolescents present with severe, acute, symptomatic tetany, intravenous calcium needs to be administered for control of symptoms, followed by oral calcium replacement, as discussed below for the treatment of hypocalcemia. Vitamin D–dependent rickets type I clinically presents similarly to vitamin D–deficiency rickets, but biochemically these patients have adequate vitamin D levels. The treatment for this type of rickets is with calcitriol or 1-alpha-hydroxy vitamin D. The recommended dosage for treatment of rickets is 2 to 8 mcg/day of 1-alpha-hydroxy vitamin D or 1 to 4 mcg/day of calcitriol.

After adequate healing of the acute condition, lifelong maintenance therapy with 1 to 3 mcg/day of 1-alpha-hydroxy vitamin D or 2 mcg/day of calcitriol is generally required. Patients in the third main group, those with vitamin D–dependent rickets type 2, are rare and mainly represent target-organ resistance to calcitriol because of a defect in the vitamin D receptor. Patients with severe defects do not respond to vitamin D therapy, are a therapeutic challenge, and need large doses of calcium supplementation. Milder and moderate levels of the defect respond to large doses of calcitriol or 1-alpha-hydroxy vitamin D with adequate calcium supplementation.

Dosages as large as 0.5 to 5 mcg/day in milder cases and up to 5 to 60 mcg/day in those with a moderate defect may be needed. Calcium supplementation of about 2 g/day is generally recommended. Adolescents on therapeutic doses of calcium and/or vitamin D should be monitored for serum levels of calcium, phosphorus, and vitamin D levels. The urine calcium/creatinine ratio is needed to avoid hypercalciuria.

3.5.2 Hypocalcemia

Hypocalcemia may be seen in the adolescents with nutritional deficiency, vitamin D deficiency, hypoparathyroidism, or pseudohypoparathyroidism; it may also be a part of an autoimmune polyglandular syndrome resulting from hypomagnesemia due to an excessive phosphate load, or it may be associated with mitochondrial disorders. Adolescents with hypocalcemia may have a wide range of clinical presentations ranging from asymptomatic hypocalcemia to severe presentation with signs and symptoms of tetany and seizures.

The acute presentation is much more dramatic, with tetany, paresthesias, muscle cramps, hyperirritability, weakness, behavioral disturbances including anxiety and depression; as well as positive Chvostek's, Erb's and Trousseau's signs. Life-threatening situations may include laryngospasm and frank seizures. The ECG may demonstrate prolonged QT and ST intervals.

Treatment

Irrespective of the underlying cause, the aim of treatment in hypocalcemia is to normalize serum calcium to at least the lower normal range and at the same time prevent hypercalcemia and hypercalciuria. Patients with acute presentations will need intravenous calcium to normalize the calcium levels quickly. This may be done by using 10 percent calcium gluconate in a dose of 1 to 2 mL/kg (max = 10 mL) repeated every 6 hours until seizures and tetany resolve. Alternatively, a continuous intravenous infusion with 1 to 3 mg/kg per hour of elemental calcium may be given after the initial intravenous dose. Subcutaneous extravasation of calcium can cause burns; therefore the greatest care must be exercised in administering intravenous calcium.

Oral calcium supplementation is started as soon as possible. In ordering oral calcium supplementation it is important to remember that doses should be expressed in terms of the amount of elemental calcium. This is very important because the amount of elemental calcium varies with the particular calcium salt in the preparation being used. For example, calcium carbonate contains 40 percent elemental calcium, therefore a 600-mg tablet of calcium carbonate will have 240 mg of elemental calcium. Dosages for oral calcium supplementation will vary depending on age as well as the severity of hypocalcemia.

The dosage range for children is about 45 to 65 mg/kg per day divided every 6 hours, while the adult dosage range is 1 to 2 g/day divided every 6 to 8 hours. It is important to monitor calcium and phosphorus levels on these relatively high doses of supplementation. Depending on the underlying cause of the hypocalcemia, additional therapy with vitamin D may be needed, as previously noted. Hypomagnesemia coexistent with hypocalcemia will need concurrent treatment for successful resolution of the hypocalcemia.

3.5.3 Hypercalcemia

Hypercalcemia in adolescents may be seen as a result of hyperparathyroidism, hypervitaminosis D, immobilization, Williams syndrome; it may also be associated with bone tumors or with activating mutations of the PTH receptor. The adolescents may present again with extremely nonspecific symptoms including muscular weakness, weight loss, sleep problems, behavioral problems, abdominal pain, pathologic fractures, nephrocalcinosis, or renal calculi. Hypercalcemia may also not uncommonly be diagnosed incidentally on a routine basic metabolic panel screening. The treatment modalities vary with the underlying cause, which must be addressed and treated as appropriate. If there is an exogenous source of the extra vitamin D, it must be discontinued immediately. Intravenous hydration is indicated for the treatment of severe hypercalcemia. A low-calcium diet is recommended.

Medical intervention may include administration of prednisone to help lower serum calcium levels, and this may have to be continued until the other dietary and preventive measures take effect. A dosage of 1 to 2 mg/kg per day of prednisone may be used. Hypercalcemia associated with hypophosphatemia may require additional phosphate repletion. The use of bisphosphonates in the treatment of hypercalcemia and hypercalciuria of immobilization and other causes with evidence of bone resorption has been found to be helpful. The treatment of the specific underlying cause will be the ultimate long-term treatment, such as removal of any parathyroid adenomas.

3.6 Disorders of Pubertal Development

3.6.1 Normal pubertal development in girls

It is important to understand normal pubertal timing for the accurate evaluation of disorders of puberty (23,24,25). The first clinical sign of pubertal onset in girls is the onset of breast development, or thelarche (23,24). Menarche (onset of menstrual periods) generally is regarded as culmination of the pubertal process and generally follows 2 to 3 years after thelarche. Pubertal staging is done by using the Tanner staging methods; breast development and pubic hair are staged separately. (See Figs. 2.1 and 2.2 in chapter 2 in Greydanus DE, Patel DR, Omar HA, Feucht C, Merrick J: Adolescent Medicine – Pharmacotherapeutics in General, Mental and Sexual Health, de Gruyter, Berlin, 2012.)

The peak growth velocity and menarche occur at Tanner stages 3 to 4. Mean age at thelarche is believed to be somewhere between 10 and 11 years of age in white girls, 9 and 10 years in black girls, and somewhere in between for Hispanic girls. The lowest normal age for the onset of breast development remains controversial: in white girls, some contend it starts at 8 years while others state 7 years; in African American girls, 7 years versus 6 years. Therefore girls having evidence of breast development prior to these time frames should be investigated further for early onset of puberty. Lack of breast development by 13 years of age would be labeled as delayed pubertal onset. Mean age of menarche, however, is more consistent and is noted to be 12.6 years in white girls, 12.1 years in black girls, and 12 .2 years in Mexican American girls. No menarche until 16 years of age is referred to as delayed menarche.

Normal pubertal development in boys is gauged by Tanner staging for pubic hair, testicular volume, and penis size. Testicular enlargement is the first clinical sign of onset of pubertal development in boys. A Prader orchidometer may be used to measure testicular size; 3 mL and less is a prepubertal volume while 25 mL is the adult testicular volume. Average age of onset of testicular enlargement and hence onset of puberty in boys is about 11 to 12 years. The average age of pubarche is between 12 and 12.5 years in white boys, with African American boys starting about a year earlier. Axillary hair generally appear 1 to 2 years after pubarche. Facial hair starting with upper lip hair usually appear around the age of 15 years. Therefore onset of pubertal development with testicular enlargement before the age of 8 to 9 years is considered early and after the age of 14 years is considered delayed.

Pubarche before the age of 10 years may also need further workup. Technically, therefore, precocious pubertal development is not seen in adolescents just based on the time frame of features seen. However, since the concerns associated with precocious puberty relate to adolescence, these are discussed here along with delayed puberty. The causes of precocious puberty are elaborated in ▶Tab. 3.4.

Central precocious puberty (CPP)

This is also referred to as gonadotropin-dependent precocious puberty. CPP signifies activation of the hypothalamo-pituitary-gonadal (HPG) axis. It is more common in girls than boys and about 95 percent of CPP in girls is idiopathic versus 50 percent of CPP in boys being idiopathic; the other 50 percent generally have an underlying pathologic etiology. Children presenting with early puberty should have a complete physical examination to stage the level of pubertal development as well as to look

Tab. 3.4: Causes of precocious puberty.

I. Central precocious puberty (CPP)/ gonadotropin-dependent precocious puberty

1. Idiopathic
   - Isolated
   - Familial
2. Central nervous system (CNS) lesions
   - Developmental abnormalities
   - Brain tumors – astrocytoma, neurofibromatosis, pinealoma, craniopharyngioma, granulomas
   - Damage or dysfunction – radiation, chemotherapy, infections, head trauma
3. Others
   - Hypothyroidism – Van Wyk–Grumbach syndrome
   - Congenital adrenal hyperplasia – untreated

II. Peripheral precocious puberty/gonadotropin-independent precocious puberty

1. McCune-Albright syndrome
2. Adrenal gland tumors – adenoma, carcinoma
3. Gonadal tumors:
   - Ovarian – ovarian cyst, granulosa cell tumors, thecoma, luteoma
   - Testicular – Leydig cell tumors
4. Human chorionic gonadotropin (hCG) – secreting tumors:
   - CNS germinoma, hepatoma, hepatoblastoma, teratoma
5. Congenital virilizing adrenal hyperplasia

for any evidence of underlying pathology. Laboratory investigations include evidence of pubertal levels of gonadotropins, namely follicle-stimulating hormone (FSH) and luteinizing hormone (LH), measured in the basal or stimulated state as well as elevated sex steroids including estrogens in girls and testosterone in boys.

Skeletal age is advanced; magnetic resonance imaging (MRI) of the pituitary and hypothalamic area should be done to rule out any space-occupying lesions; pelvic ultrasonography may be helpful for the evaluation of ovarian and uterine size and endometrial stripe. If an underlying pathology is delineated, it will have to be addressed and treated appropriately as indicated. The main issues that result from the precocity itself are a short final adult height because of a shortened window of linear growth available prior to epiphysial fusion and psychological issues arising from difficulty in social adjustment because of a physical precocity generally unassociated with behavioral or psychological maturity.

The treatment of CPP therefore involves suppression of the HPG axis by suppressing the gonadotropins. This is achieved by administration of a GnRH agonist, which interferes with the pulsatility of the endogenous GnRH, the latter being an essential for pubertal onset and progression. GnRH agonists are available in the form of aqueous preparations requiring daily subcutaneous injections or the more commonly used depot preparations such as leuprolide acetate.

Several depot preparations are available: the preparation that is effective for 28 days and hence administered every 4 weeks deep intramuscularly and is available in strengths of 7.5, 11.25, and 15 mg as a pediatric depot preparation. The dosage is usually 0.3 mg/kg per dose given every 28 days, which may be titrated up by 3.75 mg every 4 weeks if sufficient suppression for downregulation is not seen. The daily preparation is given in a dosage of 50 mcg/kg per day. Alternative depot preparations that require administration every 3 months or yearly are other options, although the preparation most commonly used is the 28-day form.

If treatment is started earlier in the course of pubertal development, regression or halting of the pubertal physical as well as biochemical changes is noted and the rate of skeletal maturation is also slowed. These patients should be followed in the clinic every 3 to 4 months for close monitoring of clinical and biochemical evidence of pubertal suppression.

3.6.2 Gonadotropin-independent or peripheral precocious puberty (PPP)

PPP signifies clinical evidence of puberty without concomitant stimulation of the HPG axis. Laboratory evaluation reveals high estrogen or testosterone levels in face of prepubertal levels of gonadotropins. Imaging should exclude tumors in the CNS, gonads, or adrenals.

Treatment is based on the underlying cause. Hypothyroidism, if present, should be appropriately treated. Underlying tumors must be removed. Benign follicular cysts usually need no treatment. In case of high androgens, antiandrogens (e.g., spironolactone), inhibitors of steroid synthesis (e.g., ketoconazole), or P-450 aromatase inhibitors (e.g., testolactone) may be useful (26,27). In case of high estrogens, as in McCune-Albright syndrome, aromatase inhibitors are noted to be useful options. Patients with PPP may also be at a higher risk for the development of secondary CPP, in which case treatment with GnRH analogues may be appropriate.

3.6.3 Delayed puberty

Delayed puberty is defined as the absence of secondary sexual characteristics in girls by 13 years of age and in boys by 14 years of age. The definition also encompasses other scenarios such as lack of pubertal progression after pubertal initiation began on time, more than 4 years between onset of breast development and menarche, and in boys, if pubertal features began but do not show evidence of adequate progression. Causes of delayed puberty are outlined in ▶Tab. 3.5.

A detailed history and physical exam is needed to establish the present status of pubertal development and pubertal progression and to note evidence of any other underlying conditions that may be responsible for the delayed puberty. Laboratory evaluation confirms the clinical impression and may include a karyotype; gonadotropin levels including FSH and LH, GnRH, or HCG stimulation tests; and imaging of the hypothalamic-pituitary areas as well as pelvic sonography.

Treatment

Treatment depends on the underlying cause. If there a pathologic underlying cause is identified, that will have to be treated as needed. Treatment for the pubertal delay itself will also have to be instituted. Constitutional delay of puberty usually results in normal but delayed growth. If there is significant anxiety, adolescents may be treated with short-term low-dose sex steroids (estrogen in females and testosterone in males). Constitutional delay of growth and development is much more common in boys and intramuscular testosterone cypionate or enanthate may be used in doses of 50 to 100 mg every 4 weeks for about 6 months. The treatment for permanent hypogonadism (hypergonadotropic or hypogonadotropic) is the same.

Treatment essentially involves replacement of testosterone in boys and of estrogen in girls. In both cases an effort is made to mimic normal physiologic pubertal development as closely as possible by starting the hormone replacement in very small doses and then making small, gradual incremental increases in doses to mimic normal pubertal progression. Therefore in boys testosterone injections may be started with about 50 mg every 4 weeks, gradually increased to the adult replacement dose of 200 to 300 mg every 2to 4 weeks over several years. The injectable forms previously noted are the ones generally used initially. Once pubertal development is complete and final adult height is attained, other forms of administration for testosterone such as gels and patches may be utilized for ongoing adult replacement.

In girls, estrogen therapy is similarly initiated in low doses to mimic very early pubertal estrogen levels and gradually increased in small increments over about 2 years. Once adequate estrogenization is attained, progesterone can be added for normal menstrual cycling. Multiple estrogen preparations are available; depending on particular needs and preferences, a specific preparation may be selected. Some of the well-known estrogens and their equivalent doses are outlined here:

- Conjugated equine estrogens: Starting with a dose of 0.15 or 0.3 mg daily for 6 months, then making small increments of 0.15 to 0.3 mg every 6 months to a full dose of 0.625 to 1.2 mg by the end of second year of treatment. The starting dose, dosing increments, and total dose required may vary depending on individual requirements.

Tab. 3.5: Causes of delayed puberty.

I. Constitutional delay of growth and puberty

II. Hypogonadotropic hypogonadism (gonadotropin deficiency)

1. Genetic causes
   - Genetic syndromes: Kallman's syndrome, Prader-Willi syndrome
   - DAX 1, SF1 mutations
   - Isolated FSH or LH deficiency
2. Acquired causes
   - CNS – tumors, post irradiation, post inflammatory
3. Endocrine disturbances
   - Hypothyroidism/hyperthyroidism
   - Hyperprolactinemia
   - Panhypopituitarism

III. Hypergonadotropic hypogonadism (primary gonadal failure)

1. In males
   - Klinefelter's syndrome (47XXY)
   - Mixed gonadal dysgenesis
   - Testicular dysgenesis
   - Cryptorchidism
   - LH resistance
   - Testicular damage: irradiation, chemotherapy, infections
2. Females
   - Turner's syndrome
   - Mixed gonadal dysgenesis
   - Ovarian dysgenesis
   - FSH and LH resistance
   - Acquired causes: chemotherapy, radiation therapy, autoimmune gonadal failure
3. In males and females
   - Functional causes
   - Chronic severe malnutrition
   - Chronic systemic illnesses
   - Excessive exercise
   - Psychogenic

SF, steroidogenic factor; DAX, dosage-sensitive sex reversal, adrenal hypoplasia critical region, on chromosome X, gene 1.

- Transdermal estrogen preparations: Usual small starting dose of 0.0625 mg/day and gradually increased over 2 years to a total daily dose of 0.05 to 0.1 mg/day. The adult replacement dose is 0.1 mg/day. The issues involved with cutting the estrogen patches to deliver a smaller dose are not clearly defined, although this is being done clinically off label with generally adequate results.
- Oral ethinyl estradiol and intramuscular depot preparations are also used, the principle again being to start at doses that may be as small as 1/10 of the adult dose and making small, gradual increments over about 2 years.

After adequate estrogenization is achieved over about 2 years, progesterone is added to achieve menstrual cycling. Various options for progesterone administration include oral medroxyprogesterone, using 10 mg/day, or micronized progesterone at 200 mg/daygiven for 10 days each month starting the twentieth day of the cycle. In some situations this cycling can be done with progesterone administered every 3 months for every-3-month menstrual cycles. To facilitate administration and timing, combined oral contraceptive pills can be used at this time to provide both estrogen and progesterone.

The hormonal therapy is continued as needed, probably lifelong. Treatment for girls with Turner's syndrome involves growth hormone administration as well as estrogen replacement. The estrogen replacement is individualized for timing of initiation as well as for dosing depending on individual needs. Overall the guidelines for estrogen replacement remain as noted above.

3.7 Growth Disorders

Disorders of growth are more commonly seen in the preadolescent period; however, abnormal growth may be an important issue in the adolescent as well. It is of the utmost importance that growth measurements be done accurately, in a consistent manner, and the evaluation of these accurate anthropometric measurements must be made using the appropriate reference data and growth charting tools.

3.7.1 Short stature

Multiple endocrine and nonendocrine causes may result in inadequate growth or short stature. Short stature may be familial or genetic; however, it is imperative to rule out familial conditions associated with underlying endocrine disorders or growth hormone deficiency (28,29,30,31,32). Adolescents with familial short stature have heights that are shorter than those of their peers but consistent with those of their parents and siblings. They have a normal growth velocity, normal underlying hormone workup, and their bone age is consistent with their chronologic age. The calculations for midparental target height are consistent with calculated predicted adult height. These adolescents do not need growth hormone replacement.

Constitutional delay of growth and development is characterized by short stature and delayed puberty and may be a cause of significant concern for adolescents and families. There may be a positive family history, the rate of growth is normal for the pubertal status, skeletal age is consistent with delayed puberty, and midparental target height is consistent with the predicted adult height range. These adolescents also do not generally need treatment. Sometimes low-dose sex steroids may be used to accelerate growth in cases of adolescents who have a very poor self-image.

Nonendocrine causes of short stature and failure to thrive must be ruled out in all these adolescents. Endocrine causes may include growth hormone deficiency, other disorders of the hypothalamo-pituitary-growth hormone-IGF1 axis (HPG), hypothyroidism, Cushing's syndrome, hypoparathyroidism, pseudohypoparathyroidism, and disorders of vitamin D metabolism. Detailed history, clinical examination, and laboratory workup may be needed for further investigation.

Endocrinology referral is warranted for the completion of endocrine workup. Common disorders of the HPG axis include hypopituitarism, panhypopituitarism, growth hormone deficiency, IGF1 deficiency, and growth hormone resistance. These disorders may result from congenital defects or may be acquired subsequent to trauma, infections, neurosurgical procedures, radiation, and chemotherapy. Some syndromic conditions – including Turner's syndrome (30), Down's syndrome, Russell-Silver syndrome, Prader-Willi syndrome, and DiGeorge syndrome – as well as osteochondrodysplasias, neurologic disorders including neurofibromatosis and neural tube defects, exposure to high doses of exogenous steroids, and psychosocial stress factors all may result in growth problems and short stature. Laboratory investigations may be undertaken as suggested in ▶Tab. 3.6.

Treatment

Growth hormone therapy may be indicated in multiple scenarios in adolescents with short stature including growth hormone deficiency, Turner's syndrome, chronic renal insufficiency (pre-transplant), and Prader-Willi syndrome (30,31,32). Idiopathic short stature is another indication approved by the U.S. Food and Drug Administration (FDA) where growth hormone may be used in children and adolescents who are below −2.25 SD, with otherwise normal workup. The range of growth hormone doses used in these different conditions are listed in ▶Tab. 3.7.

Tab. 3.6: Laboratory investigations for short stature.

1. General laboratory tests:
    a. CBC, ESR, comprehensive metabolic panel, antiendomysial antibodies
    b. Chromosome analysis (girls)
    c. Bone age
2. Endocrine laboratory tests:
    a. Free T4, TSH
    b. IGF-1, IGFBP3
    c. Further hormone testing based on clinical suspicion as needed
3. Further tests:
    a. Growth hormone stimulation test
    b. Pituitary/brain imaging – CT scan/MRI with and without contrast

CBC, complete blood count; ESR, erythrocyte sedimentation rate; free T4, free thyroxine level; TSH, thyroid-stimulating hormone; IGF1, insulin-like growth factor 1; IGFBP3, insulin-like growth factor binding protein 3.

Growth hormone therapy is continued until completion of linear growth or when the growth velocity is less than 2 cm per year. After completion of linear growth, there are various recommendations for further testing to rule out adult GHD. For individuals with adult GHD, growth hormone treatment is used if needed. A majority of children and adolescents with childhood GHD generally are not found to be hormone-deficient by adult standards.

Adolescents on growth hormone therapy should be followed in theclinic by an endocrinologist every 3 to 6 months to evaluate for the efficacy as well as safety of growth hormone therapy. IGF1 levels may be helpful in individualizing growth hormone dosing as well as monitoring for safety. Growth hormone generally is considered safe medication; some possible adverse reactions and side effects are listed in ▶Tab. 3.8. It is helpful to enroll patients on long-term databases and registries maintained by most manufacturers of growth hormone to assess for long-term safety and efficacy.

Tab. 3.7: Recommendations for growth hormone dosing.

	Mcg/kg per day	Mg/kg per week
GHD, adolescents	25–100	0.17–0.7
GHD, adults	6–25	0.02–0.17
TS	50	0.35
PWS	35–50	0.245–0.35
CRI	50	0.35

GHD, growth hormone deficiency; TS, Turner's syndrome; PWS, Prader-Willi syndrome; CRI, chronic renal insufficiency.

Tab. 3.8: Side effects of growth hormone therapy.

1. CNS: Pseudotumor cerebri
2. Musculoskeletal:
   - Slipped capital femoral epiphysis (SCFE)
   - Scoliosis/worsening scoliosis
   - Carpal tunnel syndrome
   - Arthralgias
   - Myalgias
3. Impaired carbohydrate metabolism while on treatment
4. Theoretical risk of malignancy
5. Respiratory compromise in patients with Prader-Willi syndrome who are morbidly obese and/or have preexisting respiratory compromise

Caution:
   - Hypothyroidism – may be unmasked on initiating growth hormone treatment
   - Screen for adrenal insufficiency before replacing thyroid hormone

3.7.2 Tall stature

Excessively tall stature with predicted adult height considerably above the target height based upon parental heights may have to be investigated and treated if required. Tall stature may be constitutional or familial/genetic with no evidence of any underlying pathology and may need no treatment. Tall stature may rarely be due to a pituitary growth hormone–secreting tumor. Adolescents with Klinefelter syndrome, Marfan syndrome, and homocystinuria present with tall stature. Somatic overgrowth is seen in Beckwith-Wiedemann syndrome (BWS) and Soto's syndrome during childhood, but these individuals are usually not excessively tall adolescents. Exogenous obesity may be accompanied by rapid growth but is usually associated with normal adult height.

Growth hormone–secreting tumors occurring before epiphysial fusion cause gigantism with excessive linear growth; but they cause acromegaly in older adolescents and adults once the epiphyses have fused. Clinical features of advanced acromegaly include coarsening of facial features and enlargement of tongue, mandible, hands, and feet. These features are much harder to find in the early phases. Pituitary enlargement and local impingement on the optic chiasm can cause headaches, vomiting, and visual field defects. There is elevation of IGF-1, IGFBP3, prolactin and GH levels, but there may be suppression of other pituitary hormones such as ACTH, TSH, and FSH/LH.

The HPG axis may be further assessed by a growth hormone suppression test (by measuring growth hormone levels at 30 and 60 minutes during an oral glucose tolerance test). MRI of the pituitary and peripituitary area will be helpful in delineating a pathologic anatomic lesion in the area. Chromosome analysis and relevant genetic studies may be required for specific overgrowth syndromes.

Treatment

Various modalities available for the treatment of these tumors include medical treatment with long-acting somatostatin analogues such as octreotide; surgical removal or radiation of an underlying tumor; or further more specific treatment based on the underlying cause.

3.8 Polycystic Ovarian Syndrome (PCOS)

PCOS is a syndrome with a heterogenous clinical presentation (33,34,35,36,37). The main components in adolescents result from hyperandrogenemia and oligoanovulation generally associated with overweight and insulin resistance. (See chapter 17 in Greydanus DE, Patel DR, Omar HA, Feucht C, Merrick J: Adolescent Medicine – Pharmacotherapeutics in General, Mental and Sexual Health, de Gruyter, Berlin, 2012.) The underlying etiology is not clear. There continues to be a controversy about the diagnostic criteria for PCOS. Consensus diagnostic criteria have been developed by the U.S. National Institutes of Health (NIH),the European Society of Human Reproduction and Embryology, and the American Society of Reproduction. The diagnostic criteria primarily include clinical or biochemical hyperandrogenism and menstrual irregularity, usually with oligomenorrhea or amenorrhea as a reflection of anovulation. The presence of cystic ovaries is not an essential diagnostic criterion. Clinical manifestations of hyperandrogenism include alopecia, hirsutism, and acne.

PCOS is more common in obesity, and patients may exhibit features of insulin resistance such as acanthosis nigricans. A higher incidence of type 2 diabetes may be noted. Lab findings include high levels of dehydroepiandrosterone sulfate (DHEAS), androstenedione, testosterone, and free testosterone. The LH/FSH ratio is increased; sex hormone binding globulin (SHBG) is decreased. Cystic ovaries may be seen on ultrasound but are not mandatory for establishing the diagnosis of PCOS. There may be high levels of insulin and glucose tolerance may be normal, impaired, or even consistent with a diagnosis of type 2 diabetes mellitus.

Since there are no clearly outlined diagnostic criteria, it is prudent to rule out other causes of hyperandrogenemia before making a diagnosis of PCOS. Multiple treatment options are available for PCOS depending on the predominant clinical manifestations. For insulin resistance, medications such as metformin are useful. Menstrual irregularities may be treated by use of hormone therapy with combination oral contraceptives (preferably with antiandrogenic progestin preparations). Antiandrogens, GnRH agonists, and glucocorticoids have also been used to counteract the effects of hyperandrogenemia.

3.9 Diabetes Mellitus (DM)

DM is a metabolic syndrome characterized by hyperglycemia due to an underlying insulin deficiency, insulin resistance, or a combination of both. Based on the underlying etiopathogenesis, DM may be classified broadly into type1 DM (T1DM or insulin-dependent diabetes mellitus – IDDM or juvenile diabetes); type 2 DM (T2DM or non-insulin dependent DM – NIDDM or adult-onset DM); MODY – maturity-onset diabetes of youth; and DM secondary to other causes.

3.9.1 Epidemiology

There are about 215,000 people younger than 20 years in the United States who have diabetes mellitus (both T1DM and T2DM); this represents 0.26 percent of all people in this age group. In children and adolescents less than 10 years old, the rate of new cases has been 19.7 per 100,000 each year for T1DM and 0.4 per 100,000 for type 2 diabetes; for those older than 10 years, the rate of new cases has been 18.6 per 100,000 each year for type 1 diabetes and 8.5 per 100,000 for T2DM.

3.9.2 Etiopathogenesis

The etiology of T1DM is probably a combination of genetic predisposition and the superadded effect of environmental triggers. The majority of cases of T1DM are type 1A, in which an autoimmune process is responsible for the destruction of pancreatic beta cells, resulting in an absolute deficiency of insulin. Type 1B DM is much less common and has an underlying nonimmune etiology. Maturity-onset diabetes of youth (MODY) describes diabetes mellitus due to defective beta-cell function, which causes impaired insulin secretion; the insulin sensitivity of the other tissues, however, is normal. MODY is believed to be an autosomal dominant disorder due to more than 200 mutations involving six chromosomes.

Diabetes may occur secondary to other chronic illnesses such as cystic fibrosis and Cushing's syndrome or develop secondary to exposure to exogenous toxins, drugs, or infections. Patients with type 1 DM have a higher incidence of associated autoimmune endocrinopathies. These include Hashimoto's thyroiditis, Addison's disease, celiac disease, pernicious anemia and an association with the autoimmune polyglandular syndromes. Thyroid function testing is recommended annually in type I DM patients. Type 2 DM, on the other hand, is commonly associated with obesity and the spectrum of manifestations associated with metabolic syndrome X.

3.9.3 Clinical presentation

Adolescents may present in one of three ways: in a state of acute diabetic ketoacidosis (DKA), with nausea, vomiting, abdominal pain, hyperglycemia, dehydration, Kussmaul breathing, and even altered sensorium or with the typical symptomatology of polyuria, polydipsia, nocturia, and weight loss. The third presentation is DM found incidentally on a urinalysis or basic metabolic panel done for other reasons.

3.9.4 Diagnostic criteria

The diagnostic criteria for DM include fasting blood glucose of equal to or greater than 126 mg/dL and random or 2-hour postprandial (after 75 g of glucose) blood glucose of equal to or greater than 200 mg/dL tested on two separate occasions. As of 2010, the Endocrine Society has endorsed the use of glycated hemoglobin (HbA1c) as a diagnostic parameter as well, with levels of equal to or greater than 6.4 percent being indicative of diabetes.

3.9.5 Management

DM is a chronic disease that requires long-term comprehensive management, which actually starts right at the time of diagnosis (38,39,40,41,42,43,44,45). The multidisciplinary diabetes care team approach has been found to be most effective for achieving well-rounded, comprehensive care. The team comprises the primary care physician along with the endocrinologist, who work together with the core team comprising a nurse, diabetes educator, nutritionist, and a social worker/psychologist. The importance of maintaining a good glycemic control in order to delay the onset of chronic complications has been well demonstrated in multiple long-term studies, such as the Diabetes Control and Complications Trial (DCCT).

Intensive and comprehensive diabetes education starts at the time of diagnosis and is needed to familiarize the patient, family, and close friends with "survival skills." Survival skills include education the ability to check blood sugar, give an insulin injection, calculate the right dose of insulin, count carbohydrates, and understand the need for ongoing meticulous log keeping of the self-monitored blood sugar data (40,41). The importance of self-monitoring of blood glucose to titrate the doses of insulin is emphasized.

Management of DKA

DKA comprises a clinical syndrome with hyperglycemia, ketosis, and acidosis. A state of insulin deficiency causes hepatic gluconeogenesis and decreased peripheral glucose utilization leading to hyperglycemia; lipolysis and ketogenesis causes ketouria and ketonemia; and further metabolic decompensation results in acidosis. Traditionally DKA was believed to be the hallmark for T1DM, but now it is well recognized that DKA also occurs in T2DM. The initial management of DKA is similar in patients with type I and type 2 DM but must be individualized depending on the specific presentation, degree of illness, and laboratory findings.

Adolescents with a relatively mild DKA who are otherwise not ill may be initiated directly on a subcutaneous insulin regimen; in the relatively sicker adolescents, therapy is normally initiated with an intravenous insulin drip. Patients are generally 10 percent to 15 percent dehydrated at presentation and may have electrolyte derangements. Appropriate and judicious fluid correction over 36 to 48 hours should be undertaken, along with close monitoring and appropriate replacement of sodium, potassium, phosphate, and magnesium.

An insulin drip with regular insulin is initiated at 0.1 units/kg per hour; dextrose is added to the intravenous fluid once blood sugar is below 250 to 300 mg/dL. The rates are adjusted to maintain blood sugars in the range of 100 to 200 mg/dL. Most institutions generally have their own DKA protocols in place to facilitate management, ensure close monitoring, and minimize errors. These adolescents are switched to the subcutaneous insulin regimen when they are asymptomatic, ready to eat, and generally ketone-negative.

Types of insulin

Insulin is used for the treatment for type1 DM; it may also be used in type 2 DM in addition to insulin sensitizers. The first insulin was derived from animals, primarily cattle or pigs. However, recombinant DNA technology has greatly transformed the availability of insulin. The differences between these types of recombinant human insulin are in the amino acid sequence of the human insulin. At present all available insulins are manufactured in the laboratory and are classified into groups based on their onset and duration of action. The four main types are:

- Long-acting: glargine, detemir (may be intermediate also)
- Intermediate-acting: NPH (neutral protamine Hagedorn)
- Short-acting: regular
- Rapid acting: lispro, aspart, glulisine

The timing of action of these types of insulin are summarized in ▶Tab. 3.9. Based on the timing of action of the various types of insulin, different combination regimens have been devised, all in an effort to mimic the physiologic action of insulin in the body in relation to food. Two of the commonly used regimens are detailed in ▶Tab. 3.10. The management of diabetes involves two important mechanical activities: blood glucose testing and subcutaneous insulin administration. Advances continue in the field of diabetes management with the aim of achieving near normal glycemic control and simplifying insulin administration and glucose monitoring to ensure near

Tab. 3.9: Timing of action of different typess of insulin.

Type of insulin	Onset of action	Time of peak action	Duration of action
Long-acting insulin (Glargine)	2–3 hours	Peakless	About 24 hours
Intermediate-acting insulin	2–4 hours	6–8 hours	10–14 hours
Short-acting insulin	30–60 minutes	2–3 hours	4–6 hours
Rapid-acting insulin	15 minutes	30–60 minutes	About 4 hours

normal life routines. Insulin must be still administered subcutaneously. Various insulin delivery systems available for use are listed in ▶Tab. 3.11.

Blood glucose monitoring

Blood glucose monitoring at home is done by using glucose testing meters. Technologic advances have made many different types of glucose testing meters available that offer newer features like being small and attractive, requiring very small amounts of blood, having the ability to store several days of blood glucose data and the ability to communicate with insulin delivery devices, and the ability to be downloaded with computer programs. Several continuous glucose monitoring systems are available now for further assistance in the management of patients with widely fluctuating blood sugar levels.

Glycated hemoglobin and ketone testing

HbA1c or glycated hemoglobin measures nonenzymatic binding of glucose to hemoglobin and reflects average blood sugar control over the preceding 3 months. HbA1c is measured at the time of the clinic visit and is used to monitor long-term glycemic control as well as to authenticate the self-monitoring data.

Patients are also taught to check for ketones at home when they are sick and/or have hyperglycemia (blood glucose 250–300 mg/dL). Adolescents generally test ketones (acetoacetate) in urine; blood ketones (beta-hydroxybutyric acid) can be measured by some glucometers as well. Adolescents and families are educated about "sick-day treatment regimens," which essentially include close blood glucose monitoring, ketone testing, frequent administration of rapid-acting insulin, and adequate hydration.

Role of lifestyle modifications

Adolescents with diabetes are encouraged to participate in sports and physical activity for improving insulin sensitivity, maintaining good glycemic levels, and controlling weight. Some modifications may be needed in the form of extra testing, or extra carbohydrate intake may be needed to avoid hypoglycemia, especially in T1DM. Lifestyle modifications including exercise/activity and dietary modifications are the mainstay of treatment of T2DM.

Medication therapy in T2DM

The role of medications in T2DM is complementary to these lifestyle modifications (42,43,44,45). The aim of oral medications in these adolescents is to improve insulin

Tab. 3.10: Two commonly used insulin regimens.

NPH based/regimen of three injection a day		
Insulin: Intermediate- acting insulin: NPH	Short/rapid acting insulin: Regular, Aspart, ispro, Glulisine	
3 Injections:	Prebeakfast (AM):	⅔ of total daily dose
		NPH (⅔ of AM dose) + short/rapid acting (⅓ of AM dose)
		The two types of insulin may be combined and drawn up together in one syringe
	Predinner and before bed (PM)	⅓ of PM dose is short-/rapid-acting – given predinner
		⅔ of PM dose is NPH – given before bed
Advantages:	Usually no lunchtime insulin required	
	Only three shots a day	
Disadvantages:	Consistency in meal timings required	
	Consistency in carbohydrate content of meals required	
	Meal content must be more or less similar from day to day	
Intensive flexible insulin dose regimen		
Long-acting insulin: glargine	For basal insulin coverage	
	Once a day subcutaneous (usually bedtime)	
	Comprises 50% of total daily dose	
Rapid-acting insulin:	As bolus for meal coverage	
	Given multiple times a day for meals	
	Bolus is based on a ratio of insulin:carbohydrate (I:C) ratio	
	I:C ratio calculated by:	Using rule of 500 (500 divided by total daily dose) or
		calculated based on total daily carbohydrate intake, based on carbohydrate content to be 50% of total daily caloric intake

(Continued)

Tab. 3.10: Two commonly used insulin regimens (*Continued*)

	Correction factor (CF):	Refers to the amount blood glucose lowered by one unit of insulin
		CF is used to correct for hyperglycemia usually at meal times
		Calculated by using rule of 1,800 (1,800 divided by total daily dose) or three times the I:C ratio
Advantages:	More flexible with regard to meal timings as well as content	
	Offers better glycemic control	
Disadvantages:	More shots required	
	More blood glucose testing required	

Tab. 3.11: Various insulin delivery systems.

Insulin syringes and vials

- Remain the least expensive method for insulin delivery
- Cumbersome and tedious

Insulin pen devices

- Are quicker and more convenient to use.
- Offer more precise dosing.
- Usually allow for discrete use by adolescents in social situations.

Continuous subcutaneous insulin infusion (CSII) via the insulin pump

- Enables the administration of rapid acting insulin over the 24-hour period.
- Multiple basal rates can be used to mimic intrinsic insulin secretion.
- Food intake is covered with bolus insulin, which can also be adjusted for immediate, square-wave, or dual-wave delivery depending on meal content.
- Use of CSII therefore offers great flexibility in lifestyle along with being able to maintain adequate glycemic control.
- Pumps can be placed in the suspended mode at times of prolonged intense physical activity to avoid hypoglycemia.
- Extreme motivation needed to achieve tight glycemic control.
- Patients still need to do frequent self- monitoring of blood glucose.
- Patients must acquire technical expertise to deal with the pump and be able to troubleshoot mechanical failures.
- All these patients must receive adequate education regarding nutrition and carbon carbohydrate counting

sensitivity and/or augment insulin secretion. Metformin is an insulin sensitizer and is the most common oral medication used in the adolescent age group. Metformin and insulin are the only agents approved by the FDA for the treatment of type 2 diabetes in children and are the mainstay of treatment of T2DM in adolescents under 18 years of age.

The mechanism of action of metformin includes decreasing hepatic glucose production and increasing glucose uptake in muscles and adipose tissues via actions on the insulin receptors. The main side effects include abdominal discomfort, distention, and nausea, which can be lessened by starting at a lower dose of 500 mg daily and gradually increasing it to a daily maximum of 2000 mg/day and taking the medication with meals.

However, several other medications, including sulfonylureas and meglitinides, have also been used by some physicians, primarily as off-label treatment options. The use of thiazolidinediones in pediatric patients is being investigated. Some other groups of medications that are approved for adults and older adolescents include the following:

- Sulfonylureas/meglitinides – both of which increase insulin secretion.
- Alpha-glucosidase inhibitors/acarbose – these delay the absorption of carbohydrates or lipase inhibitors, which reduce the absorption of fat.
- DPP-IV inhibitors (e.g., sitagliptin) – these increase insulin production and decrease hepatic glucose production.
- Incretin-like medications including exenatide – these cause a glucose-dependent increase in insulin secretion from beta cells.
- Amylin analogs such as pramlintide – these decrease hepatic glucose production by decreasing glucagon secretion and delaying stomach emptying.

3.10 Conclusions

Endocrine disorders in adolescents are important issues for both adolescents and their clinicians. This discussion considers normal growth and development in youth and reviews a variety of potential endocrine conditions, including hyper- and hypothyroidism, diabetes insipidus, adrenal gland disorders, parathyroid dysfunction, disorders of pubertal development, growth disorders, polycystic ovarian syndrome, and diabetes mellitus. (See chapter 17 in Greydanus DE, Patel DR, Omar HA, Feucht C, Merrick J: Adolescent Medicine – Pharmacotherapeutics in General, Mental and Sexual Health, de Gruyter, Berlin, 2012.) Important management considerations are reviewed including pharmacologic treatment.

References

1. Kappy M, Allen D, Geffner M. Pediatric Practice Endocrinology. New York: McGraw Hill; 2010.
2. Sperling MA. Pediatric Endocrinology, 3rd ed. Philadelphia: Saunders Elsevier; 2008.
3. Lifshitz F. Obesity, diabetes mellitus, insulin resistance, and hypoglycemia. In: Pediatric Endocrinology, 5th ed. Vol. 1. London: Informa Healthcare; 2006.
4. Greydanus DE, Patel D, Pratt H. Essentials of Adolescent Medicine. New York: McGraw-Hill, 2005.

5. Kamboj MK. Clinical Issues in endocrinology. In: Greydanus DE, Patel DR, Feinberg AN, Reddy VN, Hatim O. Handbook of Clinical Pediatrics. Singapore: World Scientific; 2010:195–224.

6. Kronenberg HM, Melmed S, Polonsky KS, Larsen PR. Williams Textbook of Endocrinology, 11th ed. Philadelphia: Saunders Elsevier; 2007.

7. Pescovitz OH, Eugster EA. Pediatric endocrinology: Mechanism, manifestations and management. Philadelphia: Lippincott Williams & Wilkins, 2004.

8. Cooper DS. Antithyroid drugs for the treatment of hyperthyroidism caused by Graves disease. Endocrinol Metab Clin North Am 1998;27:225–47.

9. Zimmerman D, Lteif AN. Thyrotoxicosis in children. Endocrinol Metab Clin North Am 1998;27:109–26.

10. Rivkees SA, Sklar C, Freemark M. Clinical Review 99: The management of Graves disease in children, with special emphasis on radioiodine treatment. J Clin Endocrinol Metab 1998;83:3767–76.

11. O Torring, L Tallstedt, G Wallin, G Lundell, JG Ljunggren, A Taube, et al. Graves hyperthyroidism: Treatment with antithyroid drugs, surgery, or radioiodine – a prospective, randomized study. Thyroid Study Group. J Clin Endocrinol Metab. 1996;81:2986–93.

12. Read CH, Tansey MJ, Menda TY. A 36-year retrospective analysis of the efficacy and safety of radioactive iodine in treating young Graves patients. J Clin Endocrinol Metab 2004;89:4229–33.

13. Vande Walle J, Stockner M, Raes A, Nørgaard JP. Desmopressin 30 years in clinical use: a safety review. Curr Drug Saf 2007;2:232.

14. Fjellestad-Paulsen A, Paulsen O, d'Agay-Abensour L, Lundin S, Czernichow P. Central diabetes insipidus: oral treatment with dDAVP. Regul Pept 1993; 45:303–7.

15. Merke DP, Bornstein SR. Congenital adrenal hyperplasia. Lancet 2005;365:2125–36.

16. Merke DP, Bornstein SR, Avila NA, Chrousos GP. NIH conference. Future directions in the study and management of congenital adrenal hyperplasia due to 21-hydroxylase deficiency. Ann Intern Med 2002; 136:320–24.

17. Joint LWPES/ESPE CAH Working Group. Consensus statement on 21-hydroxylase deficiency from the Lawson Wilkins Pediatric Endocrine Society and the European Society for Paediatric Endocrinology. J Clin Endocrinol Metab 2002;87:4048–53.

18. Ten S, New M, Maclaren N. Clinical Review: Addison's disease. J Clin Endocrinol Metab 2001;86:263–315.

19. Bartoszewska M, Kamboj M, Patel DR. Vitamin D, muscle function, and exercise performance. Pediatr Clin North Am 2010;57:849–61.

20. Kamboj MK. Metabolic bone disease in adolescents: recognition, evaluation, treatment, and prevention. Adolesc Med State Art Rev 2007;18:24–46.

21. Huh SY, Gordon CM. Vitamin D deficiency in children and adolescents: epidemiology, impact and treatment. Rev Endocr Metab Disord 2008;9:161–70.

22. Greydanus DE, Bricker LA. Parathyroid disorders in the adolescent. Asian J Pediatr Practice 2005;23:123–29.

23. Marshall WA, Tanner JM. Variations in pattern of pubertal changes in girls. Arch Dis Child 1969; 44:291–303.

24. Marshall WA, Tanner JM. Variations in the pattern of pubertal changes in boys. Arch Dis Child 1970;45:13–23.

25. Kaplowitz PB, Oberfield SE. Reexamination of the age limit for defining when puberty is precocious in girls in the United States: implications for evaluation and treatment. Drug and Therapeutics and Executive Committees of the Lawson Wilkins Pediatric Endocrine Society. Pediatrics 1999;104:936–41.

26. Shulman DI, Francis GL, Palmert MR, Eugster EA for the Lawson Wilkins Pediatric Endocrine Society Drug and Therapeutics Committee. Use of aromatase inhibitors in children

and adolescents with disorders of growth and adolescent development. Pediatrics. 2008;121: e975–83.

27. Feuillan P, Calis K, Hill S, Shawker T, Robey PG, Collins MT. Letrozole treatment of precocious puberty in girls with the McCune-Albright syndrome: a pilot study. J Clin Endocrinol Metab. 2007;92:2100–106.

28. GH Research Society. Consensus guidelines for the diagnosis and treatment of growth hormone deficiency in childhood and adolescence: Summary statement of the GH Research Society. J Clin Endocrinol Metab 2000;85:3990–93.

29. Wilson TA, Rose SR, Cohen P, Rogol AD, Backeljauw P, Brown R, et al. Update of guidelines for the use of growth hormone in children: The Lawson Wilkins Pediatric Endocrinology Society Drug and Therapeutics Committee. J Pediatr 2003;143(4):415–21.

30. Saenger P, Wikland KA, Conway GS, Davenport M, Gravholt CH, Hintz R, et al. Fifth International Symposium on Turner Syndrome. Recommendations for the diagnosis and management of Turner Syndrome. J Clin Endocrinol Metab 2001;86:3061–69.

31. Lee PDK, Allen DB, Angulo MA, Cappa M, Carrel AL, Castro-Magana M, et al. Consensus statement – Prader-Willi syndrome: Growth hormone (GH)/insulin-like growth factor axis deficiency and GH treatment. Endocrinologist 2000;10:71–73.

32. Fine RN. Growth hormone in children with chronic renal insufficiency and end-stage renal disease. Endocrinologist 1998;8:160–69.

33. Kamboj MK, Patel DR. Polycystic ovarian syndrome: A diagnostic and therapeutic challenge. J Pediatric Sci 2010;2:e4.

34. Rotterdam ESHRE/ASRM-Sponsored PCOS Consensus Workshop Group. Revised 2003 consensus on diagnostic criteria and long-term health risks related to polycystic ovary syndrome. Fertil Steril 2004;81:19–25.

35. Azziz R, Carmina E, Dewailly D, Diamanti-Kandarakis E, Escobar-Morreale HF, Futterweit W, et al. Criteria for defining polycystic ovary syndrome as a predominantly hyperandrogenic syndrome: An Androgen Excess Society guideline. J Clin Endocrinol Metab 2006;91:4237–45.

36. Buggs C, Rosenfield RL. Polycystic ovary syndrome in adolescence. Endocrinol Metab Clin North Am 2005;34:677–705.

37. Bricker L, Greydanus DE. The metabolic syndrome: A gathering challenge in time of abundance. Adolesc Med State Art Rev 2008; 19(3):475–97.

38. Diabetes. Accessed 2011 Jun 12. URL: http://diabetes.niddk.nih.gov/dm/pubs/statistics/#fast. accessed 022811.

39. Bantle JP, Wylie-Rosett J, Albright AL, Apovian CM, Clark NG, Franz MJ, et al. Nutrition recommendations and interventions for diabetes: a position statement of the American Diabetes Association. Diabetes Care 2008;31(Suppl 1):S61–78.

40. Kamboj MK, Draznin MB. Office management of the adolescent with diabetes mellitus. Prim Care Clin Office Pract 2006;33:581–602.

41. Kamboj MK, Draznin MB. Diabetes. In: Patel D, Greydanus D, eds. Pediatric practice: Sports medicine. New York: McGraw Hill, 2008:157–66.

42. Fleischman A, Rhodes ET. Management of obesity, insulin resistance and type 2 diabetes in children: consensus and controversy. Diabetes Metab Syndr Obes 2009; 2:185–202.

43. Zeitler P, Epstein L, Grey M, Hirst K, Kaufman F, Tamborlane W, et al. Treatment options for type 2 diabetes in adolescents and youth: a study of the comparative efficacy of metformin alone or in combination with rosiglitazone or lifestyle intervention in adolescents with type 2 diabetes. Pediatr Diabetes 2007;8:74–87.

44. Bowen ME, Rothman RL. Multidisciplinary management of type 2 diabetes in children and adolescents. J Multidiscip Health 2010 28;3:113–24.

45. Gungor N, Hannon T, Libman I, Bacha F, Arslanian S. Type 2 diabetes mellitus in youth: the complete picture to date. Pediatr Clin North Am 2005;52:1579.

4 Neurologic disorders
Madeline A. Chadehumbe and Olufemi Soyode

This chapter provides a brief overview of some of the neurologic disorders commonly encountered in adolescents: epilepsy, headaches, tics, and tremors. An emphasis is placed on the initial approach to management. The most commonly used medications in treating adolescents with neurologic presentations are reviewed. The goal of the chapter is to equip the reader with a quick reference to aid in the diagnoses and initial management of these common disorders seen in children and adolescents.

4.1 Epilepsy

A seizure is "a transient, involuntary alteration of consciousness, behavior, motor activity, sensation, or autonomic function caused by an excessive rate and hypersynchrony of discharges from a group of cerebral neurons" (1). Epilepsy is defined as more than one unprovoked seizure.

4.1.1 Epidemiology

It is estimated that 4 to 10 percent of children suffer at least one seizure by age 16 years. The lifetime risk of one seizure (febrile seizures included) is about 8 to 10 percent. The ratio of children with a first unprovoked seizure to those who develop epilepsy is about 5:1 (1,2).

4.1.2 Classification

Distinction is made between a seizure type and epilepsy syndrome. The seizure type is determined by the patient's behavior and electroencephalographic (EEG) pattern during the actual seizure event (see ▶Tabs. 4.1 and 4.2). On the other hand, the epilepsy syndrome is defined by the seizure type, natural history, EEG findings (ictal and interictal), response to anticonvulsant (AED) treatment, etiology, and outcome.

4.1.3 Differential diagnosis

The differential diagnosis includes syncope (see chapter 10), cardiac arrhythmias, migraine and its variants, behavioral events (such as nonepileptic staring spells, jitteriness, self-stimulation, or stereotypies), movement disorders (such tics, benign myoclonus, dyskinesias, or dystonias),sleep disorders (such as night terrors, narcolepsy, sleep myoclonus or confusional arousals [see chapter 8]) and psychogenic conditions (such as nonepileptic seizures, rage attacks, or panic attacks).

Tab. 4.1: ILAE Classification of seizure types.

Partial seizures

• Simple partial (consciousness retained)

  Motor

  Sensory

  Autonomic

  Psychic

• Complex partial (consciousness impaired)

  Simple partial followed by impaired consciousness

  Consciousness impaired at onset

• Partial seizures with secondary generalization

Generalized seizures

• Absences

  Typical

  Atypical

• Generalized tonic-clonic

• Tonic

• Clonic

• Myoclonic

• Atonic

• Infantile spasms

Unclassified seizures

4.1.4 Management

Only about 27 to 44 percent of patients who present with their first unprovoked seizure will have a second one (3,4,5,6,7,8,9). A majority of the recurrences occur early (within the first 1 to 2 years). Risk factors for recurrence include an abnormal EEG, focal seizure or exam, remote symptomatic seizures, positive family history, young age (first year of life), and history of prior febrile seizure (10,11,12,13,14,15,16, 17,18).

There is no evidence of a difference when treatment is started after the first seizure versus after a second seizure in achieving a 1-or 2-year seizure remission (19). Even though a decision to treat is made on an individual basis after weighing the risks versus the benefits of treatment, prophylactic treatment is generally recommended after a second unprovoked seizure since, at this point, the risk of recurrence is deemed to be higher. In most cases children who have been seizure-free on medications for 2 or more years have a higher chance of remaining seizure-free after coming off anticonvulsant therapy (20,21).

Tab. 4.2: 1989 International League Against Epilepsy (ILAE) classification of epilepsies and epileptic syndromes.

Localization-related (focal or partial) epilepsy

- Idiopathic

  Benign childhood epilepsy with centrotemporal spikes (benign rolandic epilepsy)

  Childhood epilepsy with occipital paroxysms
- Symptomatic

  The subclassification is determined by the anatomic location suggested by the clinical history, predominant seizure type, interictal and ictal EEG, and imaging studies – thus, SPSs, CPSs, or secondarily generalized seizures arising from frontal lobes, parietal, temporal, occipital, or multiple lobes or an unknown focus
- Localization related but uncertain symptomatic or idiopathic

Generalized epilepsies

- Idiopathic

  Benign neonatal familial convulsions

  Benign neonatal convulsions

  Benign myoclonic epilepsy of infancy

  Childhood absence epilepsy (pyknoepilepsy)

  Juvenile absence epilepsy

  Juvenile myoclonic epilepsy (impulsive petit mal)

  Epilepsy with grand mal seizures upon awakening

  Other generalized idiopathic epilepsies that do not conform exactly to the syndromes just described
- Cryptogenic or symptomatic generalized

  West syndrome (infantile spasms)

  Lennox-Gastaut syndrome

  Epilepsy with myoclonic astatic seizures

  Epilepsy with myoclonic absences

  Symptomatic

  Nonspecific cause

  Early myoclonic encephalopathy

  Specific disease states manifesting with seizures

Epilepsies and syndromes underdetermined as focal or generalized

- With both generalized and focal seizures

  Neonatal seizures

  Severe myoclonic epilepsy of infancy

  Epilepsy with continuous spike-and-wave patterns during slow-wave sleep

  Acquired epileptic aphasia (Landau-Kleffner syndrome)

(Continued)

Tab. 4.2: 1989 International League Against Epilepsy (ILAE) classification of epilepsies and epileptic syndromes. (*Continued*)

Without unequivocal generalized or focal features
All cases with GTCSs in which the EEG findings do not allow classification as definitely generalized or localization-related: e.g., sleep GTCSs

Special syndromes

• Situation-related seizures
Febrile convulsions
Isolated seizures or isolated status epilepticus
• Acute symptomatic seizures: e.g., alcohol withdrawal seizures, eclampsia, uremia

PS, complex partial seizures; EEG, electroencephalogram; GTCS, generalized tonic-clonic seizures; SPS, simple partial seizures.

4.1.5 Seizure prophylaxis

Identifying the right seizure type and epilepsy syndrome is important in choosing an anticonvulsant for seizure prophylaxis (see ▶Fig. 4.1). For generalized epilepsies, "broad-spectrum" anticonvulsants are the best option. In addition, ethosuximide is an excellent choice for childhood absence epilepsy. This drug, however, will not prevent other types of generalized seizures. Therefore if a patient is at risk for a generalized convulsive seizure, other broad-spectrum agents must be considered either in combination with or as a replacement for ethosuximide. The "narrow spectrum" drugs are a good choice for partial epilepsies, but they may exacerbate generalized epilepsies. Therefore when the seizure type is unclear, a broad-spectrum agent is the best choice. A number of antiseizure medications are reviewed in the following paragraphs.

Valproic acid

The initial starting dosage is 10 to 15 mg/kg per day divided into two or three daily doses. One can raise the dosage by 5 to 10 mg/kg per day with a goal maintenance range of 20 to 50mg/kg per day. The goal serum level is 50 to 100 μg/mL. Common side effects include gastrointestinal (GI) upset, weight gain, drowsiness, alopecia, tremors, pancreatitis, and thrombocytopenia. Valproic acid can cause polycystic ovarian syndrome in adolescent females. Valproate interferes with the metabolism of other anticonvulsant agents and may increase the serum levels of phenobarbital, phenytoin, carbamazepine, diazepam, clonazepam, and ethosuximide. It should be avoid in adolescent females because it can lead to weight gain, hair loss, ovarian cysts, and teratogenicity.

Topiramate

The initial starting dosage is 1 to 2 mg/kg per day divided into two daily doses. This dosage may be raised by 1 to 3 mg/kg per day with a goal maintenance range of 3 to 9 mg/kg per day. Common side effects include weight loss, poor concentration or memory

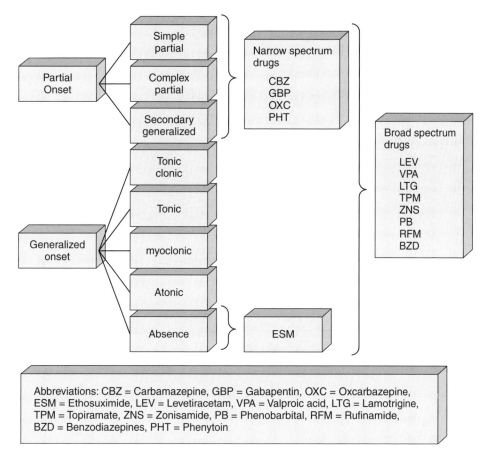

Fig. 4.1: Choosing an anticonvulsant (a medication commonly used for the treatment of generalized epilepsy).

difficulty, cognitive changes, word-finding difficulty, sedation, parasthesias, glaucoma, and kidney stones.

Levetiracetam

The initial starting dosage is 10 to 20 mg/kg per day divided into two daily doses. This may be increased by 10 to 15 mg/kg per day with a goal maintenance range of 30 to 60 mg/kg per day. The most common side effects are irritability and depression; others include headache, anorexia, fatigue, and infection (i.e., rhinitis, otitis media, gastroenteritis, and pharyngitis).

Ethosuximide

The initial starting dosage is 7.5 to 15 mg/kg per day divided into two daily doses for ages below 6 years or 125–250 mg twice a day for those above 6 years of age. This dosage may be raised by 7.5 mg/kg per day with a goal maintenance range of

20 to 40 mg/kg per day and a goal serum level of 40 to 100 µg/mL. Common side effects include GI upset, weight gain, and headache; rare effects include erythema multiforme and a lupus-like syndrome.

4.1.6 Medications commonly used for focal epilepsy

Oxcarbazepine

The initial starting dosage is 8 to 10 mg/kg per day divided into two daily doses. This may be raised by 10 mg/kg per day with a goal maintenance range of 20 to 40 mg/kg per day; the goal serum level is 10 to 35 µg/mL. Common side effects include drowsiness, blurred vision, and lethargy. Other side effects include rash, leukopenia, aplastic anemia, and hepatic toxicity. In addition to oxcarbazepine, any of the medications used for generalized epilepsies (broad-spectrum AEDs) can be useful for focal epilepsies.

4.1.7 Acute seizure management for status epilepticus
(21,22,23,24,25,26,27,28)

Initial treatment must focus on the airway, breathing, and circulation (ABCs) by establishing a patent airway, assessing the patient's need for respiratory support (which might include intubation and obtaining intravenous access), and monitoring the patient's circulatory status. Medications used in the treatment of status epilepticus include benzodiazepines (lorazepam and diazepam), phenytoin or fosphenytoin. and phenobarbital.

Benzodiazepines

These drugs act as anticonvulsants by binding to the gamma-aminobutyric acid (GABA) receptors. They are usually fast-acting and effective in the management of acute seizures. Common side effects include sedation and respiratory suppression, especially when used in combination with phenobarbital.

Lorazepam is preferred because of its longer half-life (12–24 hours) and rapid onset of action (2–5 minutes). It can be given via the intravenous or intramuscular route at 0.05 to 0.1 mg/kg per dose (maximum 4 mg/dose). The dose may be repeated after 5 to 15 minutes. Diazepam is also fast-acting but has a shorter half-life (less than 30 minutes) than lorazepam. It can be given at a dose of 0.2 to 0.4 mg/kg via the intravenous or intraosseous route with a maximum of 10 mg/dose. It can also be given rectally for the treatment of acute seizures.

Phenytoin or fosphenytoin

These agents are used if a seizure continues despite the use of a benzodiazepine. Phenytoin can only be given intravenously at a loading dose of 10 to 20 mg/kg. It has a peak effect at 10 to 20 minutes after completion of the infusion and its duration of action is 12 to 24 hours. Phenytoin must be administered slowly at a rate of 0.5 to 1.0 mg/kg per minute to a maximum of 50 mg/kg per minute. Hypotension and cardiac dysrhythmias can occur if the infusion is too fast. Also, thrombophlebitis can occur following the infusion. Tissue necrosis may occur with accidental infiltration (3,20,21,22,23).

Fosphenytoin has several safety advantages over phenytoin. It is a prodrug that is rapidly converted to phenytoin after being administered. The mode of administration can be intravenous or intramuscular. It can be administered faster than phenytoin at 3 mg/kg per minute to a maximum of 150 mg/min. It has fewer local and systemic side effects than phenytoin. Also it is dosed as phenytoin equivalents (PEs) with a loading dose of 10 to 20 mg PE/kg (3,23,28).

Phenobarbital

This drug is used if the previously noted medications fail. The initial loading dose of phenobarbital is 20 mg/kg; its onset of action is about 15 to 20 minutes and the duration of action is between 24 and 120 hours. Common side effects include significant sedation, hypotension, and respiratory depression, especially when used in conjunction with a benzodiazepine.

If seizures persist at this point, a drug-induced coma with continuous infusions of pentobarbital, midazolam, or propofol may be required. The patient will also likely have to be intubated and placed on continous EEG monitoring in an intensive care unit (ICU) setting. This step should be under the guidance of a neurologist working in conjunction with the ICU clinicians.

4.2 Headaches

4.2.1 Epidemiology

The prevalence of headache range from 37 to 51 percent in 7-year-olds; it gradually increases to about 57 to 82 percent by age 15. Recurring or frequent headaches occur in 2.5 percent of 7-year-olds and 15 percent of 15-year-olds. The prevalence of migraine headaches in children between 7 and 15 years of age is about 3.9 percent (29,30). Before puberty, boys are affected more frequently than girls; after puberty, headaches occur more frequently in girls (30).

4.2.2 Headache classification

Headaches are classified into two general categories (primary and secondary) (see ▶Tab. 4.3). Secondary headaches are associated with underlying CNS pathology. Any headache in either of these two categories can be either episodic or considered a chronic daily headache if it is present 15 or more days per month for 3 or more months. ▶Tab. 4.4 lists the differential diagnoses for headaches.

4.2.3 Management

Migraine treatment can be focused on either acute headache management (abortive therapy) or prophylactic treatment (31,32,33,34,35).

Tab. 4.3: The International Classification of Headache Disorders.

Primary headaches
• Migraines
• Tension-type headaches
• Cluster headache
• Other primary headache disorders

Secondary headaches
• Headache attributed to head or neck trauma
• Headache attributed to cranial or cervical vascular disorders
• Headache attributed to nonvascular intracranial disorders
• Headache attributed to a substance or withdrawal from substances
• Headache attributed to infection
• Headache attributed to disorders of homeostasis
• Headache attributed to disorders of the cranium, neck, eyes, ears, nose, sinuses, teeth, or other facial or cranial structures
• Headache attributed to psychiatric disorders
• Cranial neuralgia and central causes of facial pain
• Other headaches, cranial neuralgia, central or primary facial pain

Tab. 4.4: Differential diagnosis of headaches.

Acute generalized headaches
Infection, toxic exposure, seizure (postictal), hypertension, increased intracranial pressure(ICP) (ventriculoperitoneal [VP] shunt malfunction), hypoxia, metabolic (hypoglycemia, electrolyte imbalance), trauma, stroke (subarachnoid hemorrhage or sinus venous thrombosis, iatrogenic (post–lumbar puncture headache), exercise/exertion

Focal acute headaches
Trauma, infection (sinusitis, otitis media, etc), Chiari malformation, glaucoma, Tolosa-Hunt syndrome, temporomandibular joint disorder, dental pain, occipital neuralgia

Acute recurrent headaches
Migraine, hypertension, vasculitis, increased ICP (VP shunt malfunction), arteriovenous malformation, seizure (postictal), metabolic (hypoglycemia, electrolyte imbalance), exercise/exertion

Chronic progressive headaches
Increased ICP (VP shunt malfunction), hydrocephalus, subdural hematoma, pseudotumor cerebri), neoplasm, CNS and systemic infections

Abortive therapy

Medications in this category should treat acute events quickly and consistently, reducing the chances for headache recurrence. The patient's ability to function should be restored rapidly with minimal to no side effects. The presence of nausea and vomiting might limit the patient's ability to take oral medications. Therefore alternate routes of administration (intranasal, sublingual, and intravenous) and the use of antiemetics should be considered. Acetaminophen (Tylenol), ibuprofen, and sumatriptan can all be effective in treating acute headache (32,35). The first dose should be taken preferably within the first 20 to 30 minutes of headache onset (35). Overuse of over-the-counter pain medications (more than five times per week) can lead to worsening of headaches causing a rebound phenomenon. Therefore the use of short-acting analgesics should be limited to no more than two to three times weekly to prevent a headache due to medication (32,33,34). These short-acting agents include acetaminophen, ibuprofen and triptan medications such as sumatriptan.

The initial dose of acetaminophen is 10 to 15 mg/kg orally or per rectum with a maximal dose of 1 g. The same dose may be repeated in 2 to 4 hours if the headache persists and a third dose may be given within 4 to 6 hours of the second dose. The patient should not receive more than three doses in a 24-hour period. Ibuprofen is a classic NSAID. It is given in a dose of 7.5 to 10 mg/kg at the onset of the headache; a second dose may be given within 2 to 4 hours. It should be avoided in those with abdominal pain, tinnitus, or dizziness (see chapters 12 and 13 regarding NSAIDs).

Sumatriptan is a 5-hydroxytryptamine agonist. It should be used in individuals who do not respond to acetaminophen or ibuprofen and is not used in patients under 10 years of age. The initial oral dose is 25 mg, which may be repeated after 2 hours if symptoms persist. If there is no response to this dose, 50 mg, the maximal dose, may be tried. Common side effects include a feeling of warmth or flushing, chest or jaw tightness, facial burning, stinging, and numbness. Rare adverse effects include palpitations, tachyarrhythmias, and hypotension. See ▶Tab. 4.5 for additional triptan medications.

Prophylactic therapy

Headache prophylaxis should be considered in children who miss school once or twice monthly owing to headaches. A child who has more than four severe headaches monthly, especially if they affect daily activities, is also a candidate for prophylactic treatment. The goals of prophylactic treatment should include reducing headache frequency, severity, and duration. Prophylactic treatment should improve responsiveness to the treatment of acute headaches. It should also improve daily function, reduce disability, and improve the patient's quality of life.

Medications to use include topiramate, amitriptyline, and valproic acid. Topiramate is an anticonvulsant; the starting dose is 12.5 mg at night with gradual increase every 2 weeks over 2 months up to 50 mg twice a day. The dosage range is 1 to 10 mg/kg per day divided twice a day. Common side effects include weight loss, poor concentration or memory difficulty, cognitive changes, word-finding difficulty , sedation, paresthesias, glaucoma, and kidney stones. It is a good choice for obese patients and those with asthma.

Amitriptyline, a tricyclic antidepressant, is started at 1 mg/kg per day divided every 8 hours. It should be increased in increments of 0.25 mg/kg per day every 2 weeks to

Tab. 4.5: Triptan medications for the treatment of migraine headaches.

1. Sumatriptan (Imitrex)

   a. Initial dose: 25–50 mg orally; this can be repeated after 2 hours; the maximumal daily dose for adults is 200 mg.

   b. Intranasal dose: 20 mg, repeated after 2 hours if necessary.

   c. Subcutaneous dose: 6 mg, repeated after 1 hour if necessary.

2. Zolmitriptan (Zomig or Zomig ZMT [orally disintegrating pill])

   a. Initial dose: 2.5 or 5.0 mg orally; can be repeated after 2 hours; maximal daily dose for adults is 10 mg.

   b. Intranasal dose: 5 mg; can be repeated after 2 hours if necessary.

3. Rizatriptan (Maxalt, Maxalt-MLT [orally disintegrating pill])

   a. Oral dose: 5 or 10 mg to be repeated after 2 h if necessary; maximum dose is 30 mg

4. Naratriptan (Amerge)
   Oral: 2.5 mg; can be repeated after 4 hours if necessary

5. Almotriptan (Axert)
   Oral: 12.5 mg that can be repeated after 2 hours if necessary

6. Frovatriptan (Frova)
   Oral: 2.5 mg; can be repeated after 2 hours if necessary (maximal daily dose: 7.5 mg)

7. Eletriptan (Relpax)
   Oral: 20 or 40 mg; can be repeated after 2 hours if necessary (maximal daily dose: 80 mg)

Used with permission from Greydanus DE, Van Dyke DH: Neurologic disorders. In: DE Greydanus, DR Patel, HD Pratt, eds. Essential Adolescent Medicine. New York: McGraw-Hill; 2006:257.

a maximum of 1.5 mg/kg per day. One can also start with 5 mg orally at night and titrate upward as noted. The maintenance dose is 5 to 25 mg orally at night. Common side effects include sedation and weight gain; others include nonspecific ECG changes and changes in atrioventricular conduction. One should monitor for cardiac conduction abnormalities, dry mouth, constipation, drowsiness, and confusion.

Valproic acid, an anticonvulsant medication,is started at 10 mg/kg per day divided twice a day; it is increased by 5 mg/kg per day every week to a maximal dose of 30 to 40 mg/kg per day. While the patient is on this medication, the complete blood count and liver function tests should be monitored. Common side effects include gastrointestinal upset, weight gain, somnolence, dizziness, and tremor. Other adverse effects include thrombocytopenia, leukopenia, and bruising. Serum concentrations should be measured every 3 to 6 months; the level of drug in serum should be between 50 and 100 mg/dL. Valproic acid is to be avoided in adolescent females owing to the risk of weight gain, hair loss, ovarian cysts, and teratogenicity.

4.3 Tic disorders

Tics are stereotyped, patterned, repetitive movements or vocalizations. They can be classified as simple or complex. Simple motor tics are brief, sudden movements

Tab. 4.6: Diagnostic criteria for Tourette's syndrome from DSM-IV-TR (307.23) (2).

- Both multiple motor and 1 or more vocal tics must be present at some time during the illness, although not necessarily concurrently.

- The tics occur many times a day (usually in bouts) nearly every day or intermittently over more than 1 year, during which time there must not have been a tic-free period of more than 3 consecutive months.

- The age at onset is younger than 18 years.

- The disturbance is not due to the direct physiological effects of a substance (e.g., stimulants) or a general medical condition (e.g., Huntington disease or postviral encephalitis).

---

involving only a few muscle groups. Examples include eyeblinks, shoulder jerks, and repetitive throat clearing. Complex motor tics are more involved, comprising unusual movements of several muscle groups; examples include jerking the head to the left with an associated tongue lick and shoulder shrug. Complex vocal tics include phrases and may be exemplified by coprolalia (uttering swear words) or echolalia (repeating the words or phrases of others).

Tics are the main symptom in Tourette's syndrome (TS). TS is a childhood neuropsychiatric disorder characterized by motor and vocal tics. It has a high association with comorbidities such as obsessive-compulsive disorder (OCD) and attention deficit hyperactivity disorder (ADHD) and other learning disorders. It is thought to run in families, although a specific gene locus is yet to be found (36,37). The definition of TS as noted in *The Diagnostic and Statistical Manual of Mental Disorders*, Fourth Edition, Text Revision (DSM-IV-TR) is given in ▶Tab. 4.6 (37).

4.3.1 Epidemiology

The prevalence estimates for TS vary from 10 to 700 per 100,000 depending on the study. Typically tics have their onset at school age, at about 7 years, with a peak in the middle teen years and significant improvement in most by the late teens and early adulthood. About 10 percent of such children will have a progressive and disabling course that lasts into adulthood. There is a strong male preponderance and familial tendency. The tics change in type, severity and frequency over time.

4.3.2 Differential diagnosis/diagnostic evaluation

Youths with tics or TS should have a completely normal neurologic examination aside from the presence of tics. A good developmental history is important to exclude underlying genetic disorders such as Down's syndrome, Fragile X, or autistic spectrum disorders. On the physical examination, one should exclude dysmorphic features, neurocutaneous disorders, and signs of neurodegenerative disorders such as Kayser-Fleischer rings in the eyes (diagnostic of Wilson's disease), spasticity, and chorea (suggestive of Huntington's disease, pantothenate kinase–associated disease, or neuroacanthocytosis). A thorough assessment of gait and tone should capture most of these (see ▶Tab. 4.7). TS is typically a clinical diagnosis and therefore no specific laboratory or genetic testing exists. Routine

Tab. 4.7: Differential diagnosis of tics.

Disease	Brief description
Wilson's disease	Autosomal recessive disorder with dysarthria, dystonia, tremor, rigidity and drooling Kayser-Fleischer rings on eye exam
Juvenile Huntington's chorea	Autosomal dominant disorder with progressive dementia and choreoathetosis and hyperkinesis Abnormal rigidity on physical exam
Neuroacanthocytosis	Familial progressive disorder of chorea and psychiatric symptoms Progressive dementia and seizures with loss of deep tendon reflexes
Benign familial chorea	Rare disorder of autosomal dominant inheritance Intention tremor, dysarthria, hypotonia, and athetosis with preserved intelligence
Tardive dyskinesia	Drug-induced choreiform movements, often involving facial and buccal muscles, occurring in the course of drug therapy*

*Drugs most associated include neuroleptics such as haloperidol, antiemetics such as metoclopramide, and xanthenes such as theophylline.

imaging studies are not recommended since they are usually normal and should be utilized only in those individuals with specific neurologic abnormalities.

4.3.3 Treatment

The management of TS requires a multidisciplinary approach with psychological and medical supports. A collaborative effort of the primary care physician, neurologist, psychiatrist, psychologist, family members, and school professionals is often needed. Medical therapies are reserved only for tics that interfere with social interactions, school performance, or activities of daily living. There is no one medication that benefits all patients and none of the medications will completely abolish symptoms associated with tic disorders. The goal of treatment is to control the tics such that the child can encounter less social interference and discomfort from the tics (38,39).

Clinicians should take into account coexisting behavioral symptoms such as ADHD as well as anxiety and obsessive compulsive traits and treat these accordingly. General principles of treatment include setting realistic expectations of therapy and treating existing comorbidities first. Medications should be initiated at low doses and gradually titrated upward with frequent evaluations for efficacy and toxicity. In treating, avoid combination therapy if possible; once nonneuroleptic therapy has failed, consider referral to a specialist.

Alpha-2 adrenergic agonists (clonidine, guanfacine) are considered first-line agents in the treatment of tic disorders, followed by nondopamine blocking agents (atomoxetine, baclofen, clonazepam) as second-line treatment. Third-line agents (because of adverse effects) include both typical and atypical dopamine blocking agents (haloperidol, pimozide, fluphenazine, risperidone, ziprasidone, and tetrabenazine) (40,41,42, 43,44,45,46,47).

Less commonly used treatments include botulinum toxin type A and deep brain stimulation for more painful and intractable tics (48,49). Selective serotonin reuptake inhibitors can be useful when patients have comorbid anxiety, depression, or OCD and topiramate in patients with comorbid obesity, migraines, or bipolar disorder.

Alpha-2 adrenergic agonists

Clonidine and guanfacine are both alpha-2 adrenergic agonists that reduce norepinephrine release. Guanfacine has a longer duration of action and is more selective for postsynaptic 2a receptors within the prefrontal cortex. These are considered first-line agents, especially in those with milder tics, concomitant ADHD, aggressive outbursts, difficulty sleeping, or who are easily frustrated (see ▶Tab. 4.8). Treatment is initiated at a low dose at bedtime and gradually titrated at 3- to 14-day intervals. Response to treatment may take 2 to 6 weeks. Common adverse effects include dry mouth and eyes, sedation, orthostatic hypotension, and headache. Owing to the risk of rebound (including hypertension, tics, and anxiety), clonidine should be tapered. Guanfacine is often preferred because of its less sedating properties; it is also less likely to produce withdrawal effects. These agents may be safely combined with stimulants.

Nondopamine receptor blocking agents

These second-line agents (see ▶Tab. 4.9) include atomoxetine, baclofen, and clonazepam. Atomoxetine inhibits the reuptake of norepinephrine and is useful when patients have concomitant ADHD (40). Common side effects may include gastrointestinal (GI) upset, insomnia, reduced appetite, and increased blood pressure.

Baclofen acts as a GABA analogue and inhibits transmission of monosynaptic and polysynaptic reflexes at the spinal cord level (see ▶Tab. 4.9). Common adverse effects include sedation, dizziness, ataxia, decreased blood pressure, and gastrointestinal disturbances. One placebo-controlled crossover clinical trial demonstrated that baclofen (60 mg daily) produced a statistically significant improvement in patients' overall

Tab. 4.8: Alpha-2 agonists (first line treatment) (51,52,53).

	Clonidine	Guanfacine
Initial dose	0.05 mg daily Titrate by 0.05 mg every 3–7 days	0.5 mg daily Titrate every 3–14 days to usual dose of 1.5–3 mg daily
Maximal dose	0.4 mg daily in divided doses	4 mg daily in three divided doses
Common side effects	Sedation Dry mouth Dizziness Headache Orthostatic hypotension	
Comments	Upon discontinuation, taper to avoid withdrawal effects	Less likely to produce withdrawal symptoms Longer half-life; more selective

Tab. 4.9: Nondopamine blocking agents (second line treatment) (51,52,53).

	Atomoxetine	Baclofen	Clonazepam
Initial dose	0.5mg/kg per day in two divided doses >70 kg: 40 mg/day	10–15 mg daily in three divided doses	0.5–12 mg daily in divided doses
Maximal dose	1.8mg/kg per day with max 100 mg/day Max 80 mg/day if concomitant potent CYP 2D6 inhibitor	60–80 mg daily in three divided doses	0.5–12 mg daily in divided doses
Side effects	Insomnia Decreased appetite GI upset Headache Hypertension	Sedation Fatigue Dizziness Ataxia Hypotension GI upset	Sedation Depression Cognitive impairment Behavioral problems Dizziness Fatigue
Comments	CV assessment prior to initiation Provide second dose in late afternoon or early evening	Avoid abrupt discontinuation	Gradually taper to avoid withdrawal Controlled substance Physical & psychological dependence

CYP, cytochrome; GI, gastrointestinal; CV, cardiovascular.

well-being without decreasing motor or vocal tic burden (41). If baclofen is discontinued, it should be gradually tapered; abrupt discontinuation should be avoided.

Clonazepam enhances the activity of GABA by binding to benzodiazepine sites on the GABA receptor complex. Clonazepam has been widely used for suppressing tics and is beneficial in those patients who have concomitant anxiety disorders (▶Tab. 4.9). Common side effects may include sedation, cognitive impairment, depression, ataxia, behavioral problems, and fatigue. Cautionary use should be considered owing to clonazepam's ability to cause physical and psychological dependence.

Dopamine receptor blocking medications (third-line treatment)

Third-line agents include typical and atypical antipsychotics as well as tetrabenazine. Typical antipsychotics include haloperidol, pimozide, and fluphenazine, which have potent dopamine (D2) receptor blockade (45,46,47). All three block alpha-adrenergic receptors, 5-HT (5-hydroxytryptamine/serotonin) 2 receptors, and fluphenazine also antagonize histamine-1 receptors (see ▶Tab. 4.10).

Common side effects may include sedation, weight gain, hypotension, tachycardia, and extrapyramidal symptoms. All three can cause QTc prolongation and hyperprolactinemia, and can lower the seizure threshold. Caution should be used in patients with cardiovascular disease, prolonged QTc intervals, and those with seizure disorders. Caution should also be used when these agents are given in combination with other medications that prolong the QTc interval (they are contraindicated with pimozide).

Tab. 4.10: Typical antipsychotics (third-line treatment) (15,16,17).

	Haloperidol	Pimozide	Fluphenazine
Initial dose	0.25–0.5 mg daily	0.05 mg/kg per day; max 1 mg daily Give at bedtime	1 mg at bedtime
Maximal dose	0.05–0.075 mg/kg per day in two to three divided doses	0.2 mg/kg per day; max 10 mg daily	4 mg daily in divided doses
Side effects	Hypotension Tachycardia QTc prolongation Sedation Depression EPS NMS Hyperprolactinemia	Sedation Hypotension QTC prolongation Constipation Xerostomia EPS NMS Hyperprolactinemia	Sedation Hypotension Tachycardia Arrhythmia EPS NMS Hyperprolactinemia
Comments	May lower seizure threshold Taper to prevent withdrawal dyskinesias EPS dose- and duration-dependent	May lower seizure threshold Taper to prevent withdrawal dyskinesias Monitor ECG at baseline & periodically CI with potent CYP 3A4 inhibitors & QTc prolonging agents	May lower seizure threshold Greater risk for EPS Lower risk for ACH side effects

ACH, anticholinergic; CI, contraindicated; CYP, cytochrome P; EPS, extrapyramidal; NMS, neuroleptic malignant syndrome.

The manufacturer of pimozide recommends baseline and periodic monitoring of the ECG. All three agents can be associated with drug interactions due to their effects on CYP 450 enzyme metabolism and inhibition. Pimozide is contraindicated with potent CYP 450 3A4 inhibitors such as macrolide antibiotics (clarithromycin, erythromycin), azole antifungals (itraconazole, others), and protease inhibitors (ritonavir, others). Owing to pimozide's ability to antagonize the acetylcholine receptor, additional side effects include constipation and xerostomia. These medications increase the risk for neuroleptic malignant syndrome and tapering is recommended when discontinuing haloperidol and pimozide to prevent withdrawal dyskinesias.

Atypical antipsychotics used in the treatment of tic disorders include risperidone and ziprasidone (▶Tab. 4.11). (See chapter 15 in Greydanus DE, Patel DR, Omar HA, Feucht C, Merrick J: Adolescent Medicine – Pharmacotherapeutics in General, Mental and Sexual Health. Berlin: de Gruyter; 2012.) Risperidone acts by blocking the D2 and 5-HT2 (as well as other) serotonin receptors and H1 and alpha-adrenergic receptors. It is thought that this atypical antipsychotic agent is likely superior to typical antipsychotics and should be considered in patients with comorbid OCD (47).

Ziprasidone acts by blocking D2 and D3, alpha-1 adrenergic, H1, and multiple 5-HT receptors. Common side effects include sedation, dizziness, orthostatic hypotension, GI

Tab. 4.11: Typical antipsychotic and monoamine-depleting agents (third-line treatment) (51,52,53).

	Risperidone	Ziprasidone	Tetrabenazine
Initial dose	0.25–0.5 mg at bedtime Titrate at weekly intervals	5 mg at bedtime Titrate at weekly intervals	6.25 mg twice daily Gradual titration to effective dosage
Maximal dose	4 mg daily in divided doses	40 mg daily in divided doses	2D6 (PM) or receiving potent 2D6 inhibitor: 25 mg/dose and 50 mg daily (adult) 2D6 (EM): 37.5 mg/dose & 100 mg daily (adult)
Side effects	Sedation Dizziness OSH GI upset Weight gain Hyperprolactinemia EPS/NMS	Sedation Dizziness GI upset OSH QTc prolongation Rash Hyperprolactinemia EPS/NMS	Depression Fatigue Seation GI upset Parkinsonism EPS/NMS Hyperprolactinemia
Comments	Monitor BMI, fasting glucose and fasting lipid profile EPS dose-dependent	Monitor BMI, fasting glucose, and fasting lipid profile Monitor ECG Less risk for weight gain	Perform CYP 2D6 genotype testing at baseline Evaluate for drug interactions Monitor for depression Avoid use in untreated or inadequately treated depression or active suicidal ideations

BMI, body mass index; CYP, cytochrome; EM, extensive metabolizer; EPS, extrapyramidal; NMS, neuroleptic malignant syndrome; OSH, orthostatic hypotension; PM, poor metabolizer.

upset and hyperprolactinemia. These agents can also result in EPS (less than typical antipsychotics) and NMS. Ziprasidone can increase the QTc interval; ECG monitoring is therefore recommended. Ziprasidone is also contraindicated in patients with a prolonged QT interval and in combination with QTc-prolonging agents. Owing to the risk for metabolic complications, fasting lipid profile, fasting blood glucose, and body mass index (BMI)/weight should be routinely monitored.

Tetrabenazine is unique in that it depletes catecholamines at the presynapse and blocks dopamine receptors at the postsynapse (▶Tab. 4.11). Patients should undergo CYP2D6 genotype testing at baseline in order to determine the maximal dosage that can be used. Those who are poor CYP 2D6 metabolizers (or those taking potent CYP 2D6 inhibitors) should receive a maximal dose of 50 mg daily (adult dose) compared with 100 mg daily (adult dosage), which is to be used in those who are extensive CYP 2D6 metabolizers.

Common side effects include depression, anxiety, fatigue, sedation, GI upset, and parkinsonian symptoms. Tetrabenazine should not be used in those with untreated or inadequately treated depression or who are actively suicidal. If depression occurs on therapy, the tetrabenazine dosage should be reduced and an antidepressant considered. If symptoms fail to resolve, tetrabenazine may have to be discontinued. Tetrabenazine has been associated with QTc prolongation, neuroleptic malignant syndrome (NMS), and hyperprolactinemia.

4.4 Tremor

This is an involuntary somewhat rhythmic, reciprocal, oscillatory (back and forth) movement of a part of the body. It usually occurs around a joint and can affect a limb, eyes, head, face, vocal cords, or trunk. It most often affects the hands.

4.4.1 Epidemiology

This movement disorder is seen in about 5 percent of the normal adult population; of these adults, about 5 to 30 percent had onset in childhood. There are several types of tremor, the most commonly encountered being essential tremor (50,51,52,53,54).

4.4.2 Differential diagnosis

Physiological tremor

This is present in all individuals but is not usually evident to the observing eye unless the person is engaging in exercise or is anxious, fatigued, or being treated by certain pharmacologic therapies such as adrenergic agonists, nicotine, thyroid hormones, or caffeine. In the absence of any drug use, it is reasonable to exclude thyrotoxicosis and pheochromocytoma. This is a low-amplitude tremor occurring at 6 to 12 Hz. It is usually accentuated by maintaining a frozen or still posture (see ▶Tab. 4.12) and requires no treatment.

Parkinsonian tremor

This tremor is rarely seen in adolescence unless associated with the use of certain pharmacologic therapies such as neuroleptics or in association with structural lesions within the basal ganglia; it may also be seen in neurodegenerative conditions such as Wilson's disease. The tremor is often coarse and seen at rest with a frequency of 4 to 6 Hz. See ▶Tabs. 4.13 and 4.14.

Intention tremor

This is also a rare tremor that in seen in association with cerebellar dysfunction. This tremor may be seen with the use of certain pharmacologic therapies, such as valproic acid and lithium. This tremor interferes with directed movements such as finger-to-nose testing. Usually removal of the pharmacologic agent will resolve the tremor. Neuroimaging is often required to exclude a cerebellar pathology.

Tab. 4.12: Descriptions and differential diagnosis of tremors.

Tremor	Definition	Example
Rest	Tremor of a body part that is not being moved voluntarily	Parkinson's disease Anxiety Alcohol or drugs such as valproic acid Benign essential tremor Wilson's disease Mercury poisoning Neurosyphilis
Action		
Postural	Tremor that is present while holding a position against gravity (outstretched arms)	Essential tremor Peripheral neuropathy (usually associated weakness and atrophy) Parkinson's disease
Kinetic	Tremor that occurs during a voluntary movement	Essential tremor Parkinson's disease
Intention	Tremor worsened by goal-directed movements (past pointing)	Cerebellar pathology Wilson's disease

Tab. 4.13: Common types of tremor.

Tremor type	Frequency (Hz)	Description	Pathology
Physiologic	6–12	Low amplitude Usually not visible unless fatigued, strenuous exercise, caffeine Postural tremor	No lesion Usually enhanced by drugs like adrenergic agonists or caffeine
Parkinsonian	4–6	Coarse, large amplitude tremor, usually at rest Rare in childhood	Basal ganglia Drugs such as neuroleptics
Intention	<5	Tremor that is accentuated by approaching a target. For example, finger to nose testing Kinetic (action) tremor	Cerebellar lesion Region of Red Nucleus
Psychogenic	Variable	Inconsistent Distractable	
Essential	4–11	Fairly low amplitude in childhood with worsening with age Kinetic (action) and postural	Dysfunction of olivocerebellar circuit

Tab. 4.14: Drugs associated with tremor.

Class	Example
Anticonvulsants	Valproic acid Phenytoin Carbamazepine Lacosamide
Antidepressants	Lithium Tricyclic antidepressants Bupropion
Beta-adrenergic agonists	Terburtaline Meteproterenol Epinephrine Theophylline
Neuroleptics	Haloperidol Atypical neuroleptics
Xanthines or derivatives	Coffee, tea
Chemotherapeutic agents	Vincristine Ara-C Cyclosporine

Psychogenic tremor

This is often of sudden onset with a variable frequency and distribution, and it is distractible. It often involves a combination of action, postural, and rest tremors.

Essential tremor

This is the most common type of tremor and a likely reason for evaluation. It usually has a gradual onset in late adolescence or early adulthood. Early presentations in patients as young as 2 years have been reported. This tremor is usually not severe in adolescence but may worsen with age, with noted increases in amplitude and diminished frequency. It has a frequency of 4 to 8 Hz. It is thought to be as a result of dysfunction within the olivocerebellar circuit (55). There are no associated gold-standard tests; hence the diagnosis is clinical. The consensus statement of the Movement Disorder Society on Tremor requires the presence of an action tremor of greater severity than that of an enhanced physiologic tremor with no other causes identified (56). The investigation group of the Movement Disorder Society and Tremor defines it with these core criteria: bilateral action tremor of the hands and forearms (but not at rest) or isolated head tremor with no signs of dystonia. Secondary or supportive criteria include long duration of symptoms over 3 years, positive family history, and responsiveness to or improvement with use of alcohol (57).

Essential tremor usually involves the hands or the head. Most commonly it is brought to attention when handwriting or eating is affected. It is enhanced by action or postural maneuvers (e.g., handwriting and drinking liquids). It is not present at rest and is rarely disabling under the age of 15 years. It most commonly affects both upper limbs, although there may be some side to-side asymmetry. It is more common among males in children or adolescents; in adults it usually affects women more often (58,59). There is a strong genetic tendency with a family history noted in about 60 to 80 percent of patients (60).

Essential tremor is often worsened by anxiety, fatigue, or caffeine and improves with the use of alcohol in adults; alcohol is not used in adolescents. This tremor is usually lifelong, although waxing and waning may be noted. There is increased documentation of the association with subtle or soft neurologic signs such as cognitive delays, hearing abnormalities, gait and balance abnormalities, olfaction, hand–eye coordination, and mood disorders (61,62,63,64).

Management of essential tremor

The following pharmacologic therapies are outlined for use in essential tremor (ET), although not all ETs require medications. In mild forms, just reassurance will usually alleviate the stress and anxiety that may be exacerbating the tremor. If that does not help, referral to occupational therapy may be considered for coping mechanisms, such as wearing a weighted wrist band while writing. If the tremor is interfering with the activities of daily living, pharmacologic therapies including propranolol, primidone, gabapentin, and topiramate may be considered. Other considerations may include alprazolam or clonazepam. Botox and surgical interventions such as deep brain stimulation are best reserved for more resistant cases.

Propranolol

This beta-adrenergic receptor antagonist was recognized as early as the 1970s to be useful in controlling tremor (64). The mechanism of action is thought to be mediated through peripheral beta-2-adrenergic receptors located in the muscle spindles (65). Propanolol has been the most studied beta-adrenergic agent, but similar efficacy has been noted with similar agents, with the absence of cardiac beta-1 selectivity being preferred (66). Treatment is started at a dosage of 5 mg once a day, which may be titrated upward as tolerated to 4mg/kg per day divided twice daily.

Once a therapeutic dosage has been reached, an extended-release formulation should be considered so as to improve compliance. Higher doses may be required with time as the tremor tends to worsen with age. The side effects include hypotension, bradycardia, syncope, and erectile dysfunction. It is important to note that propranolol may worsen depression or asthma and also to mask the symptoms of hypoglycemia.

Primidone

This anticonvulsant is a desoxybarbiturate whose usefulness in ET was discovered in the 1980s (67). The mechanism of action is not understood; in epilepsy, however, it is known to alter the sodium and calcium channel ion fluxes across membranes (68). It is metabolized to phenobarbitone but its metabolite has not proven as effective as primidone (69). In adults, the efficacy of primidone is similar to that of propanolol (70). It is recommended to start at dosage of 25 mg/day, increasing as tolerated to about 250 mg three times a day.

The side effects include sedation, nausea, dizziness, and ataxia. It has been suggested to limit the side effects by pretreating with phenobarbital for 3 to 4 days to induce the metabolism of the drug (68). Its use in adolescents is limited by the documented concern of cognitive impairment with phenobarbital in children and adolescents with epilepsy.

Gabapentin

This antiepileptic medication is often used in the treatment of neuropathic pain. Its mechanism of action in the use with ET is not known. Several trials have shown mixed results, with some noting efficacy comparable with that of propanolol (71,72). The recommended starting dosage is 100 mg once a day increasing as tolerated to about 30mg/kg per day divided into two or three daily doses. The side effects include drowsiness, dizziness, headache, and weight gain.

Topiramate

This antiepileptic agent is also used in the treatment of migraine headaches as well as essential tremor. It has a complex mechanism of action including sodium channel blockade, GABAergic effect, and carbonic anhydrase inhibition (73). Its mechanism of action in ET is not known. In a large multicenter trial, topiramate showed benefit in tremor reduction as well as functional improvements in motor tasks, writing, and speaking. This study was associated with high withdrawal rates secondary to side effects (32% as compared with 9.5% with placebo) (74). The recommended starting dosage is 25 mg once a day increasing as tolerated to about 4mg/kg per day divided into two daily doses. Common side effects include anorexia, weight loss, parasthesias, and concentration and attention difficulties.

4.5 Conclusions

This chapter provides a brief overview of some of the neurologic disorders commonly encountered in adolescents: epilepsy, headaches, tics, and tremors. The most commonly used medications when treating adolescents with neurologic presentations are reviewed. Primary care clinicians can become familiar with these commonly used drugs and, by using them judiciously, provide considerable benefit to their adolescent patients with these neurologic conditions. Consultation with experts in neurology is essential for adolescents with epilepsy and for those with complex or refractive headaches, tics, or tremors.

References

1. Friedman MJ. Seizures in children. Pediatr Clin North Am 2006;53: 257–77.
2. Hauser WA, Rich SS, Lee JR, Annegers JF, Anderson VE. Risk of recurrent seizures after two unprovoked seizures. N Engl J Med 1998;338(7):429–34.
3. McAbee GN, Wark JE. A practical approach to uncomplicated seizures in children. Am Fam Physician 2000;62(5):1109–16.

4. Shinnar S, Berg AT, Moshe SL, Petix M, Maytal J, Kang H, et al. Risk of seizure recurrence following a first unprovoked seizure in childhood.: a prospective study. Pediatrics 1990; 85:1076–85.
5. Shinnar S, Berg AT, Moshe SL, O'Dell C, Alemany M, Newstein D, et al. The risk of recurrence following a first unprovoked afebrile seizure in childhood: an extended followup. Pediatrics;1996:98:216–25.
6. Berg A, Shinnar S. The risk of recurrence following a first unprovoked afebrile seizure in childhood: a quantitative review. Neurology 1991;41:965–72.
7. Hauser WA, Anderson E, Loewenson RB, McRoberts SM. Seizure recurrence after a first unprovoked seizure. N Engl J Med 1982;307:522–28.
8. Hauser WA, Anderson VE, Loewenson RB, McRoberts SM. Seizure recurrence after a first unprovoked seizure: an extended followup. Neurology 1990;40:1163–70.
9. Shinnar S, Berg AT, O'Dell C, Newstein D, Moshe SL, Hauser WA. Predictors of multiple seizures in a cohort of children prospectively followed from the time of their first unprovoked seizure. Ann Neurol 2000;48:140–47.
10. Shinnar S, Kang H, Berg AT, Goldensohn ES, Hauser WA, Moshé SL. EEG abnormalities in children with a first unprovoked seizure. Epilepsia 1994;35(3):471–76.
11. Winckler MI, Rotta NT. Clinical and electroencephalographic follow-up after a first unprovoked seizure. Pediatr Neurol 2004;30(3):201–6.
12. Stroink H, Brouwer OF, Arts WF, Geerts AT, Peters AC, van Donselaar CA. The first unprovoked, untreated seizure in childhood: a hospital based study of the accuracy of the diagnosis, rate of recurrence, and long term outcome after recurrence. Dutch Study of Epilepsy in Childhood. J Neurol Neurosurg Psychiatry 1998;64:595–600.
13. Shinnar S, Berg AT, O'Dell C, Newstein D, Moshe SL, Hauser WA. Predictors of multiple seizures in a cohort of children prospectively followed from the time of their first unprovoked seizure. Ann Neurol 2000;48:140–47.
14. Boulloche J, Leloup P, Mallet E, Parain D, Tron P. Risk of recurrence after a single, unprovoked, generalized tonic-clonic seizure. Dev Med Child Neurol 1989;31:626–32.
15. Camfield PR, Camfield CS, Dooley JM, Tibbles JAR, Fung T, Garner B. Epilepsy after a first unprovoked seizure in childhood. Neurology 1985;35:1657–60.
16. Annegers JF, Shirts SB, Hauser WA, Kurland LT. Risk of recurrence after an initial unprovoked seizure. Epilepsia 1986;27:43–50.
17. Hart YM, Sander JWAS, Johnson AL, Shorvon SD. National general practice study of epilepsy: recurrence after a first seizure. Lancet 1990; 336:1271–74.
18. Martinovic Z, Jovic N. Seizure recurrence after a first generalized tonicclonic seizure in children, adolescents and young adults. Seizure 1997; 6:461–65.
19. Hirtz D, Berg A, Bettis D, Camfield C, Camfield P, Crumrine P, et al. Practice parameter: Treatment of the child with a first unprovoked seizure: Report of the Quality Standards Subcommittee of the American Academy of Neurology and the Practice Committee of the Child Neurology Society. Neurology 2003;60(2):166–75.
20. Freeman JM, Tibbles J, Camfield C, Camfield P. Benign epilepsy of childhood: a speculation and its ramications. Pediatrics 1987;79:864–68.
21. Panayiotopoulos CP. The epilepsies: Seizures, syndromes and management. Oxford: Bladon, 2005.
22. Lowenstein DH, Alldredge BK. Status epilepticus. N Engl J Med 1998;338:970–76.
23. Wolf SM, Ochoa JG, Conway EE. Seizure management in pediatric patients for the nineties. Pediatr Ann 1998;27:653–64.
24. Fitzgerald BJ, Okos AJ, Miller JW. Treatment of out of hospital status epilepticus with diazepam rectal gel. Seizure 2003;12:52–55.

25. Scott RC, Besag FM, Neville BG. Buccal midazolam and rectal diazepam for treatment of prolonged seizures in childhood and adolescence: a randomized trial. Lancet 1999; 353:623–26.
26. Chamberlain JM, Altieri MA, Futterman C, Young GM, Ochsenschlager DW, Waisman Y. A prospective, randomized study comparing intramuscular midazolam with intravenous diazepam for the treatment of seizures in children. Pediatr Emerg Care 1997;13: 92–94.
27. Vilke GM, Sharieff GQ, Marino A, Gerhart AE, Chan TC. Midazolam for the treatment of out of hospital pediatric seizures. Prehosp Emerg Care 2002;6:215–17.
28. Reuter D, Brownstein D. Common emergent pediatric neurologic problems. Emerg Med Clin North Am 2002;20(1):155–76.
29. Bille B: Migraine in school children. Acta Paediatr 1962;51(Suppl 136):1.
30. Dalsgaard-Nielsen T: Some aspects of the epidemiology of migraine in Denmark. Headache 1970;10:14.
31. Lewis D, Ashwal S, Hershey A, Hirtz D, Yonker M, Silberstein S, et al. Practice parameter: Pharmacological treatment of migraine headache in children and adolescents: report of the American Academy of Neurology Quality Standards Subcommittee and the Practice Committee of the Child Neurology Society. Neurology 2004;63(12):2215–24.
32. Reimschisel T. Breaking the cycle of medication overuse headache. Contemp Pediatr 2003;20:101.
33. Rothner A, Guo Y. An analysis of headache types, over-the counter (OTC) medication overuse and school absences in a pediatric/adolescent headache clinic. Headache 2004;44:490.
34. Lewis DW. Headaches in children and adolescents. Curr Probl Pediatr Adolesc Health Care 2007;37:207–46.
35. Alsobrook JP2nd, Pauls DL. The genetics of Tourette syndrome. Neurol Clin 1997;15 (2):381–93.
36. American Psychiatric Association. DSM-IV-TR. Washington, DC: American Psychiatric Association, 2000.
37. Gilbert DL. Treatment of children and adolescents with tics and Tourette syndrome. J Child Neurol 2006;21:690–700.
38. Tourette Syndrome Study Group. Treatment of ADHD in children with tics: A randomized controlled trial. Neurology 2002;58:527–36.
39. Allen AJ, Kurlan RM, Gilbert DL, Coffey BJ, Linder SL, Lewis DW, et al. Atomoxetine treatment in children and adolescents with ADHD and comorbid tic disorders. Neurology 2005;65:1941–49.
40. Singer HS, Wendlandt J, Krieger M, Giuliano J. Baclofen treatment in Tourette syndrome: A double-blind, placebo-controlled, crossover trial. Neurology 2001;56:599–604.
41. Gilbert D, Singer HS: Commentary. Risperidone was as effective as pimozide for Tourette's disorder. Evid Based Ment Health 2001; 4:75.
42. Gilbert DL, Dure L, Sethuraman G, Raab D, Lane J, Sallee FR. Tic reduction with pergolide in a randomized controlled trial in children. Neurology 2003;60:606–11.
43. Chapel JL, Brown N, Jenkins RL: Tourette's disease. Symptomatic relief with haloperidol. Am J Psychiatry 1964;121:608–10.
44. Gilbert DL, Batterson JR, Sethuraman G, Salle FR. Tic reduction with risperidone vs. pimozide in a randomized, double-blind, crossover trial. J Am Acad Child Adolesc Psychiatry 2004;43:206–14.
45. Bruggeman R, van der Linden C, Buitelaar JK, Gericke GS, Hawkridge SM, Temlett JA. Risperidone versus pimozide in Tourettes's disorder: A comparative double-blind parallel-group study. J Clin Psychiatry 2001;62:50–56.

46. Ratzoni G, Gothelf D, Brand-Gothelf A, Reidman J, Kikinzon L, Gal G, et .Weight gain associated with olanzapine and risperidone in adolescent patients: A comparative prospective study. J Am Acad Child Adolesc Psychiatry 2002;41:337–43.

47. Marras C, Andrews D, Sime E, Lang AE. Botulinum toxin for simple motor tics: a randomized, double-blind controlled clinical trial. Neurology 2001;56(5):605–10.

48. Visser-Vandewalle V, Ackermans L, van der Linden C, Temel Y, Tijssen MA, Schruers KR, et al. Deep brain stimulation in Gilles de la Tourettes's syndrome. Neurosurgery 2006;58(3):E590.

49. Facts and Comparisons. Drug information full monographs. Wolters Kluwer Health, Incorporated. Accessed 2011 Jun 01. URL: http://0-online.factsandcomparisons.com. libcat.ferris.edu/index.aspx.

50. Wenning GK, Kiechl S, Seppi K, Müller J, Högl B, Saletu M, et al. Prevalence of movement disorders in men and women aged 50–89 years (Bruneck Study cohort): a population-based study. Lancet Neurol 2005;4(12):815–20.

51. Lou JS, Jankovic J. Essential tremor: Clinical correlates in 350 patients. Neurology 1991;41:234–38.

52. Koller WC, Busenbark K, Miner K. The relationship of essential tremor to other movement disorders: report on 678 patients. Essential Tremor Study Group. Ann Neurol 1994;35:717–23.

53. Paulson GW. Benign essential tremor in childhood: symptoms, pathogenesis, treatment. Clin Pediatr (Phila) 1976;15:67–70.

54. Deuschl G, Bergman H. Pathophysiology of non-parkinsonian tremors. Mov Disord 2002;17(Suppl 3):S41–48.

55. Deuschl G, Bain P, Brin M. Consensus statement of the Movement Disorder Society on tremor: Ad hoc scientific committee. Mov Disord 1998;13(Suppl 3):2–23.

56. Bain P, Brin M, Deuschl G, Elble R, Jankovic J, Findley L, et al. Criteria for the diagnosis of essential tremor. Neurology 2000;54(Suppl 4): S7.

57. Louis ED, Fernandez-Alvarez E, Dure LS 4th, Frucht S, Ford B. Association between male gender and pediatric essential tremor. Mov Disord 2005;20:904–6.

58. Hardesty DE, Marangnore DM, Matsumoto JY, Louis ED. Increased risk of head tremor in women with essential tremor: longitudinal data from the Rochester Epidemiology Project. Mov Disord 2004;19: 529–33.

59. Jankovic J, Madisetty J, Vuong KD. Essential tremor among children. Pediatrics 2004;114:1203–5.

60. Gasparini M, Bonifati V, Fabrizio E, Fabbrini G, Brusa L, Lenzi GL, et al. Frontal lobe dysfunction in essential tremor: a preliminary study. J Neurol 2001;248:399–402.

61. Benito-Leon J, Louis ED, Bermejo-Pareja F. Population-based case control study of cognitive function in essential tremor. Neurological Disorders in Central Spain (NEDICES) Study Group. Neurology 2006;66:69–74.

62. Louis ED, Benito-Leon J, Bermejo-Pareja F. self-reported depression and anti-depression medication use in essential tremor: cross-sectional and prospective analyses in a population-based study. Neurological Disorders in Central Spain (NEDICES) Study Group. Eur J Neurol 2007;14:1138–46.

63. Winkler GF, Young RR. The control of essential tremor by propanolol. Trans Am Neurol Assoc 1971;96:66–68.

64. Abila B, Wilson JF, Marshall RW, Richens A. The tremorolytic action of beta-adrenoceptor blockers in essential, physiological and isoprenaline-induced tremor is mediated by beta-adrenoceptors located in a deep peripheral compartment. Br J Clin Pharmacol 1985;20:369–76.

65. Calzetti S, Findley LJ, Gresty MA, Perucca E, Richens A. Metoprolol and propanolol in essential tremor: a double-blind, controlled study. J Neurol Neurosurg Psychiatry 1981;44(9):814–19.
66. Koller WC, Vetere-Overfield B. Acute and chronic effects of propanolol and primidone in essential tremor. Neurology 1989;39(12):1587–88.
67. Handley R, Stewart AS. Mysoline: a new drug in the treatment of epilepsy. Lancet 1952;1:742–44.
68. Ondo WG. Essential tremor: treatment options. Curr Treat Options Neurol 2006;8 (3):256–67.
69. Sasso E, Perucca E, Calzetti S. Double-blind comparison of primidone and Phenobarbital in essential tremor. Neurology 1988; 38:808–10.
70. Zesiewicz TA, Elble R, Louis ED, Hauser RA, Sullivan KL, Dewey RB Jr, et al. Practice parameter: therapies for essential tremor: report of the Quality Standards Subcommittee of the American Academy of Neurology. Neurology 2005;64:2008–20.
71. Ondo W, Hunter C, Vuong KD, Schwartz K, Jankovic J. Gabapentin for essential tremor: a multiple-dose, double blind, placebo-controlled trial. Mov Disord 2000;15(4):678–82.
72. Pahwa R, Lyons K, Hubble JP, Busenbark K, Rienerth JD, Pahwa A, et al. Double-blind controlled trial of gabapentin in essential tremor. Mov Disord 1998;13(3):465–67.
73. Galvez-Jimenez N, Hargreave M. Topiramate and essential tremor. Ann Neurol 2000;47 (6):837–38.
74. Ondo WG, Jankovic J, Connor GS, Pahwa R, Elble R, Stacy MA, et al.Ondo WG, Jankovic J, Connor GS, et al. Topiramate in essential tremor: a double blind, placebo-controlled trial. Neurology 2006;66(5):672–77.

5 Gastrointestinal disorders

Orhan K. Atay

A number of gastroenterologic conditions are found in the adolescent and their proper management is important to the overall physicologic and psychologic health of this individual. This chapter looks at such issues as irritable bowel syndrome, constipation, gastroesophageal reflux, esinophilic esophagitis, celiac disease, inflammatory bowel disease, hepatitis, and pancreatitis.

5.1 Irritable bowel syndrome

The Rome III diagnostic criteria for irritable bowel syndrome (IBS) include recurrent abdominal pain or discomfort at least 3 days per month in the last 3 months associated with two or more of the following: (a) improvement with defecation, (b) onset associated with a change in the frequency of stool, and (c) onset associated with a change in form (appearance) of stool (1). Prior to making the diagnosis of IBS, there should be no clinical evidence of an organic cause.

IBS is divided into three general categories: IBS constipation-predominant (IBS-C), IBS diarrhea-predominant (IBS-D), and a mixed or alternating stool pattern (IBS-M).

Visceral hypersensitivity is a term used in describing functional abdominal pain. Anorectal manometry is a test that uses a catheter with pressure sensors to detect both anal sphincter and rectal pressure. A balloon is attached to the tip of the catheter and used to distend the rectum, simulating the distention caused by the descent of stool into the rectal vault. Studies have shown that patients with IBS have decreased thresholds for sensation and discomfort when the balloon is inflated. This evidence suggests that patients with IBS have a hypersensitive enteral nervous system leading to more intense abdominal discomfort (2).

Previous gastrointestinal infection (viral, bacterial, or parasitic) may predispose patients to postinfectious IBS. Typically these patients have a better prognosis in regard to symptom resolution. Research suggests that enteral flora play a pivotal role in the development of symptoms associated with IBS, especially IBS-D.

5.1.1 Epidemiology

IBS is a debilitating disorder that is estimated to cost $1.35 billion per year in the United States. Up to 15 percent of the population in North America meets the criteria for IBS. An estimated 25 to 50 percent of referrals to gastroenterologists are for patients with IBS. Women outnumber men 2:1, especially for IBS-C (3).

5.1.2 Differential diagnosis

A thorough history and physical exam can usually lead to an accurate diagnosis of IBS without ordering expensive and potentially invasive testing. Specific concerns identified during the office visit (i.e., weight loss, focal abdominal pain, hematochezia) should prompt further investigation into other possible etiologies for the patient's symptoms.

5.1.3 Management

IBS affects not only the patient but also the family as a whole. In order to effectively manage the symptoms of IBS, the patient as well as the family must be accepting of the diagnosis. Because genetics plays a role, it is not unusual to learn of other family members sharing a diagnosis of IBS. It is tempting for the clinician to "rule out" other disorders by ordering a multitude of tests. Testing can be invasive, expensive, unnecessary, and avoidable if the time is taken to obtain a complete and thorough history and physical examination. Understanding the specific triggers that elicit symptoms is central to treating this condition.

Pharmacologic treatment should be tailored toward the individual's symptoms. Given that an imbalance of intestinal flora may lead to symptoms of IBS, probiotic therapy has been found to be beneficial. Even more encouraging, the use of a 2-week course of rifaximin, a nonabsorbable antimicrobial agent, has been shown to be efficacious in IBS without constipation and with long-duration of response. More importantly, the drug itself is well tolerated with few adverse reactions (4).

Narcotics should be avoided in patients with IBS. Narcotic bowel syndrome occurs when narcotics are used to treat symptoms of IBS, with a subsequent to worsening of symptoms and likely narcotic dependency. Once this cycle begins, it is very difficult to break and often requires psychotherapy and the involvement of a pain clinic (5).

Antispasmodics (e.g., dicyclomine, hyoscyamine) have been beneficial, but mostly in the setting of intermittent symptoms of pain. Long-term use has been associated with the development of significant constipation due to their anticholinergic properties. Therefore, patients and their families should be advised about this potential side effect.

IBS-C requires the use of laxative therapy. A thorough physical exam can identify this as the cause of abdominal discomfort. For those patients who may not cooperate with a rectal exam, an abdominal x-ray can help to clarify this diagnosis. It is the author's experience that compliance with laxative therapy tends to be poor, especially in the adolescent population. Dietary fiber may be beneficial for some patients with IBS-C but in excess may cause bloating and possible exacerbation of symptoms. Antidepressant medication, specifically tricyclic (low-dose) and possibly selective serotonin reuptake inhibitors, have been effective in the treatment of IBS. Cognitive-behavioral therapy in conjunction with medical treatment may be beneficial in some patients.

5.2 Constipation

The Rome III criteria for functional constipation in children and adolescents include at least two of the following present for a least 2 months: (a) two or fewer defecations per week, (b) at least one episode of fecal incontinence per week, (c) history of retentive posturing or excessive volitional stool retention, (d) history of painful or hard bowel movements, (e) presence of a large fecal mass in the rectum, (f) history of large-diameter stools that may obstruct the toilet (6). The Bristol stool chart can be helpful in acquiring a descriptive history of the patient's bowel habits (see ▶Fig. 5.1).

5.2.1 Epidemiology

Constipation is a common pediatric condition thought to occur in up to 8 percent of children (7). It typically starts with withholding behavior in two pivotal points in a child's development. Potty training has been linked with withholding behavior as the child strives to gain control of his or her environment. In addition, the new responsibility of the child to discontinue whatever activity he or she may be engaged in in order to utilize the toilet can be arduous. The entrance into grade school also poses a challenge when the child is faced with using public restrooms. Anxiety related to this is quite common and can lead to withholding behavior in which the child will wait until he or she returns home in order to have a bowel movement.

5.2.2 Differential diagnosis

The vast majority of constipation is functional, meaning no specific organic etiology is identified. It is important, however, to consider hypothyroidism, celiac disease, pseudo-obstruction, and congenital abnormalities (i.e., short-segment Hirschsprung's disease, anteriorly displaced anus) when a patient is refractory to standard medical management.

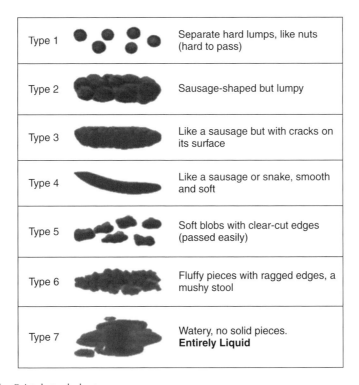

Type 1	Separate hard lumps, like nuts (hard to pass)
Type 2	Sausage-shaped but lumpy
Type 3	Like a sausage but with cracks on its surface
Type 4	Like a sausage or snake, smooth and soft
Type 5	Soft blobs with clear-cut edges (passed easily)
Type 6	Fluffy pieces with ragged edges, a mushy stool
Type 7	Watery, no solid pieces. **Entirely Liquid**

Fig. 5.1: The Bristol stool chart.

5.2.3 Management

Laxatives are the mainstay of treatment for constipation. Laxatives are divided into osmotic agents and stimulants. Examples of osmotic agents include lactulose, PEG 3350, milk of magnesia, and magnesium citrate. Lactulose has been associated with flatulence and abdominal discomfort. Magnesium citrate and milk of magnesia have both been implicated in electrolyte disturbances, especially magnesium toxicity. PEG 3350 has an excellent safety profile and is well tolerated, which makes it an appealing drug for long-term use.

High-dose PEG 3350 in combination with bisacodyl can be a safe and effective method used for the purpose of bowel preparation prior to colonoscopy (8). In the author's practice, we use 4 tablets of bisacodyl in combination with 15 capfuls (17 g per capful) of PEG 3350 mixed in 64 oz of Gatorade to disimpact severely constipated patients. This treatment is well tolerated; therefore compliance is good.

Stimulant laxatives include bisacodyl and senna. Stimulants can cause abdominal cramping and when utilized daily can result in laxative abuse and eventual reliance on therapy to maintain bowel function. Suppositories and rectal enemas have not been proven to be superior to oral therapy alone (9). Long-term use of suppositories and enemas should be avoided if possible. Patients with anatomic or spinal cord abnormalities (e.g., myelomeningocele) are the exception. These patients may benefit from a cecostomy button or appendicocecostomy procedure in order to receive antegrade enemas.

A common problem in patients with chronic constipation is dyssynergia or paradoxical puborectalis contractions. These patients have uncoordinated muscle contractions during the process of defecation. Even though they may generate adequate rectal pressure to expel stool from the rectal vault, they will simultaneously contract the anal sphincter, thereby leading to incomplete stool evacuation. Anorectal manometry with biofeedback can help identify this problem and with repeated sessions potentially correct it as well.

Encopresis is the act of fecal soiling, generally in the setting of leakage of liquid stool around hard impacted stool. Patients are not aware of the soiling episode until after it has occurred. This unfortunate problem can cause significant emotional distress. In adolescents, it usually indicates chronic, long=standing constipation with rectal dilation and an associated decrease in rectal sensory threshold. Resolution of encopresis requires motivation in the patient and realistic expectations in terms of length of therapy.

5.3 Gastroesophageal reflux disease

Gastroesophageal reflux (GER) is a normal physiologic process in which gastric contents are expelled into the esophagus. Gastroesophageal reflux disease (GERD), however, is the very same process in association with pain and/or mucosal injury. Nonerosive reflux disease is a condition in which GERD occurs in the absence of esophagitis. The distinction between these conditions may require endoscopic and/or impedance/pH testing.

5.3.1 Epidemiology

GER occurs in up to 30 percent of infants at 3 months of age and typically resolves by 15 months. GER that persists beyond 18 months may require endoscopic, radiologic, and/or impedance/pH testing. Certain populations are at high risk for lifelong GERD. This includes patients with neurologic impairment, hiatal hernia, or a history of esophageal atresia. The development of Barrett's esophagus, a metaplastic condition that can progress to esophageal malignancy, is very rare in pediatrics, occurring in 5 percent of patients with severe chronic GERD (10).

5.3.2 Differential diagnosis

In evaluating a patient with suspected GERD, it is important to recognize other conditions that may present with similar symptoms consistent with GERD. Eosinophilic Esophagitis is an inflammatory condition of the esophagus that can be distinguished from GERD only through endoscopic and histologic evaluation. This disease is discussed more extensively in the next section of this chapter. Rumination disorder is a condition in which the patient will effortlessly regurgitate gastric contents back into the oral cavity. The patient will proceed to chew and reswallow the food. Patients will display this behavior immediately after eating and have no evidence of GER at night while sleeping.

5.3.3 Management

Lifestyle changes are the most benign interventions that may improve symptoms of GERD. Dietary modification, including avoidance of caffeine, spicy foods, carbonated beverages and chocolate, may be beneficial. Obesity has a clear association with GERD and thus weight reduction should be encouraged in these patients (11).

Acid suppressant medication is the mainstay of medical therapy. These drugs are divided into histamine-2 (H2) blockers and proton pump inhibitors (PPIs). H2 blockers (i.e., ranitidine, cimetidine) inhibit both basal and food-stimulated acid secretion and are considered effective but less effective than PPIs. H2 blockers have been used successfully for the treatment of mild esophagitis. They have traditionally been used as the first-line agents in the "step-up" approach to treating GERD. All are generally well tolerated and are available over the counter. Cimetidine can increase the concentration of other medications through inhibition of the cytochrome P450 enzyme system; when used chronically, they can have antiadrogenic effects (i.e., gynecomastia, impotence). Tachyphylaxis (development of tolerance) has been an issue for H2 blockers but not with PPIs. PPIs (e.g., esomeprazole, pantoprazole) inhibit the secretion of hydrogen ion into the gastric lumen by binding to the parietal cell proton pump. PPIs can lower serum concentrations of drugs that require acid for absorption (e.g., itraconazole) and two are now available over the counter (omeprazole and lansoprazole). PPI therapy is the gold standard in treating moderate to severe esophagitis. A PPI may be used for up to 12 weeks in order to facilitate healing of the esophageal mucosa (12).

With the widespread use of long-term acid suppressant therapy, prescribing clinicians are more aware of the potential side effects. Postmenopausal women receiving acid suppressant therapy have a higher incidence of hip fracture, suggesting a possible link with calcium deficiency (13). Vitamin B12 may potentially be deficient in patients on acid suppressant therapy (particularly the elderly) owing to the dependence of vitamin B12 absorption on gastric pH. In addition, acid-suppressed patients may be more susceptible to small intestinal bacterial overgrowth and *Clostridium difficile* infection due to the lack of gastric acid acting as a protective barrier (14).

Gastroparesis confirmed using scintigraphy (gastric emptying study) may warrant the use of prokinetic therapy. There is a lack of strong evidence to support the role of prokinetic therapy in the treatment of GERD. In addition, severe side effects have been associated with currently available prokinetic drugs. Metoclopramide, for example, has been linked to extrapyramidal symptoms, including tardive dyskinesia, a permanent neurologic side effect. Erythromycin, an antibiotic with prokinetic properties affecting motilin receptors, also lacks evidence to support its use in the treatment of GERD.

It is imperative to identify patients at high risk for chronic GERD in order to prevent the development of Barrett's esophagus, a metaplastic condition that may lead to adenocarcinoma of the esophagus. Those patients refractory to acid suppressant medication may require surgical intervention (i.e. Nissen fundoplication). (see chapter 8 in Greydanus DE, Patel DR, Omar HA, Feucht C, Merrick J: Adolescent Medicine – Pharmacotherapeutics in General, Mental and Sexual Health. Berlin: de Gruyter, 2012). It is important to discuss with your patient the risks and possible failure of a Nissen fundoplication. In follow-up studies, 25 percent of patients have reported operative failure, which was confirmed by pH testing (15). In addition, up to one third of patients reported adverse events including gas-bloat syndrome, dumping syndrome and persistent gagging/retching (16).

5.4 Eosinophilic esophagitis

Eosinophilic esophagitis (EoE) is an allergy-mediated disorder characterized by infiltration of the esophageal mucosa by eosinophils. The histologic criteria for number of eosinophils per high-power field is greater than 15. Interleukin-5 is an important cytokine that causes the release of eosinophils from the bone marrow into the bloodstream. Eotaxin-1 maintains baseline levels of eosinophils in the gastrointestinal tract and therefore may play an significant role in the pathogenesis of EoE (17). A common presenting symptom of EoE in the adolescent population is dysphagia. The esophageal mucosa over time becomes fibrotic, which can lead to stricturing of the esophageal lumen. Esophageal dysmotility may occur in addition to esophageal strictures.

5.4.1 Epidemiology

The estimated prevalence of EoE in the United States is 52 per 100,000 (18). There is a male predominance of 3 to 1. A genetic association has been identified, since many patients have family members afflicted with the same disease. The presentation is dependent on age. Younger patients, namely children, tend to present with nonspecific symptoms including abdominal pain, GER, and failure to thrive. Older patients (adolescents and adults) present with dysphagia. A substantial number of patients with esophageal food impaction are later diagnosed with EoE.

5.4.2 Differential diagnosis

Symptoms of EoE may be difficult to distinguish from GERD. Typically patients with EoE will have symptoms refractory to acid suppressant therapy. The diagnosis can be clarified with endoscopy and the use of an impedance/pH probe. It is important to rule out anatomic abnormalities including esophageal ring and web, both of which can present with symptoms of dysphagia and esophageal food impaction. Although esophageal dysmotility is a component of EoE, other causes of dysmotility may include achalasia, which can be distinguished by endoscopic and manometric evaluation.

5.4.3 Management

EoE is a chronic disease with no cure. Fortunately, effective management is available. The optimal approach is to identify a food allergen and implement allergen avoidance. Evaluation for allergies is best performed by an allergist familiar with this disease. A radioallergosorbent test, skin-prick test, and patch testing can help identify specific food allergens to be avoided in the patient's diet.

Topical steroids in the form of fluticasone or viscous budesonide are commonly used, with age-dependent dosing. With the fluticasone 220-mcg inhaler, two puffs swallowed twice daily is an accepted dose in patients older than age 10. A lower dose in younger children, two puffs of 110 mcg swallowed twice daily, may be more appropriate. Budesonide is compounded with sucralose to add viscosity. The usual ratio is 5 g of sucralose for every 2 mL of budesonide. Budesonide 500 mcg swallowed twice daily is given to children under 10 years of age and 1 mg swallowed twice daily for those over 10 years of age.

It is important to instruct your patients to swish and rinse their mouths with water after swallowing the steroid in order to avoid the development of thrush. Patients should not eat or drink for 30 minutes after ingesting the steroid in order to increase contact time with the esophageal surface. Although GERD is a separate disease, it is well documented that acid-suppressant therapy in conjunction with topical steroids may be beneficial in patients with EoE.

If steroid therapy is ineffective, the patient may require a six-food elimination diet, removing milk, soy, egg, wheat, peanuts, and seafood. A gradual reintroduction of food under close endoscopic surveillance is required. An alternative to the six-food elimination diet is the implementation of an elemental diet, although many patients may find this difficult and subsequently require gastrostomy tube placement (19).

5.5 Celiac disease

Celiac disease is a chronic condition characterized by gluten-induced enteropathy. The offending protein, gluten, is found in food products containing wheat, rye, or barley. Although oats do not contain gluten, they have historically been avoided in patients with celiac disease owing to cross-contamination with other gluten-containing food products.

With the advent of convenient and noninvasive serologic screening, primary care physicians are playing a larger role in the detection of this disease. Deamidated gliadin and tissue transglutaminase antibodies are both sensitive and specific as part of the initial screening for celiac disease (20). Endoscopic evaluation with duodenal biopsies is still the gold standard for confirming the diagnosis. Patients should not be instructed to initiate a gluten-free diet until the endoscopy is performed so as to avoid masking the histologic evidence of celiac disease.

Common gastrointestinal manifestations include abdominal pain, weight loss, diarrhea, and/or constipation. Extraintestinal manifestations of this disease include anemia, dental enamel defects, arthralgia, neuropsychiatric abnormalities, dermatitis herpetiformis, osteopenia, and hepatitis.

5.5.1 Epidemiology

Celiac disease is an autoimmune disorder with an underlying genetic predisposition (DQ2/DQ8) and likely environmental trigger. It occurs in approximately 1 percent of the population, although this statistic may be higher given the increasingly well recognized group of asymptomatic patients (21). High-risk groups include patients with Down's syndrome, Turner's syndrome, Williams syndrome, and IgA deficiency. There is also an association with type 1 diabetes mellitus and thyroid disease.

5.5.2 Differential diagnosis

Crohn's disease, autoimmune enteropathy and protein-losing enteropathy may present with similar symptoms. Endoscopic, histologic, and serologic testing can distinguish celiac disease from these other conditions.

5.5.3 Management

All patients, including clinically asymptomatic patients, diagnosed with celiac disease should initiate and comply with a gluten-free diet. As little as 10 mg of gluten consumed daily can lead to mucosal damage (22). A dietitian with expertise in celiac disease should be consulted to help provide dietary guidance for the family.

Fortunately repeated endoscopy is not necessary since dietary compliance can be monitored using serologic testing. After several months on a gluten-free diet, serology should be significantly improved if not normalized. Acquired lactose intolerance is not uncommon, since lactase is found in the villi of the small intestine. As the villi regenerate, most patients will begin to tolerate lactose in their diets.

A multivitamin supplement should be given and vitamin and trace mineral levels monitored in patients who present with significant malnutrition. A recent study has revealed promising results in the use of wheat flour fermented with sourdough lactobacilli and fungal proteases. This process decreases the concentration of gluten. Ingestion of this wheat product was well tolerated by patients with celiac disease. This initial study will require further validation prior to making definitive recommendations (23).

5.6 Inflammatory bowel disease

Inflammatory bowel disease (IBD) is a condition thought to be caused by dysregulated activity of the immune system, resulting in inflammation throughout various regions of the gastrointestinal (GI) tract. Genetics and environmental triggers play an important role in the pathogenesis of this disease.

IBD can be divided into two groups: Crohn's disease (CD) and ulcerative colitis (UC). The fundamental distinction is related to the site of inflammation in the GI tract. For instance, ulcerative colitis is limited to the colon; it almost always starts at the rectum and extends to various lengths throughout the colon. The inflammation is continuous without skip areas of healthy-appearing mucosa. CD, on the other hand, can affect any region of the GI tract from the mouth to the anus. The inflammation is transmural, with the occasional finding of noncaseating granulomas. Other features that distinguish UC from CD are listed in ▶Tab. 5.1.

There are many extraintestinal manifestations of IBD. Primary sclerosing cholangitis (PSC) is an inflammatory condition of the biliary tract causing scarring, which can subsequently lead to cirrhosis. It occurs in less than 5 percent of UC patients; however, the majority of patients with PSC have UC. Although it can occur in CD, it is far less common when compared with the incidence in UC. Magnetic resonance cholangiopancreatography can help in the diagnosis. The development of PSC has a high association with colon cancer; thus dysplasia screening should be performed yearly starting at the time that PSC is diagnosed.

Arthralgia and arthritis are common manifestations of IBD. The type of joint involvement, axillary versus peripheral, can be clinically significant. The severity of peripheral arthritis is dependent on intestinal disease activity. In contrast, axillary arthritis or ankylosing spondylitis is independent of intestinal disease activity.

The integument system can also be involved. Erythema nodusum (painful erythematous lesions occurring on the skin) and pyoderma gangrenosum (ulcerating lesions of the extremities and/or trunk) are both responsive to immunosuppressant therapy.

5.6.1 Epidemiology

The incidence of IBD in children is increasing. An estimated incidence in one study was 7.05 per 100,000, with twice as many cases of CD than of UC (24). The peak onset of IBD is between 15 and 25 years of age. Interestingly, industrialized nations have a higher incidence of IBD. The hygiene hypothesis may explain this, as nonindustrialized nations tend to have a higher incidence of endemic parasitic infections. Genetics plays a strong role in the development of IBD. The relative risk of developing IBD in siblings of patients with this disease compared with the general population is 36.5 and 16.6 in CD and UC respectively (25).

Tab. 5.1: Other features that distinguish UC from CD.

Symptom	Crohn's disease (%)	Ulcerative colitis (%)
Abdominal Pain	50	90
Diarrhea	60	95
Weight loss	95	40
Fever	20	15
Rectal bleeding	25	95
Arthritis	10	5
Perianal Fissure/fistulas	25	0
Growth failure	40	5

5.6.2 Differential diagnosis

It is important to exclude an infectious etiology in evaluating a patient for IBD. Bacterial GI infections can have symtoms similar to those of IBD. *Clostridium difficile*, a cause of infectious colitis, was previously thought to be predominantly nosocomial and associated with antibiotic use. The frequency is now increasing in the community setting and is not always associated with antibiotic use. Initial testing should include stool culture and *C. difficile* stool toxin or testing by the polymerase chain reaction (PCR). Histologic features can help distinguish acute from chronic inflammation. Serologic panels may also be useful in the diagnosis of IBD but do not replace standard testing (i.e., endoscopy).

5.6.3 Management

Conventional medical therapy for IBD consists of the step-up approach (26). This treatment paradigm starts with the use of steroids and mesalamine-based products. Steroids have significant side effects leading to osteopenia, growth retardation, hypertension, glucose intolerance, mood changes, and cosmetic concerns (cushingoid appearance, acne). Therefore, steroids should only be used as an induction agent or during a flare. Maintenance therapy using steroids is to be avoided.

Mesalamine's (also referred to as 5-aminosalicylate) anti-inflammatory properties may be due to a variety of pathways including leukotriene and prostaglandin inhibition as well as antioxidant properties. In order for mesalamine to reach the colon for activity, a variety of formulations exist, including prodrugs (sulfasalazine, balsalazide, olsalazine) and delayed-release (i.e., pH-sensitive film coating [Asacol], ethylcellulose-coated [Pentasa]) agents. Mesalamine is generally effective in mild to moderate UC and only modestly more effective than placebo in CD. For distal UC, rectal formulations (enemas [Rowasa] or suppositories [Canasa]) may be more effective than oral preparations (27).

The next class of drugs in the step-up model of medical management is the use of immunomodulators (azathioprine, 6-mercaptopurine, methotrexate). These drugs suppress the immune system by decreasing the bone marrow production of white blood cells and can take up to 3 months to achieve maximal benefit. It is suggested that thiopurine methyltransferase enzyme activity be tested prior to initiating azathioprine and 6-mercaptopurine, since patients who have a deficiency in this enzyme are at risk for developing severe and possibly fatal pancytopenia.

The most effective drugs fall into the category of biologic agents (infliximab, adalimumab, certolizumab). Biologic agents are antibodies that target tumor necrosis factor alpha (TNF-A), a protein responsible for the immune cascade that causes the inflammation in IBD. This medication is given either intravenously or via subcutaneous injection. Studies have shown that in combination, immunomodulators and biologic agents are superior to monotherapy in the treatment of CD (28). Unfortunately, malignancies, including lymphoma (and the incidence of a rare and deadly form of lymphoma, heaptosplenic T-cell lymphoma) have been associated with this combination. It is recommended that patients undergo hepatitis B and tuberculin skin testing prior to the initiation of therapy owing to the potential of reactivation of latent tuberculosis and chronic hepatitis B. TNF-blocking agents have also been associated with serious infections, including sepsis, pneumonia, and opportunistic infections. Vaccine status should be up to date prior to starting therapy and live vaccines should be avoided during therapy.

Surgical therapy can be curative in UC. (see chapter 8 in Greydanus DE, Patel DR, Omar HA, Feucht C, Merrick J: Adolescent Medicine – Pharmacotherapeutics in General, Mental and Sexual Health. Berlin: de Gruyter, 2012). An ileal pouch anal anastomosis is a procedure in which the colon is removed with the exception of a short segment of rectal cuff. A pouch is created from the ileum and later attached to the rectal cuff. In CD, surgery is never a cure. It is almost inevitable that disease will recur at the surgical margin. Long-term postoperative immunosuppressant management may reduce the likelihood of disease reoccurrence.

The top-down approach, starting with biologic agents, is becoming more accepted for the treatment of IBD. A more aggressive medical approach initially may potentially alter the course of the disease and reduce the likelihood of future surgery (29).

Unfortunately IBD is a life-long condition with no cure. However, medical therapy continues to advance. Genetics will play a larger role in predicting disease presentation, progression, and optimal treatment.

5.7 Hepatitis

Hepatitis is a nonspecific term used to define inflammation of the liver. There are multiple causes, including infectious, metabolic, autoimmune, and drug-induced. It is beyond the scope of this chapter to discuss each etiology in detail.

Viral infection is a common cause of elevated liver enzymes. Hepatitis types B and C are well known causes of chronic hepatitis. Hepatitis B infection occurs in various phases. The immune-tolerant phase is defined by active viral replication in the setting of relatively normal liver enzymes. Patients typically test positive for hepatitis B surface antigen (HBsAg) and hepatitis Be antigen (HBeAG). Hepatitis B surface antibody (HBsAb) is negative during this phase. This phase can last for years. The immune active phase is defined as liver enzyme elevation greater than two times the upper limit of normal. If the virus is cleared by treatment or spontaneous remission, the HBsAg and HBeAg will both become negative and HBsAb will become positive.

The disease course of hepatitis C virus is dependent on the route of acquisition. Patients who acquired hepatitis C via vertical transmission have a lower rate of spontaneous seroconversion. Regardless, the disease has a slow insidious course with harmful consequences, in particular hepatocellular carcinoma, usually occurring decades after initial acquisition of the infection.

Nonalcoholic fatty liver disease (NAFLD) ranges from simple steatosis (fatty infiltration of the liver) to nonacoholic steatohepatitis (NASH). NASH can progress from inflammation of the liver to cirrhosis. Cirrhosis secondary to NASH is a growing indication for liver transplantation (30).

Autoimmune hepatitis (AIH) is classified as either type 1 or 2, depending on the specific serologic markers. Type 1 is associated with antinuclear antibodies and anti-smooth muscle antibodies. Type 2 is associated with antiliver andantikidney microsome antibodies. As in many diseases, there is a genetic component along with an environmental trigger. The severity of the disease can vary from mild liver enzyme elevation to fulminant hepatic failure.

An unfortunate cause of hepatitis is acetaminophen toxicity. In the adolescent population, this may occur intentionally in the setting of attempted suicide. It is cruicial that this diagnosis be made quickly, since the patient's prognosis is dependent on the timeliness of starting medical therapy (with N-acetylcysteine). The Rumack-Matthew nomogram (▶Fig. 5.2) is a useful diagram for clinicians to use in order to predict prognosis and help determine if treatment is indicated. It does require a serum concentration of acetaminophen and knowledge of the time of acetaminophen ingestion.

5.7.1 Epidemiology

The incidence of hepatitis B continues to decline, likely related to the implementation of hepatitis B vaccination. In 2007, the Centers for Disease Control (CDC)reported the incidence of hepatitis B in children less than 15 years of age to be 0.03 per 100,000. Rates were highest among non-Hispanic blacks.

Approximately 3.2 million people in the United States are infected with hepatitis C. Fortunately, despite this impressive number, hepatitis C infection is uncommon in the pediatric population. The overall incidence of hepatitis C has declined since 1995 (31).

NAFLD is a leading cause of liver disease in the adolescent population. It can affect up to one third of the general population. NASH can affect up to 20 percent of the

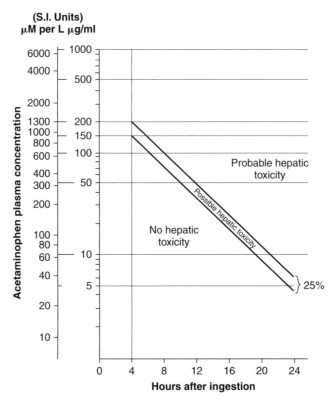

Fig. 5.2: The Rumack-Matthew nomogram.

obese population (32). There is a clear association with NASH and metabolic syndrome (hypertriglyceridemia and type 2 diabetes mellitus). Hispanics have a higher frequency of NASH compared with other ethnic groups (33).

Type 1 AIH has a less severe course compared with type 2 and tends to affect adults. Type 2 AIH may present with a more severe and rapidly progressive course. Type 2 AIH also tends to affect females more than males.

In the pediatric population, close to 50 percent of acetaminophen toxicity is the result of intentional overdose (34). The majority of acetaminophen-induced hepatocellular injury is found in those who intentionally overdose compared with unintentional overdose. The rate of unintentional overdose in the pediatric population will hopefully decline with removal of infant over-the-counter acetaminophen and regulated standard concentrations (milligram/milliter).

5.7.2 Differential diagnosis

There are a variety of causes of hepatitis. Clinical history, laboratory, and radiologic studies can aid in the diagnosis. Liver biopsy may be required to confirm the suspected diagnosis prior to initiating treatment. In the case of suspected acetaminophen poisoning, obtaining acetaminophen levels can be both diagnostic and prognostic.

5.7.3 Management

Treatment for infectious hepatitis has evolved over the past few decades. The standard approach for the treatment of pediatric patients with hepatitis B is based on age and the current status. For patients 1 to 12 years of age, interferon alpha-2b is the standard therapy. Nucleoside analogues inhibit HBV DNA polymerase and are also available if the patient meets age criteria. Nucleoside analogues approved by the U.S. Food and Drug Administration (FDA) for treating hepatitis B include lamivudine (age equal to or greater than 2), adefovir (age equal to or greater than 12), entecavir (age equal to or greater than 16), and telbivudine (age equal to or greater than 16). These agents are fairly well tolerated but have been associated with exacerbations of hepatitis B upon discontinuation and rare reports of lactic acidosis and hepatomegaly with steatosis. Adefovir when used at higher than recommended doses and in patients with preexisting renal insufficiency is associated with renal toxicity. Resistance to lamivudine has been seen within the first year and increases with duration of therapy, telbivudine is associated with cross-resistance. Adefovir and entacavir maintain some activity against lamivudine-resistant HBV (35,36). If the patient is suspected to be in the immune-active phase, it is reasonable to monitor him or her for up to 6 months for possible spontaneous seroconversion.

Genotype plays a major role in the decision to treat hepatitis C. Genotypes 2 and 3 have a high response rate to pegylated interferon in combination with ribavirin. This is in contrast to a lower response rate with the use of combination therapy in genotype 1. The treatment duration is 48 weeks for genotype 1 and 24 weeks for genotypes 2 and 3 (37). Recently boceprevir and telaprevir (protease inhibitors that inhibit viral replication) in combination with pegylated interferon and ribavirin have been approved by the FDA for the treatment of hepatitis C genotype 1 in adults. Pegylated interferon is associated with a wide array of side effects including an influenza-like syndrome, fatigue, myalgias, anorexia, hypo- or hyperthyroidism, psychiatric syndromes including depression and anxiety, alopecia, injection-site reactions, and bone marrow suppression. Ribavirin is associated with cough, rash, and hemolytic anemia. Granulocyte-colony stimulating factor and erythyropoietin are utilized to treat the bone marrow suppression. Side effects associated with therapy can make adherence challenging. The addition of a protease inhibitor has resulted in more patients achieving a sustained virologic response compared with standard therapy alone (35,36). The most successful treatment for NAFLD is weight reduction (38). A low-fructose diet and vitamin E antioxidant therapy may be of some benefit, although studies have shown mixed results. For those with metabolic syndrome, metformin may also have some beneficial effect.

The mainstay of treatment for AIH is immunosuppressant drugs. Steroids are used initially, and an immunomodulator (azathioprine) is used for long-term management. Type 2 AIH has a lower response rate to therapy compared with type 1. The decision to discontinue immunosuppressant therapy depends on the degree of liver damage (i.e., cirrhosis), disease activity, and type 2 status (39).

Treatment success for acetaminophen toxicity depends on the promptness of medical care. If ingestion occurred within 4 hours, activated charcoal can be administered at a dose of 1 mg/kg. N-acetylcysteine should be administered if the serum acetaminophen levels plot above the possible hepatic toxicity line on the Rumack-Matthew nomogram or if the ingestion is greater than 150 mg/kg in children or greater than 7.5 g in adolescents and adults. The duration of treatment is dependent on the route (intravenous is for 21 hours versus 72 hours for oral administration) and the clinical status of the patient (i.e., increasing liver enzymes, coagulopathy). If liver enzymes are found to be elevated, treatment should be continued until the liver enzymes are clearly declining.

Either oral or intravenous administration is effective. Oral dosing is 140 mg/kg as an initial dose; this is followed by 17 doses of 70 mg/kg administered every 4 hours. The oral route is associated with an unpleasant odor, which can make it less palatable. If the patient is uncooperative or vomiting, N-acetylcysteine should be given via the intravenous route. Intravenous N-acetylcysteine is given at a dose of 150 mg/kg over 1 hour, followed by a 4-hour infusion of 50 mg/kg, followed by a 16-hour infusion of 100 mg/kg. The total dose infused over 21 hours should equal 300 mg/kg. Patients suspected of developing acute liver failure should be transferred to a hospital capable of performing a liver transplant.

5.8 Pancreatitis

The typical presentation of pancreatitis includes epigastric pain with radiation to the back, nausea, and vomiting with or without jaundice. Amylase and lipase levels greater than three times the upper limit of normal are very sensitive and specific for pancreatitis.

Acute prancreatitis is a reversible inflammatory process occurring in the pancreatic parenchyma with no lasting effects on pancreatic exocrine and endocrine function. In contrast, chronic pancreatitis is an irreversible process in which the pancreatic endocrine and/or exocrine function is permanently deficient. The distinction between acute and chronic pancreatitis is independent of the frequency of episodes of pancreatitis.

There are many causes of pancreatitis and, as with most conditions, the etiology is usually dependent on the patient's age. In the adult population, pancreatitis commonly occurs as result of alcohol use or biliary tract disease. The patient is given the diagnosis of idiopathic pancreatitis if no cause is found. The etiology of pancreatitis in pediatrics may include infection, trauma, drug toxicity, congenital abnormalities, cystic fibrosis, hereditary pancreatitis, autoimmune pancreatitis, hypertriglyceridemia and hypercalcemia.

Infectious organisms may include bacterial (*Mycoplasma, Salmonella*), viral (mumps, coxsackievirus, cytomegalovirus) or parasitic (*Toxoplasma*) types. Several drugs have been association with pancreatitis, including an antiepileptic medication (valproic acid) and immunosuppressant agents (mercaptopurine, azathioprine, L-asparginase).

5.8.1 Epidemiology

Studies at major pediatric tertiary centers have shown a rising incidence of acute pancreatitis in the pediatric population. A study performed at the Children's Hospital of Pittsburgh found that the number of cases of acute pancreatitis in children increased from 28 in 1993 to 141 total cases in 2004 (40).

5.8.2 Differential diagnosis

Patients that present with symptoms of pancreatitis in the setting of normal pancreatic enzymes should be evaluated for peptic ulcer disease and hepatobiliary disease. If the clinical history and physical exam findings are consistent with pancreatitis, the author would recommend repeating the pancreatic enzymes 12 to 24 hours after the initial laboratory studies were drawn.

There are other causes of elevated amylase levels that should be considered. Amylase is produced in the salivary glands and fallopian tubes. An amylase isoenzyme may help distinguish pancreatic from nonpancreatic disease. In addition, macroamylasemia is a condition that leads to chronic elevation of serum amylase levels.

5.8.3 Management

Fluid resuscitation is the mainstay of initial treatment (41). Bolus intravenous fluids (IVF) followed by large volumes of continuous intravenous fluids should be administered. In adults, IVF up to 300 mL/hr or more may be required. Pain management is very important and using morphine is an acceptable approach. Previously, clinicians were hesitant to use morphine in patients with pancreatitis owing to concerns regarding increased pressure on the sphincter of Oddi. There is no definitive evidence associating morphine with exacerbation of pancreatitis.

Traditionally, enteral nutrition was held until pancreatic enzymes declined to near normal levels. Recently, however, enteral nutrition has been found to be safe and beneficial. Total parenteral nutrition should be reserved for patients unable to tolerate enteral nutrition. Feeding tubes may be required initially. There is no absolute contraindication to using gastric feedings, although jejunal feedings may reduce pancreatic stimulation by bypassing the sphincter of Oddi. In addition, feeding a patient low-fat versus a regular diet does not seem to make any significant clinical difference.

Octreotide, a somatostatin analogue, was previously used in the treatment of pancrea-titis. Recent studies have shown no substantial benefit in patients treated with octreotide compared with a control group (42).

5.9 Conclusions

The gastrointestinal tract is an important organ system; its dysfunction can lead to considerable medical and psychological problems. This chapter reviews important gas-trointestinal tract disorders, including irritable bowel syndrome, constipation, gastroe-sophageal reflux, esinophilic esophagitis, celiac disease, inflammatory bowel disease, hepatitis, and pancreatitis.

References

1. Clouse RE, Mayer EA, Aziz Q, Drossman DA, Dumitrascu DL, Mönnikes H, Naliboff BD. Functional abdominal pain syndrome. Gastroenterology 2006;130(5):1492.
2. Prior A, Maxton DG, Whorwell PJ. Anorectal manometry in irritable bowel syndrome: differences between diarrhoea and constipation predominant subjects. Gut 1990;31 (4):458–62.
3. Saito YA, Schoenfeld P, Locke GR 3rd. The epidemiology of irritable bowel syndrome in North America: a systematic review. Am J Gastroenterol 2002;97(8):1910–15.
4. Pimentel M, Lembo A, Chey WD, Zakko S, Ringel Y, Yu J, et al. Rifaximin therapy for patients with irritable bowel syndrome without constipation. N Engl J Med 2011;364 (1):22–32.
5. Grunkemeier DM, Cassara JE, Dalton CB, Drossman DA. The narcotic bowel syndrome: clinical features, pathophysiology, and management. Clin Gastroenterol Hepatol 2007;5 (10):1126–39.
6. Rasquin A, Di Lorenzo C, Forbes D, Guiraldes E, Hyams JS, Staiano A, Walker LS. Child-hood functional gastrointestinal disorders: child/adolescent. Gastroenterology 2006;130 (5):1527–37.
7. Loening-Baucke V. Constipation in early childhood: patient characteristics, treatment, and longterm follow up. Gut 1993; 34(10):1400–404.
8. Enestvedt BK, Fennerty MB, Eisen GM. Randomised clinical trial: MiraLAX vs. Golytely – a controlled study of efficacy and patient tolerability in bowel preparation for colono-scopy. Aliment Pharmacol Ther 2011;33(1):33–40.
9. Bongers ME, van den Berg MM, Reitsma JB, Voskuijl WP, Benninga MA. A randomized controlled trial of enemas in combination with oral laxative therapy for children with chronic constipation. Clin Gastroenterol Hepatol 2009;7(10):1069–74.
10. Vandenplas Y, Rudolph CD, Di Lorenzo C, Hassall E, Liptak G, Mazur L, et al. North American Society for Pediatric Gastroenterology Hepatology and Nutrition, European Society for Pediatric Gastroenterology Hepatology and Nutrition. Pediatric gastroesopha-geal reflux clinical practice guidelines: joint recommendations of the North American Society for Pediatric Gastroenterology, Hepatology, and Nutrition (NASPGHAN) and the European Society for Pediatric Gastroenterology, Hepatology, and Nutrition (ESPGHAN). J Pediatr Gastroenterol Nutr 2009; 49(4):498–547.
11. El-Serag H. The association between obesity and GERD: a review of the epidemiological evidence. Dig Dis Sci 2008;53(9):2307–12.
12. Treatment of peptic ulcers and GERD. Treatment Guidelines 2008;6(72):55–60.

13. Corley DA, Kubo A, Zhao W, Quesenberry C. Proton pump inhibitors and histamine-2 receptor antagonists are associated with hip fractures among at-risk patients. Gastroenterology 2010;139(1):93–101.
14. Cunningham R, Dale B, Undy B, Gaunt N. Proton pump inhibitors as a risk factor for Clostridium difficile diarrhoea. J Hosp Infect 2003;54(3):243–45.
15. van der Zee DC, Arends NJ, Bax NM. The value of 24-h pH study in evaluating the results of laparoscopic antireflux surgery in children. Surg Endosc 1999;13:918–21.
16. Harnsberger JK, Corey JJ, Johnson DG, Herbst JJ. Long-term followup of surgery for gastroesophageal reflux in infants and children. J Pediatr 1983;102:505–8.
17. Nielsen RG, Husby S. Eosinophilic oesophagitis: epidemiology, clinical aspects, and association to allergy. J Pediatr Gastroenterol Nutr 2007;45(3):281–89.
18. Spergel JM, Book WM, Mays E, Song L, Shah SS, Talley NJ, Bonis PA. Variation in prevalence, diagnostic criteria, and initial management options for eosinophilic gastrointestinal diseases in the United States. J Pediatr Gastroenterol Nutr 2011;52(3):300–6.
19. Furuta GT, Forbes D, Boey C, Dupont C. Putnam P, Roy SK, et al. EGIDs Working Group: Eosinophilic gastrointestinal diseases (EGIDs). J Pediatr Gastroenterol Nutr 2008;47(2):234–38.
20. Rozenberg O, Lerner A, Pacht A, Grinberg M, Reginashvili D, Henig C, Barak M. A novel algorithm for the diagnosis of celiac disease and a comprehensive review of celiac disease diagnostics. Clin Rev Allergy Immunol 2011 Jan 30. [EPub ahead of print]
21. Dubé C, Rostom A, Sy R, Cranney A, Saloojee N, Garritty C, et al. The prevalence of celiac disease in average-risk and at-risk Western European populations: a systematic review. Gastroenterology 2005; 128(4 Suppl 1):S57–67.
22. Hischenhuber C, Crevel R, Jarry B, Mäki M, Moneret-Vautrin DA, Romano A, et al. Review article: safe amounts of gluten for patients with wheat allergy or coeliac disease. Aliment Pharmacol Ther 2006;23(5):559–75.
23. Greco L, Gobbetti M, Auricchio R, Di Mase R, Landolfo F, Paparo F, et al. Safety for patients with celiac disease of baked goods made of wheat flour hydrolyzed during food processing. Clin Gastroenterol Hepatol 2011;9(1):24–29.
24. Kugathasan S, Judd RH, Hoffmann RG, Heikenen J, Telega G, Khan F, et al. Wisconsin Pediatric Inflammatory Bowel Disease Alliance. Epidemiologic and clinical characteristics of children with newly diagnosed inflammatory bowel disease in Wisconsin: a statewide population-based study. J Pediatr 2003;143(4):525–31.
25. Satsangi J, Parkes M, Jewell DP, Bell JI. Genetics of inflammatory bowel disease. Clin Sci (Lond) 1998;94(5):473–78.
26. Burger D, Travis S. Conventional medical management of inflammatory bowel disease. Gastroenterology. 2011;140(6):1827–37.
27. Drugs for inflammatory bowel disease. Treatment Guidelines 2009;7(85):65–74.
28. Colombel JF, Sandborn WJ, Reinisch W, Mantzaris GJ, Kornbluth A, Rachmilewitz D, et al. SONIC Study Group. Infliximab, azathioprine, or combination therapy for Crohn's disease. N Engl J Med 2010;362(15):1383–95.
29. D'Haens GR. Top-down therapy for Crohn's disease: rationale and evidence. Acta Clin Belg 2009;64(6):540–46.
30. Feldstein AE, Charatcharoenwitthaya P, Treeprasertsuk S, Benson JT, Enders FB, Angulo P. The natural history of non-alcoholic fatty liver disease in children: a follow-up study for up to 20 years. Gut 2009;58(11):1538–44.
31. Daniels D, Grytdal S, Wasley A. Centers for Disease Control and Prevention (CDC). Surveillance for acute viral hepatitis. United States, 2007. MMWR Surveill Summ 2009;58(3):1–27.
32. Farrell GC, Larter CZ. Nonalcoholic fatty liver disease: from steatosis to cirrhosis. Hepatology 2006;43(2 Suppl 1):S99–S112.

33. Browning JD, Szczepaniak LS, Dobbins R, Nuremberg P, Horton JD, Cohen JC, et al. Prevalence of hepatic steatosis in an urban population in the United States: impact of ethnicity. Hepatology 2004;40(6):1387–95.
34. Alander SW, Dowd MD, Bratton SL, Kearns GL. Pediatric acetaminophen overdose: risk factors associated with hepatocellular injury. Arch Pediatr Adolesc Med 2000;154 (4):346–50.
35. Lexi-Drugs®. Lexi-Comp, 2011 Jun 6.
36. Drugs for non-HIV viral infections. Treatment Guidelines 2007;5(59):59–70.
37. Ghany MG, Strader DB, Thomas DL, Seeff LB; American Association for the Study of Liver Diseases. Diagnosis, management, and treatment of hepatitis C: an update. Hepatology. 2009;49(4):1335–74.
38. Nobili V, Manco M, Devito R, Di Ciommo V, Comparcola D, Sartorelli MR, et al. Lifestyle intervention and antioxidant therapy in children with nonalcoholic fatty liver disease: a randomized, controlled trial. Hepatology 2008;48(1):119–28.
39. Oo YH, Hubscher SG, Adams DH. Autoimmune hepatitis: new paradigms in the pathogenesis, diagnosis, and management. Hepatol Int 2010;4(2):475–93.
40. Morinville VD, Barmada MM, Lowe ME. Increasing incidence of acute pancreatitis at an American pediatric tertiary care center: is greater awareness among physicians responsible? Pancreas 2010; 39(1):5–8.
41. Forsmark CE, Baillie J. AGA Institute Clinical Practice and Economics Committee; AGA Institute Governing Board. AGA Institute technical review on acute pancreatitis. Gastroenterology 2007;132(5):2022–44.
42. Uhl W, Büchler MW, Malfertheiner P, Beger HG, Adler G, Gaus W. A randomised, double blind, multicentre trial of octreotide in moderate to severe acute pancreatitis. Gut 1999;45(1):97–104.

6 Adolescent hematology

Renuka Gera, Elna Z. Saah, Anjali Pawar, Satheesh Chonat,
Ajovi B. Scott-Emuakpor, and Roshni Kulkarni

The most common nonmalignant blood disorders in adolescents include the various forms of cytopenias, anemias, bleeding and clotting disorders, and hemoglobinopathies. The public health impact of these disorders is enormous and recognition is important not only for prevention of complications but also for treatments to improve quality of life. Early recognition also provides an opportunity to address preconception care during adolescence and education. Management often requires comprehensive care that includes plans for transition of care to adults, especially in those disorders that are inherited. This chapter reviews the common nonmalignant hematologic disorders and pharmacologic approaches for treatment and prevention of complications (such as factor concentrate prophylaxis in hemophilia, use of hydroxyurea in sickle cell disease, and chelation therapy in hemoglobinopathies).

6.1 Anemia

Anemia is the most common hematologic problem seen in adolescence. The physiologic definition of anemia is a decrease in the oxygen-carrying capacity of the blood. However, for all practical purposes, anemia is defined as hemoglobin values two standard deviations below the mean. As the child matures and attains Tanner 4 maturation, the red blood cell (RBC) volume and the RBC mass reach adult normal values (1). In addition to Tanner stage, the hemoglobin values are also affected by race, gender, hereditary factors, and altitude (2). Hemoglobin values are lower in females (normal range 11.2–13.6g/dL) than males (normal range 11.5–14.8g/dL) and are also lower in African Americans than Caucasians. The normal values are procedure-dependent. Consult with a lab for the normal value. Adolescents with chronic hypoxic cardiopulmonary conditions have higher hemoglobin and show symptoms of anemia at a higher hemoglobin level.

6.1.1 Mechanism of anemia

Erythropoiesis is a very tightly regulated process. Erythropoietin, one of the RBC growth factors, is produced by the kidney and plays a critical role in the proliferation and maturation of RBCs. Under physiologic conditions RBCs endowed with hemoglobin are released in the circulation as reticulocytes. Reticulocytes take 1 day in the peripheral circulation to mature to RBCs. The normal life span of a mature RBC is 120 days. Senescent RBCs are removed from the circulation by reticuloendothelial cells in the spleen and other organs. A delicate balance between RBC production and normal senescence maintains normal hemoglobin and oxygen delivery. Normal hematopoietic progenitors have tremendous ability to compensate for the loss of RBCs provided that there is an adequate supply of nutrients such as iron, B12, and folic acid. Failure of the bone marrow to respond to blood loss, either owing to normal senescence or other pathologic processes, results in an imbalance leading to anemia (3).

The reticulocyte count is a good measure of RBC kinetics, the bone marrow's ability to produce RBCs. Most routine laboratories use a hematology analyzer and report an absolute reticulocyte count. Anemia associated with an increase in the absolute reticulocyte count is the result of increased RBC destruction; whereas a low or normal reticulocyte count in a patient with anemia is suggestive of decreased RBC production. A comprehensive classification of anemia (▶Tab. 6.1) uses this RBC kinetics.

Reticulocyte count is not part of a routine complete blood count (CBC). Most laboratories will do a reticulocyte count on the blood drawn for a CBC if the test is requested within the first 24 hours of blood draw. RBC indices such as mean corpuscular volume (MCV), mean corpuscular hemoglobin concentration (MCHC), and RBC distribution width (RDW) are part of a CBC and are used to classify anemia based on MCV (▶Tab. 6.2).

Tab. 6.1: Classification of anemia based on RBC production.

A. Anemia due to decreased RBC production (normal to decreased reticulocyte count)

    1. Bone marrow failure

        a. Aplastic anemia

           • Acquired aplastic anemia

           • Inherited bone marrow failure syndrome: Fanconi's anemia, congenital dyskeratosis

        b. Pure RBC aplasia

           • Acquired: parvovirus infection, autoimmune pure RBC aplasia

           • Inherited: Diamond-Blackfan syndrome

        c. Bone marrow replacement

           • Leukemia

           • Myelodysplastic syndrome

           • Metastatic tumors

    2. Decreased erythropoietin production

        • Chronic renal failure

        • Chronic inflammation

        • Hypothyroidism

        • Malnutrition: anorexia nervosa

B. Anemia due to inefficient production

    1. Abnormal RBC cytoplasm maturation

        • Iron deficiency

        • Thalassemia

        • Lead poisoning

        • Sideroblastic anemia

(Continued)

Tab. 6.1: Classification of anemia based on RBC production. (*Continued*)

   2. Abnormal nuclear maturation (megaloblastic anemia)

      • B12 deficiency

      • Folic acid deficiency

      • Antineoplastic agents

      • Orotic aciduria

   3. Erythropoietic protoporphyria

   4. Dyserythropoietic anemia

C. Anemia due to increased RBC destruction (increased reticulocyte count), hemolytic anemia

   1. Acquired

      • Autoimmune hemolytic anemia

      • Mechanical injury

      • Thermal injury

   2. Congenital

      • Thalassemia

      • Hemoglobinopathies

      • Hereditary spherocytosis

      • Hereditary elliptocytosis

      • G6PD* deficiency

      • Pyruvate kinase deficiency

*glucose-6-phosphate dehydrogenase.

Tab. 6.2: Classification of anemia based on MCV.

Microcytic anemia	Normocytic anemia	Macrocytic anemia
1. Iron deficiency	1. Bone marrow failure	1. B12 deficiency
a. Nutritional	2. Hemolytic anemia	2. Folic acid deficiency
b. Blood loss	a. Acquired	3. Antineoplastic drugs
• Gastrointestinal	• Immune	4. Hypothyroidism
• Pulmonary	• Thermal or mechanical	5. Liver disease
• Menorrhagia	injury	6. Diamond-Blackfan syndrome
• Epistaxis	b. Congenital	7. Down's syndrome
2. Thalassemia	• Hemoglobinopathies	8. Valproic acid
3. Hemoglobin E disease	• Hereditary spherocytosis	
4. Hemoglobin C disease	• Hereditary elliptocytosis	
5. Chronic inflammation/	• G6PD deficiency	
infection	• Pyruvate kinase deficiency	
6. Chronic renal failure	3. Acute blood loss	
7. Sideroblastic anemia	4. Splenic sequestration	

Although the classification of anemia based on RBC kinetics provides a better understanding of the underlying process, the classification based on RBC indices is easier to apply in a clinical setting. Review of peripheral smear provides very useful information regarding RBC morphology and may help establish the diagnosis. Peripheral smear is not part of a routine CBC. Indications for peripheral smear are listed in the following box. In cases of normocytic anemia with low reticulocyte count or macrocytic anemia, a bone marrow evaluation is required to establish the diagnosis.

Clinical Indications for evaluation of a peripheral smear

1. Jaundice
2. Pallor
3. Hepatomegaly
4. Splenomegaly
5. Toxic patients
6. Malaria

6.1.2 Clinical evaluation

Anemia either is primary or often is a part of another systemic process. Anemia may cause fatigue or decreased exercise tolerance. The complaints may be as vague as not being able to perform well, excess sleeping, and palpitation, but they may also be major symptoms caused by the underlying disease. Nutritional history is a valuable part of the evaluation. Adolescent diets often lack nutrients such as iron to meet increased demands placed by increased growth velocity. Menorrhagia is an important cause of anemia in adolescent girls. Teen pregnancy may further complicate the picture. Past history of jaundice may be relevant in cases of congenital hemolytic anemias. Drugs may either cause bone marrow suppression or trigger an immune hemolysis. History of either prescription or nonprescription medication use is a crucial part of evaluation. Ethnicity and family history of anemia, cholelithiasis, cholecystectomy and splenectomy should be obtained as it may indicate a hemoglobinopathy or a hemolytic disease. Important aspects of history, physical examination, and laboratory evaluation are highlighted in ▶Tab. 6.3.

6.1.3 Causes of Anemia

Iron deficiency

Iron deficiency is the most important cause of anemia in all age groups. Iron is a part of many proteins and enzymes. Two thirds of the iron in the body is in hemoglobin and 15 percent is in the muscle as myoglobin. The average diet in developed countries provides 10 to 15 mg of elemental iron daily. On average 1 to 2 mg of iron is absorbed daily to compensate for 1 mg of daily nonmenstrual iron loss. This places adolescent girls at very high risk for iron deficiency. Nine percent of adolescent girls are iron deficient and 2 percent are anemic. Iron deficiency is also common among athletes (4).

Iron from nonheme food sources is absorbed in the duodenum in ferrous (Fe2) form. Only a small portion taken up by enterocytes enters the portal circulation at both the apical and basolateral membrane. This process is regulated by a peptide hormone called

Tab. 6.3: Clinical evaluation.

History

1. Symptoms: pallor, jaundice, fever, weight loss, aches, pains, GI blood loss, hematochezia, melena, epistaxis, menorrhagia, hemoptysis, hematuria, underlying chronic illness
2. Dietary history: vegan diet
3. Family history: anemia, cholelithiasis, jaundice, splenomegaly or splenectomy
4. Race and ethnicity

Physical examination

1. Height and weight
2. Skin and conjunctivae: pallor
3. Sclerae: icterus
4. Mouth: glossitis
5. Lymph nodes
6. Cardiovascular system: tachycardia, murmur
7. Abdomen: hepatosplenomegaly
8. Skin: hyperpigmentation, vascular malformation

Laboratory evaluation

- Screening test: CBC and reticulocyte count
- Specific test: Iron studies, stool for blood, hemoglobin electrophoresis, B12, folate, direct antiglobin test (DAT), and bone marrow evaluation if indicated

hepcidin. An increased level of hepcidin plays a role in the pathogenesis of anemia of inflammation (5). Iron failing to enter the blood is lost from the body when the senescent enterocytes are sloughed into the gut lumen. Iron absorption is affected by other substances in the diet. Whereas ascorbic acid improves the absorption, tannins found in tea, phytates, phosphates, antacids, and competing metals such as zinc decrease iron absorption. Heme iron is absorbed through a distinct pathway and appears to be more efficient and less sensitive to regulatory mechanisms such as hepcidin. Causes of iron deficiency are listed in ▶Tab. 6.4.

Laboratory diagnosis

Iron-deficiency anemia is the most common cause of microcytic anemia. Other causes of microcytic anemia are listed in ▶Tab. 6.5. Laboratory tests to evaluate iron status include serum ferritin, total iron-binding capacity (TIBC), transferrin saturation, free erythrocyte porphyrins (FEPs), and soluble transferrin receptors (sTfRs). There is no single reliable laboratory test for iron deficiency. Serum ferritin, a storage form of iron, is usually low. Ferritin is an acute-phase reactant and may be elevated in patients with infection or inflammation. C-reactive protein (CRP) with ferritin is measured to evaluate for inflammation. TIBC is usually elevated; transferrin saturation index (serum iron/TIBC) × 100 is low, and FEP is elevated. sTfR and

Tab. 6.4: Causes of iron deficiency.

Increased iron requirement

1. Growth
2. Pregnancy and lactation
3. Blood loss
    a. Genitourinary tract: menorrhagia, hemoglobinuria
    b. Pulmonary : hemoptysis, pulmonary hemosiderosis
    c. Gastrointestinal tract: inflammatory bowel disease, Meckel's diverticulum, peptic ulcer disease

Inadequate iron supply

1. Nutritional deficiency
2. Iron malabsorption
3. Gastric surgery
4. Chronic illness

Tab. 6.5: Causes of microcytic anemia.

Common

1. Iron deficiency
2. Thalassemia trait (alpha or beta thalassemia)

Less common

1. Anemia of chronic illness (inflammation, renal failure)
2. Hemoglobinopathy (hemoglobin E or C disease)
3. Thalassemia, intermedia and major
4. Lead toxicity
5. Sideroblastic anemia

reticulocyte hemoglobin concentration (CHr) are new tests for the diagnosis of iron deficiency.

Transferrin receptor is a cell membrane intrinsic protein that binds transferrin and facilitates the delivery of iron into the cell. Cells deficient in iron express more sTfR to maximize iron delivery to the cell. sTfR is elevated in iron deficiency but not in anemia of inflammation. CHr in iron-deficient reticulocyte decreases before anemia develops. The test is done by flow cytometry, and many autoanalyzers used by laboratories for CBC can do CHr. Hemoglobin electrophoresis done after a trial of iron therapy will help differentiate iron deficiency from beta thalassemia trait. A combination of these tests helps differentiate between other causes of microcytic anemia (▶Tab. 6.6). Evaluation of bone marrow iron stores, although reliable, is not routinely recommended.

Anemia, microcytosis, decreased MCH, decreased RBC count, decreased reticulocyte count, increased platelet count, increased RDW, normal WBC count, and Mentzer index (MCV/RBC) greater than 13 are consistent with a diagnosis of iron-deficiency anemia. For an asymptomatic adolescent with a typical history of iron-deficient diet

Tab. 6.6: Laboratory profiles of microcytic anemia.

Test	Iron deficiency	Beta thalassemia trait	Chronic illness
MCV	↓	↓	↓
RBC count	↓	↑	↓
Mentzer index MCV/RBC	>13	<13	<13
Platelet count	↑	N	N
Ferritin	↓	N	↑
Transferrin saturation (Serum iron/TIBC) × 100	<16	N	<16
Soluble transferrin receptors	↑	NA	N↓
Hemoglobin electrophoresis	N	↑HbA2 and ±HbF	N
C-reactive protein	N	N	↑

MCV, mean corpuscular volume; N, normal; TIBC, total iron-binding capacity, HbA2, hemoglobin A2; HbF, fetal hemoglobin.

or blood loss, additional laboratory tests may not be necessary. Iron replacement therapy should be started with oral ferrous salt providing 150 to 200 mg of elemental iron given in two to three divided doses daily. To ensure adequate iron absorption, the iron should be taken with a juice that has a high ascorbic acid content and should not be taken with meals.

A reticulocyte response is usually observed in 72 hours. An increase of 2g/dL in hemoglobin level after 3 weeks of replacement therapy is considered a therapeutic response and is the most definitive evidence of iron deficiency. A sustained increase in hemoglobin is maintained until the hemoglobin normalizes. Tests to document the source of blood loss should be done. Symptomatic patients with severe anemia, conflicting CBC results, or failure of response to a trial of iron need further laboratory evaluation.

Treatment

The majority of patients with iron deficiency can be treated with oral iron. There is very little difference in the acceptability, response rates, and side-effect profile of various iron salts (▶Tab. 6.7). Juices containing vitamin C can enhance the absorption of iron. Nutritional counseling, consumption of iron-rich foods such as meats, and iron-fortified cereals is desirable. Iron treatment should be continued for 2 to 3 months after the hemoglobin normalizes provided that the underlying cause has resolved. Oral iron is well tolerated by the majority of patients. A small number of patients complain of nausea or abdominal discomfort. These symptoms can usually be managed by reducing the dose or giving iron with meals. Patients with severe GI discomfort may tolerate a single nighttime dose. Sustained-release iron preparation or more expensive polysaccharide complexes have not proven to be superior.

Parenteral iron preparations are used to treat patients with severe iron deficiency, iron malabsorption, or ongoing blood losses and those on dialysis. Parenteral preparations may cause life-threatening anaphylaxis. Serum sickness including fever, urticaria,

Tab. 6.7: Oral iron preparations.

Preparation	Elemental iron (%)	Usual tablet size (mg)	Amount of elemental iron/tablet	Absorption	Side effects
Ferrous sulfate	20	325	65	+ + +	+
Ferrous gluconate	12	300	36	+ + +	+
Ferrous fumarate	33	200	66	+ + +	+
Iron carbonyl	100	15	15	+ +	+ −
Iron polysaccharide	100	150	150	+ +	+ −

Tab. 6.8: Parenteral iron preparations.

	Iron dextran	Iron sucrose	Sodium ferric gluconate
Test dose	Indicated	Physician discretion	Physician discretion
Serious anaphylaxis	0.6%–0.7%	0.002%	0.04%
Hypersensitivity rate	0.2%–3%	0.005%	0.4%
Bioavailability	+	+ +	+ +
Administration	IM/IV	IV	IV
Concentration	50 mg/mL	20 mg/mL	12.5 mg/mL

myalgia, and arthralgia may develop in some patients. Iron dextran was the only preparation available in the past. New parenteral iron preparations such as iron sucrose and iron gluconate (▶Tab. 6.8) pose a lower risk of hypersensitivity reactions and other side effects (6). The total dose of iron to correct the anemia is calculated. Iron dextran total dose can be administered as single dose. For iron sucrose and gluconate the total is divided into three or four doses and administered over 3 to 7 days.

Megaloblastic anemia

Megaloblastic anemia is a macrocytic anemia, resulting from a global problem of DNA synthesis and affecting all proliferating cells. All three hematopoietic cell lines – white cells, RBCs, and platelets – are affected. Defective DNA synthesis in RBC precursors results in asynchrony between nuclear and cytoplasmic maturation and apoptosis. The bone marrow is hypercellular but the cells undergo apoptosis before they are released into the circulation; this ineffective hematopoiesis causes anemia, leukopenia, thrombocytopenia, and elevated levels of lactate dehydrogenase and bilirubin. Folate and B12 deficiency are two major causes of megaloblastic anemia.

Folic acid deficiency

Folic acid (folate) deficiency is the second most common micronutrient deficiency after iron deficiency. The daily folate requirement for an adolescent is 3 µg/kg per day.

A variety of food sources such as cereal, bread, fruits, vegetables, meats, and fish contain folates. Liver, kidney, orange juice, and spinach are very rich sources of folate. Nutritional deficiency in adolescence is due to diet fads, slimming diets, or chronic debilitating conditions. Folic acid malabsorption in patients with tropical and nontropical sprue, poor nutrition during periods of increased requirements such as pregnancy and lactation, hemolytic anemia such as thalassemia or sickle cell disease, or medications such as trimethoprim, pyrimethamine, or phenytoin may also cause folic acid deficiency. Megaloblastic anemia, low serum folate level, and response to 5 mg of oral folic acid daily is consistent with a diagnosis of folic acid deficiency. Treatment consists of nutritional counseling and a daily dose of 1 mg folic acid given orally. Patients with malabsorption need 5 mg of folic acid daily.

B12 (cobalamin) deficiency

Vitamin B12 is essential for cell growth and myelin synthesis. Animal proteins are a major source of cobalamin. The daily cobalamin requirement is 1 to 3 µg. B12 is absorbed in the ileum. Intrinsic factor is required for B12 absorption. An average western nonvegetarian diet contains 5 to 7 µg of cobalamin daily. A vegetarian diet supplies 0.2 to 0.5 µg of cobalamin daily. Most vegetarians are at higher risk for cobalamin deficiency. Cobalamin in the diet binds with intrinsic factor and is absorbed in the ileum. Causes of cobalamin deficiency include vegetarian diet, gastrectomy, regional ileitis (Crohn's disease), tropical and nontropical sprue, and resection of the small bowel. Pernicious anemia is an autoimmune condition and is rare in children and adolescents. Megaloblastic anemia, low serum cobalamin level, elevated methylmalonic acid, and response to B12 administration are diagnostic of cobalamin deficiency. Neurologic complications of cobalamin deficiency may precede anemia.

Parenteral cyanocobalamin is rapidly absorbed from site of intramuscular or subcutaneous injection. It is bound to plasma proteins and stored in the liver. It also undergoes enterohepatic recycling. Anemia and gastrointestinal symptoms completely respond to parenteral B12 administration. Improvement in neurologic symptoms depends onthe duration and severity of the deficiency. Cyanocobalamin nasal spray 500 µg per spay is available for the maintenance of normal hematologic status in patients with pernicious anemia who do not have any neurologic symptoms. One spray in each nostril once a week will maintain normal hematologic status.

Aplastic anemia

Aplastic anemia is a disease of the young. Most patients present between 15 and 25 years of age. The incidence of aplastic anemia is higher in developing countries. Aplastic anemia is defined as peripheral blood pancytopenia. A combination of normocytic normochromic anemia with reticulocytopenia, leukopenia, neutropenia, thrombocytopenia, and hypoplastic bone marrow is the hallmark of this disease. The degree of involvement of these cell lines may vary. The bone marrow failure may be due to inherited causes such as Fanconi's anemia or dyskeratosis congenita or it may be secondary to bone marrow suppression caused by radiation, cytotoxic drugs, benzene, or gold and other heavy metals. Sometimes an idiosyncratic bone marrow response to a drug, such as chloramphenicol, or to infectious hepatitis may cause aplastic anemia. Most cases of acquired aplastic anemia, however, are idiopathic. Idiopathic aplastic anemia is an immune-mediated disease. Immune dysregulation causes T-cell activation and destruction of hematopoietic progenitors.

The clinical presentation is variable. Most patients present with various degrees of bleeding symptoms. Thrombocytopenia usually causes easy bruising, petechiae, and mucosal bleeding from the mouth, nose, or gastrointestinal or genitourinary tracts. Life-threatening bleeding usually does not occur until late in the disease. Fatigue, lassitude, and decreased exercise tolerance is common. Infections and sore throat due to severe neutropenia are unusual at the time of presentation. Physical examination shows pallor, bruises, and ecchymosis or petechiae. Scleral icterus, lymphadenopathy and hepatosplenomegaly are absent. Liver function, renal function, and electrolytes are normal. The bone marrow aspiration and biopsy show hypoplasia and replacement by fat cells. Immune phenotype and bone marrow cytogenetics are usually normal.

Treatment

Allogeneic hematopoietic stem cell transplantation from HLA-matched sibling donor cures the majority of patients (7). A patient with a sibling donor should proceed to transplant without delay. Judicious use of transfusions and supportive therapy while waiting for a transplant is recommended. Some patients with congenital bone marrow failure syndrome may present in adolescence with symptoms of aplastic anemia. Since these diagnoses have therapeutic implications, it is imperative to test the patient for these conditions before definitive treatment with bone marrow transplant and/or immune suppression is started. The majority of patients, however, do not have HLA-matched donors. Immune suppression with antithymocyte globulin (ATG) and cyclosporine is the combination most often used. Horse ATG was used in the past. Rabbit ATG has recently been approved for use in the United States. Methyl prednisolone is used to decrease allergic reactions and serum sickness caused by ATG. Long-term disease-free survival is seen in 70 percent of patients treated with immune suppression. Patients failing to respond to immune suppression are candidates for bone marrow transplant from HLA-matched unrelated donors.

Hemolytic anemia

Hemolytic anemia is characterized by shortened RBC survival. The bone marrow tries to compensate by increasing the production of RBCs, thus elevating the reticulocyte count. Hemolytic anemia usually presents with the triad of anemia, reticulocytosis, and a variable degree of jaundice. Some patients may also have splenomegaly or hemoglobinuria. Lactic dehydrogenase (LDH) is elevated and haptoglobin decreased. Shortened RBC survival could be a result of inherited defects in the cell membrane, RBC enzyme, hemoglobin synthesis, or some acquired conditions. The most common cause of acquired hemolytic anemia is immune-mediated RBC destruction and a direct anti globulin test (DAT), also known as direct Coomb's test, is positive in such cases. Evaluation of an adolescent with hemolysis is shown in ▶Fig. 6.1.

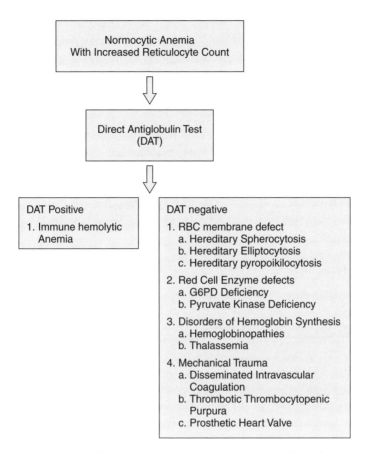

Fig. 6.1: Algorithm for the evaluation of an adolescent with suspected hemolytic anemia.

Immune hemolytic anemia

Immune-mediated hemolytic anemia in adolescence is often autoimmune in nature, hence the name autoimmune hemolytic anemia (AIHA). Anemia is the only abnormality in primary immune hemolytic anemia. Secondary immune hemolytic anemia is part of a multisystem immune process. In most cases of AIHA the autoantibody is IgG and reacts with RBCs at a warm temperature (37°C). Antibody-coated RBCs are cleared by the reticuloendothelial system and anemia ensues. In some cases the IgG binds to RBC membranes at a cold temperature and then activates complement. This complement-mediated hemolysis is intravascular and is associated with hemoglobinuria and called paroxysmal cold hemoglobinuria (PCH).

The third type of primary AIHA is caused by IgM antibodies that react with the RBCs at cold temperatures (below 37°C). Secondary AIHA is seen in the presence of other autoimmune disorders, malignancy, or infections. Drugs such as penicillins, cephalosporins, erythromycin, and tetracyclines may also cause drug induced hemolytic anemia. Although most patients present with symptoms of pallor, fatigue, and occasional jaundice, the hemolysis in AIHA is very rapid and may result in cardiorespiratory collapse.

The patients usually present with significant normocytic normochromic anemia, hemoglobin that ranges between 4 and 7 g/dL, and an elevated reticulocyte count. Several spherocytes are present in warm reacting AIHA, mimicking spherocytosis. Serum haptoglobin is low and LDH elevated. The most important test for the diagnosis of AIHA is the DAT, which demonstrates the presence of antibodies and/or a complement component on the RBCs' surface.

Treatment depends on severity or rapidity of hemolysis. Patients with mild anemia (hemoglobin 9–12 g/dL) may be observed closely. Patients with more severe anemia and rapidly falling hemoglobins need immediate therapy consisting of a packed RBC transfusion to maintain hemoglobin at 6 to 8 g/dL and corticosteroid (prednisone or methyl prednisolone) 1 to 2 mg/kg per day every 6 hours. It is often difficult to type and cross match a patient's antibody-coated RBCs. Some patients may respond to intravenous immune globulin (IVIG). In the case of drug-induced hemolysis, the offending agent should be removed.

Hereditary spherocytosis

Hereditary spherocytosis (HS) affects all races and ethnic groups. It is particularly common in people of northern European descent and is the leading cause of congenital hemolytic anemia. The mode of inheritance is autosomal dominant in 75 percent of the cases, while 25 percent are either new mutations or autosomal recessive. Molecular abnormalities responsible for defects have been well described. They involve mutations in the genes that code for RBC membrane proteins, spectrin, ankyrin, or band 3. A defect in one of these proteins results in the loss of RBC membrane integrity. As a result the cells become spherical and are prematurely destroyed in the spleen. Anemia, jaundice, splenomegaly, and a positive family history are present in the majority of cases.

Most patients with HS present in infancy or early childhood. Occasionally the diagnosis, especially when there is no family history, is delayed until adolescence, when the patient presents with abdominal pain due to splenomegaly or cholelithiasis. Patients with HS are at high risk for cholelithiasis due to high RBC turnover. Viral infections, especially parvovirus infection, may result in decreased RBC production and aplastic crisis. A complete blood count (CBC) will show normocytic normochromic anemia. The mean corpuscular hemoglobin concentration (MCHC) and reticulocyte count are elevated and spherocytes are seen on peripheral smear. Differential diagnosis includes other causes of spherocytosis (see ▶Tab. 6.9).

Tab. 6.9: Causes of spherocytosis.

1. Hereditary spherocytosis
2. Immune hemolytic anemia
   • ABO and Rh incompatibility
   • Autoimmune hemolytic anemia
3. Damage to RBC membrane
   • Burn
   • Clostridial toxins
   • Wilson's disease

The DAT is negative and helps to differentiate between HS and immune hemolytic anemia. Increased osmotic fragility on fresh and incubated blood confirms the diagnosis.

Management depends on clinical severity. Occasionally anemia is severe enough to require the transfusion of packed RBCs by age 6 to 12 weeks. Folic acid supplementation, 1 mg daily, is helpful. Baseline hemoglobin, reticulocyte count, and bilirubin should be monitored and repeated if the patient has a viral infection or appears tired. Hemoglobin may drop to 50 percent of baseline during aplastic crisis and the patient may require packed RBC transfusion. Splenectomy although curative, is recommended for moderate to severe disease. Prior to splenectomy the patient should receive *Haemophilus influenzae*, 23-valent *Streptococcuspneumoniae*, and *Neisseria meningitides* vaccines. Penicillin prophylaxis following splenectomy is recommended.

RBC enzyme deficiency

Adenosine triphosphate (ATP) generated by glycolytic pathways in erythrocytes is necessary to meet the energy requirement of RBCs. The mature erythrocyte is endowed with an adequate amount of glycolytic enzymes to last for the life of the RBC. Deficiency of any of these enzymes could result in shortened RBC survival and hemolysis. Glycolytic enzyme deficiencies with the exception of glucose-6-phosphate dehydrogenase (G6PD) and pyruvate kinase (PK) deficiencies are rare.

Glucose-6 phosphate dehydrogenase (G6PD) deficiency is an X-linked anemia usually seen in males of Mediterranean or African ancestry. Most patients usually have normal baseline hemoglobins and do not have any evidence of hemolysis. When the patient is challenged by exogenous agents (▶Tab. 6.10 offers a partial list), hemolysis and anemia develop (4). G6PD-deficient RBCs are unable to generate enough "reduced" nicotinamide adenine dinucleotide phosphate (NADPH). NADPH is closely

Tab. 6.10: Factors causing hemolysis in G6PD deficiency.

1. Food
   - Fava beans
2. Analgesics
   - Aspirin
3. Antibacterial agents
   - Sulfonamides and sulfones
   - Nitrofurantoin
4. Antimalarials
   - Primaquine
5. Miscellaneous
   - Vitamin K analogues
   - Naphthalene
   - Dimercaprol
   - Methylene blue
6. Infections

related to glutathione metabolism. Glutathione protects the cells from oxidative damage. Since RBCs carry oxygen, they are at very high risk for damage by oxygen radicals. The inability of G6PD-deficient RBCs to sustain reduced glutathione when exposed to oxidative stress results in oxidative damage to hemoglobin. The hemoglobin is precipitated as Heinz bodies. Heinz bodies damage the RBC membrane, resulting in hemolysis.

Patients with hemolysis on exposure to oxidative stress present with anemia, hemoglobinuria (tea-colored urine), jaundice, and bite cells on peripheral smear. Chronic anemia due to G6PD deficiency is rare. The diagnosis is confirmed by G6PD assay done on RBCs. Patients with high reticulocyte counts may have G6PD levels in the normal range and will need a repeat assay after the hemoglobin level normalizes.

The treatment is supportive and consists of removal of offending agents and cardiovascular stabilization with fluids and transfusion of packed RBCs if necessary. A list of offending agents should be given to these patients.

Pyruvate kinase deficiency

Pyruvate kinase deficiency is the most common glycolytic enzyme deficiency associated with anemia. Most patients are of northern European origin. Sporadic cases are seen in other ethnic groups. Inheritance of PK deficiency is autosomal recessive. Homozygous PK deficiency results in anemia, reticulocytosis, and jaundice. The clinical severity is variable from severe anemia presenting in utero or at birth to relatively minor anemia that is not discovered until adolescence. Spiculated erythrocytes and acanthocytes are seen on peripheral smear. Occasionally jaundice is the only clinical abnormality. Heterozygous PK deficiency may result in mild hemolysis. Cholelithiasis is common and leg ulcers may develop. There is little correlation between the severity of anemia and erythrocyte pyruvate kinase level. Patients with severe anemia require repeated transfusions. Splenectomy may eliminate or decrease the need for transfusions and is reserved for patients with transfusion-dependent anemia.

6.2 Hemoglobinopathies

Hemoglobinopathies are a group genetic disorders of globin (polypeptide) chain synthesis. The inheritance of each of these disorders is autosomal recessive. Each hemoglobin molecule has an alpha chain coded by two gene loci on chromosome 16 and a beta chain coded by a single gene on chromosome 11. These disorders can be either qualitative, resulting in synthesis of abnormal hemoglobin such as sickle hemoglobin (HbS), or quantitative, resulting in a decrease in globin chains as is seen in thalassemias.

6.2.1 Sickle cell disease (SCD)

Sickle cell disease is a clinicopathologic syndrome resulting from the inheritance of two abnormal beta chains, one of which must be the "sickle (ßS)." Sickle cell gene mutation is the substitution of an amino acid, valine, for glutamic acid on position 6 of beta globin (8). Sickle hemoglobin under conditions of hypoxia polymerizes and the RBC assumes a sickle shape, which can cause it to obstruct the blood flow in small blood vessels. This produces a wide spectrum of severity of disease, the hallmarks being a hemolytic anemia and painful vaso-occlusive crisis. Other major features are susceptibility to infection and chronic organ damage in older patients. A patient can be homozygous when both beta chains have this substitution (SS) or compound heterozygotes, which occurs when the patient has a sickle cell mutation in association with another mutation on a corresponding beta-chain gene, as in beta thalassemia or hemoglobin C disease. Hemoglobin SS, SC and sickle/beta-thalassemia are the major types of sickle cell disease.

Treatment of sickle cell disease

Occlusion of the blood vessels caused by sickle cells may cause repeated episodes of severe pain, infection due to poor splenic function, stroke, acute chest syndrome, pulmonary hypertension, and renal failure. With the recognition of infection as a cause of early mortality, the institution (in developed countries) of newborn screening, penicillin prophylaxis, and prompt antibiotic therapy when infection is suspected have significantly improved survival. The pharmacologic management of acute and chronic pain in these patients improves the quality of life. A disease-modifying agent, hydroxyurea, decreases not only the episodes of pain but also other SCD-related morbidities. Chelation therapy is the treatment for iron overload caused by repeated RBC transfusions.

Treatment of pain in SCD

The hallmark of SCD is the acute painful episode or vaso-occlusive crisis. The onset of pain is sudden and unpredictable and the locations are variable. Pain crisis is the most common cause for truancy and hospitalization. An increase in the frequency of pain crises during adolescence is common. Inadequate assessment of pain and physicians' discomfort with narcotic analgesics are major barriers to adequate pain control. Management of both acute and chronic pain indirectly affects the patient's overall well-being and functional capacity.

Analgesics form the backbone of SCD-related pain management. Anxiolytics and sedatives should be used in conjunction and never alone since they mask but do not eliminate pain.

For acute pain, a home trial of nonsteroidal anti-inflammatory drugs (NSAIDs; e.g., ibuprofen) and oral opioid analgesics such as acetaminophen/codeine/hydrocodone/oxycodone are recommended, with liberal fluid intake (9). Following the failure of such a home regimen, patients may require parenteral NSAIDs and narcotic analgesics. Along with parenteral administration comes the clinical responsibility of frequent reassessment and retitration accordingly, thereby decreasing the risk of cardiorespiratory complications of parenteral narcotics.

Treatment of chronic pain

As these patients age, chronic pain lasting for greater than 3 to 6 months becomes increasingly common. Avascular necrosis, arthropathies, arthritis, vertebral collapse, and chronic leg ulcers are some of the causes of chronic pain. Severe arthritis requiring joint replacement in adolescence is not uncommon. Even more confounding is that acute pain episodes superimposed on chronic pain continue to occur, resulting in a mixed picture. Combinations of the oral agents listed above are employed to maintain acceptable pain control and function. Usually a long-acting (sustained-release) agent is used twice daily in combination with a short-acting immediate release agent on an as-needed basis for breakthrough pain. Comorbidities such as depression and neuropathy also have to be addressed.

Managing chronic pain usually requires a multidisciplinary approach including social workers, psychologists and psychiatrists, surgeons, and pain specialists and is clearly beyond the scope of this text. The major barrier to optimizing sickle cell pain management is the general lack of knowledge, and hence fears, of opioid tolerance, dependence, and addiction issues. Tolerance and dependence are both physiologic responses to exogenous opioid exposure, whereas addiction is a complex psychological dependence. Patients with SCD have not been known to have a higher opioid addiction tendency than the general population and therefore should not be denied adequate, safe analgesia.

Disease-modifying agents: hydroxyurea

Following the pivotal adult multicenter study of hydroxyurea in 1995 (10), it has become the standard of care (see chapter 13). Adolescents with moderate to severe homozygous sickle cell disease (SS) and compound heterozygotes, with the genotype Sß°, are candidates for treatment with hydroxyurea.

The mechanism of hydroxyurea in SCD has not been fully delineated. Elevated fetal hemoglobin is associated with a decrease in RBC polymerization and hence reduction in painful crises and progression of organ dysfunction. Hydroxyurea was initially used for its effect in raising fetal hemoglobin in the RBC. A low count of white blood cells (particularly neutrophils) and reticulocytes caused by hydroxyurea may further decrease adhesiveness and episodes vaso-occlusion and thus decrease sickle cell (WBC)–related morbidities.

Hydroxyurea is given orally once a day as a capsule (at a dose of 20–30 mg/kg) and titrated to effect and tolerable myelosuppressive parameters. The effect is seen within a few days as the WBC counts begin to drop and fetal hemoglobin rises (11). The side effects include (a) GI upset, such as nausea; (b) myelosuppression with a low enough absolute neutrophil count and platelets that may warrant interruption of dose; and (c) some degree of hair loss, which patients find very undesirable.The causes of greatest apprehension are the potential for teratogenicity and risk of secondary malignancies. Hence there are strict guidelines for initiation of its use and for monitoring its effect. Use of effective contraception while on hydroxyurea is of utmost importance in pubertal adolescents.

Iron overload

Acute or chronic RBC transfusions are used to either prevent or treat sickle cell–related complications. Chronic transfusion is used for the primary or secondary prevention of stroke. Following a study of stroke prevention in patients with abnormal transcranial Doppler scans (12), prophylactic chronic transfusions have become standard. Furthermore, follow up of the STOP study (13) did not reveal an endpoint where discontinuation of transfusions could be safe. Iron overload is becoming increasingly a challenge in this population. Chelation, parenteral and oral, is the only modality for the elimination of iron in these patients. The agents used for this purpose are discussed further in the following section on thalassemia.

6.2.2 Thalassemia

The human adult hemoglobin, designated A, is made up of tetramers of two alpha and two beta globin polypeptides (14). The thalassemias are a heterogenous group of inherited disorders resulting from mutations in either the alpha or beta globin gene, causing decreased or absent production of either alpha or beta chains. This imbalance between alpha and beta chain production causes premature RBC demise (ineffective erythropoiesis). The clinical spectrum is one of microcytosis, varying degrees of anemia, and the compensatory effects of ineffective erythropoiesis. The milder forms are asymptomatic and the severe forms are transfusion-dependent.

Of pharmacotherapeutic significance and for the purpose of this text, we discuss beta thalassemia major (severe beta thalassemia, or Cooley's anemia). Beta-thalassemia major results when there is significantly decreased or absent expression of the beta globin gene (B+ or B0). This condition presents after the fourth month of life, when the hemoglobin switch from fetal to adult is advanced, with severe transfusion-dependent anemia. Because, as stated earlier, there is no deficiency of alpha chains, the imbalance results in a compensatory ineffective erythropoiesis, which in addition leads to increased iron absorption from the GI tract. Hence there is evidence of extramedullary hematopoiesis (hepatosplenomegaly and bone marrow expansion), growth retardation, and endocrine disorders.

Chelation therapy

The mainstay of management in severe thalassemia is the transfusion of RBCs. Over the years the general practice has been that of hypertransfusion (15). Hypertransfusion to maintain a pretransfusion hemoglobin of 10 g/dL is recommended. Most patients start receiving regular transfusions by the age 6 months. The iron overload encountered in these patients is both transfusional and from increased GI iron absorption. Except in times of excess or repeated blood loss, humans have no intrinsic mechanism for iron excretion; therefore any excess must be chelated to prevent the cardiac, liver, and endocrine complications of iron overload (hemosiderosis). Lifelong compliance with oral or parenteral chelating agents can reduce the morbidity caused by transfusional iron overload and is the major determinant of long-term survival. Compliance with chelation during adolescence can be challenging. Chelation therapy is discussed below.

Deferoxamine: This parenteral iron chelator is very effective. It enters the cells, binds to iron, and is renally excreted. It can be given by the intramuscular, intravenous, or subcutaneous route 5 to 7 days a week. With time, the subcutaneous route has become preferred. The drug is administered overnight at home by the patient or caregiver. In noncompliant patients, intravenous administration may be used. The main complications arising are local reactions at the subcutaneous site of administration. Others include neuro- and ototoxicity (there may be a high-frequency hearing loss) (16).

Deferiprone: This was the first oral chelator to be used extensively; it is licensed in parts of Europe and Asia (but not in the United States). It must be taken by mouth thre times a day; the "chelator product" is excreted in the urine. The main side effects are GI disturbances and neutropenia (17).

Deferasirox: With the approval of deferasirox in the United States came much relief. Because of its longer half-life as compared with deferiprone, it is taken once a day. It comes as a large chalky tablet that must be dissolved in water or juice. Its chalky, gritty taste is the major cause of noncompliance. Other main side effects are GI disturbances and both renal toxicity and ototoxicity (18).

6.3 Disorders of neutrophils

Neutrophils are part of innate immunity and are the first line of defense against bacterial invasion. A decrease in the number of neutrophils or their abnormal function increase the risk of infection.

Neutropenia is defined as a decrease in absolute neutrophil count (ANC) below 1,500 (19,20). Some racial groups, such as African Americans, tend to have low-normal ANCs of 1,000 to 1,500 with no deleterious effects. The risk of infection is inversely proportional to the ANC. Based on the ANC, the classification of neutropenia is presented in ▶Tab. 6.11. Patients with severe neutropenia may not show classic signs of infection such as fever, warmth, swelling, or pus formation. Often, neutropenic patients are infected with endogenous flora of the skin and gut.

6.3.1 Mechanism

Neutropenia results from decreased neutrophil production, accelerated utilization, a shift in compartments of neutrophils, or a combination of these factors. Infections and myelosuppression are the major cause of neutropenia. Isolated neutropenia due to bone marrow failure or replacement by a malignant process such as leukemia or lymphoma is rare. ▶Tab. 6.12 shows the mechanism and treatment of common type of neutropenia caused by infection in this age group.

Secondary neutropenia can also be induced by drugs or toxins (▶Tab. 6.13). The duration of drug-induced neutropenia is variable. Idiosyncratic drug reactions usually last for a few days; occasionally they may last for months. Immune-mediated neutropenia usually resolves within 6 to 8 days after the drug is withdrawn. Rebound leukocytosis with immature cells in the peripheral blood can occur.

Tab. 6.11: Clinical classification of neutropenia.

ANC	Clinical severity	Risk of infection
1000–1500	Mild	Minimal
500–1000	Moderate	Mild
200–500	Severe	Moderate to severe Usually mucocutaneous infections
Less than 200	Very severe	Fatal sepsis, systemic infections Typhlitis

Tab. 6.12: Infections associated with neutropenia.

Condition	Mechanism	Causation	Signs and symptoms	Treatment
Infection-associated neutropenia	1. Increased utilization 2. Margination 3. Direct suppression of marrow	Viruses: EBV, CMV, influenza, RSV, HIV, Influenza, Hepatitis A & B, RSV Bacteria GNC sepsis, brucellosis, tularemia, typhoid Fungal: *Histoplasma* Rickettsia: Rocky Mountain spotted fever	Will have associated symptoms of infection	Treat the infection

CMV, cytomegalovirus; EBV, Ebstein-Barr virus; GNC, Gram-negative cocci; HIV, human immunodeficiency virus; RSV, respiratory syncytial virus.

Tab. 6.13: Drug-induced neutropenia.

Drug	Mechanism	Signs and symptoms	Treatment
Penicillin, cephalosporins	Acts as a hapten, induces immune reaction Antibody-positive	Acute symptoms, may recur with even small dose	Withdraw drug G-CSF if severe infection
Phenothiazine	Directly toxic to neutrophils	Insidious. May relapse after latent period	Rechallenge with high doses Eliminate toxins G-CSF if severe infection
Dilantin Phenobarbitone	Hypersensitivity	Insidious associated rash, fever	Withdraw drug G-CSF if severe infection

G-CSF, granulocyte colony-stimulating factor.

Neutropenia can also be seen as autoimmune phenomenon as part of systemic auto-immune process such as lupus, scleroderma, Felty's syndrome, Sjögren's syndrome, HIV, EBV and Hodgkin's disease or as an isolated process. The immune destruction is mediated via antibody. The autoantibody is usually targeted against neutrophil-specific cell-surface antigens. Daily administration of a small dose of G-CSF increases the absolute neutrophil count (ANC) to the normal range within 1 to 2 weeks.

Inherited neutropenia

Inherited or congenital neutropenia (▶Tab. 6.14) is rare but causes prolonged problems and is associated with a higher risk of infection-related morbidity and mortality. Most cases of inherited neutropenia are diagnosed early in childhood; however, milder

Tab. 6.14: Inherited neutropenia.

Condition	Inheritance/ defect	Mechanism	Clinical findings	Treatment	Comments
Kostman's syndrome	AR/HAX 1 mutation	Promyelocyte arrest	Severe neutropenia early in infancy Skin soft tissue infections, Gingivitis, Pneumonias	Aggressive antibiotic therapy G-CSF 3–100 µg/Kg	2.3% per year risk of MDS after 10 years of being on G-CSF (1) BMT for G-CSF–resistant cases Annual BM exam
Severe congenital neutropenia	AD or sporadic ELA2 mutation	Accelerated apoptosis	Same as Kostman's	Same as Kostman's	Same as Kostman's
Cyclic neutropenia	AD ELA2 mutation	Maturation arrest Increased apoptosis in precursors	Cycles of about 21 days Recurrent fevers, aphthous ulcers, odontitis	G-CSF 5 µg/kg daily or alternate day	Not preleukemic
Shwachman-Diamond syndrome	AR SBDS gene	*FAS-* associated apoptosis of precursors	Recurrent infections Pancreatic insufficiency Short stature	Pancreatic enzyme replacement G-CSF for severe infections	25% develop MDS, 25% develop marrow aplasia BMT for severe complications

AD, autosomal dominant; AR, autosomal recessive; BM, bone marrow; BMT, bone marrow transplant; G-CSF, granulocyte colony-stimulating factor; MDS, myelodysplastic syndrome.

cases can be missed until adolescence. Recombinant G-CSF, improvement in supportive care, early detection of infection and treatment has improved the survival as well as quality of life of these patients.

6.3.2 Management of neutropenia

General measures

1. Maintain good oral hygiene.
2. Promptly clean cuts, abrasions on skin surface with antiseptics.
3. Schedule regular dental cleaning.
4. Routine immunizations are encouraged unless neutropenia is a manifestation of an underlying immune disorder or the patient is immunodeficient.

5. Any fevers above 100.4°F (38°C) lasting more than 1 hour or a fever of 101°F should be promptly evaluated by a health care provider. If the source of fever is unclear after obtaining blood cultures, the patient should be started on prophylactic antibiotics. Those with severe neutropenia will require hospitalization and broad-spectrum antibiotics empirically. Fourth-generation cephalosporins or beta-lactam antibiotics along with an aminoglycoside are good choices. Because of risk of vancomycin resistance, its empiric use is controversial. The duration of antibiotic therapy will depend on the response to medication, culture results, and severity of neutropenia.

6.3.3 Specific treatment

G-CSF (filgrastim) is a human G-CSF. It is produced by recombinant technology. G-CSF stimulates granulocyte progenitor proliferation, differentiation, and selected cell function such as activation and phagocytic activity. There is a linear dose response. It is used to shorten the duration and severity of chemotherapy-induced neutropenia. The usual dose for chemotherapy-induced neutropenia is 5 µg/kg per day subcutaneously daily for 7 to 10 days. It can be given prophylactically multiple times a week to maintain the ANC over 1,000 in patients with non–chemotherapy induced neutropenia. The dose and frequency may be titrated between 1 and 5 µg/kg per day one to three times a week in patients with severe chronic neutropenia.

Patients with congenital severe neutropenia require a very high dose to maintain the ANC in a safe range. G-CSF use has improved the survival and quality of life of patients with congenital severe neutropenia. Common side effects are a mild flu-like illness as well as aches and pains. Acute respiratory distress has been reported. Prolonged use of G-CSF may cause splenomegaly. Splenic rupture has been reported. Patients with congenital neutropenia should be monitored for myelodysplastic syndromes and those who are being treated with G-CSF should be monitored for leukemias (21). Pegfilgrastim is a longer-acting G-CSF. It has been used for both chemotherapy-induced and congenital severe neutropenia.

Recombinant human granulocyte and macrophage colony stimulating factor (rhu GM-CSF) is prepared by recombinant technology in a yeast expression system. It is a hematopoietic growth factor and stimulates the proliferation as well as differentiation of hematopoietic progenitor cells along granulocyte macrophage cell lines. In addition, this is used in enhancing granulocyte macrophage reconstitution after autologous and allogeneic hematopoietic stem cell transplantation (HSCT). It is also used for mobilization and collection of hematopoietic cells for autologous HSCT (22).

6.4 Disorders of platelets

Platelets play a vital role in hemostasis. Disorders of platelet number and function both cause increased mucocutaneous bleeding. A decrease in the number or function of platelets results in superficial skin and mucosal bleeding, such as ecchymoses, purpura, petechiae, epistaxis, bleeding from the gums, and menorrhagia. A normal platelet count is 150 to 400,000/mm^3. The risk of bleeding is inversely proportional to platelet number (▶Tab. 6.15).

Tab. 6.15: Relationship between platelet count and bleeding.

Platelet count	Severity	Symptoms
>100,000	Nil	None
50–100,000	Minimal	Minimal after major trauma or surgery
20–50,000	Mild	Mild cutaneous bruising
5–20,000	Moderate	Cutaneous and mucosal bleeding
<5,000	Severe	Spontaneous mucosal and CNS bleeds

Tab. 6.16: Causes and mechanisms of thrombocytopenia.

Decreased platelet production	Increased destruction	Miscellaneous
Inherited	Immune thrombocytopenia	Dilutional
• Familial thrombocytopenia	• Primary or secondary	• Massive transfusion
• Fanconi's anemia	Drugs	Sequestration
Drugs	HIT	• Splenomegaly
• Cytotoxic drugs	Infections	
• Valproic acid	• HIV	
Bone marrow replacement	• EBV	
Ineffective hematopoiesis	Posttransfusional purpura	
B12 and folic acid deficiency Infections	Consumption	
	• TTP	
	• DIC	

HIT, heparin-induced thrombocytopenia; HIV, human immunodeficiency virus; EBV, Epstein-Barr virus; DIC, disseminated intravascular coagulation; TTP, thrombotic thrombocytopenic purpura.

Qualitative platelet function abnormalities can be primary – that is, inherited – or they may be secondary. The commonest cause of the latter is the use of NSAIDs, such as aspirin. Inherited anomalies are rare.

Quantitative platelet disorders or thrombocytopenias are common. Thrombocytopenia or a low platelet count is a result of either increased platelet destruction or decreased platelet production. The causes and mechanisms of thrombocytopenia are shown in ▶Tab. 6.16.

6.4.1 Immune thrombocytopenia (ITP)

Thrombocytopenia caused by the immune-mediated destruction of platelets is called immune thrombocytopenia (ITP). ITP is further classified as primary ITP, where immune-mediated thrombocytopenia is the only clinical abnormality and there is no other associated condition or explanation for thrombocytopenia. In secondary ITP, thrombocytopenia is associated with other disorders (▶Tab. 6.17). Thrombocytopenia improves with treatment and resolution of associated condition. Occasionally specific treatment for thrombocytopenia is required.

Tab. 6.17: Causes of secondary ITP (23,24)

Antiphospholipid syndrome
Autoimmune thrombocytopenia
Common variable deficiency
Side effects of drugs
Secondary to infections with CMV, *Helicobacter pylori,* hepatitis C, HIV, varicella zoster
Lymphoproliferative disorders
Side effects of bone marrow transplantation
Side effects of vaccinations
Systemic lupus erythematosus

Primary immune thrombocytopenia: The exact incidence of ITP in adolescents is not known. The incidence of ITP in children below 15 years of age is 4.5 to 5 per 100,000. In adults the incidence decreases to 2 to 3 per 100,000. The incidence in adolescents perhaps falls between children and adults.

Clinical presentation

Patients usually present with easy bruising, petechiae, and purpura. Mucosal bleeding such as epistaxis, gum bleeding, or menorrhagia may be seen in some. Severe bleeding is rare. Spontaneous intracranial hemorrhage is seen in less than 1 percent and can develop at any time during the course of the illness. The onset of bleeding symptoms in the majority of cases is sudden. A history of smoldering symptoms with acute exacerbation is not unusual. The physical examination shows bruises, purpura, and petechiae. There may be some mucosal bleeding; lymphadenopathy and splenomegaly are rare. The CBC shows isolated low platelets with counts well below 100,000/mL. A peripheral blood smear may show rare giant platelets, while the RBC and the WBC counts are normal. Diagnosis is based on clinical presentation and physical examination. Bone marrow evaluation is seldom required.

Pathogenesis

Platelet destruction by antiplatelet autoantibodies causes thrombocytopenia. In some cases the autoantibody is targeted against platelet glycoprotein receptor GPIIb/IIIa. Antibody-coated platelets are removed by Fc receptor – mediated phagocytosis in the spleen and liver. Impaired T-cell function and cytokines may also contribute. There is now evidence that ineffective platelet production also plays a role in the pathogenesis of thrombocytopenia. The clinical course of primary ITP is unpredictable. Most cases resolve in weeks to years. The following classification has been recommended by the international ITP working group (23):

- Newly diagnosed ITP: diagnosis to 3 months
- Persistent ITP: 3 months to 12 months
- Chronic ITP: persistently low platelet count beyond 12 months since onset
- Refractory: persistence of thrombocytopenia after splenectomy

Chronic ITP: About 15 to 20 percent of acute ITP cases fail to resolve and become chronic. At a platelet count of 30,000 to 80,000/µL spontaneous bleeding is rare and the patient may live a nearly normal life. However, contact sports ares to be avoided. These patients need therapy to raise the platelet count prior to any surgery or following trauma. Adolescents with chronic ITP who fail to respond to the treatments listed for acute and persistent ITP and/or those with significant symptoms of bleeding are candidates for splenectomy. Some 60 to 80 percent of patients respond to splenectomy.

Treatment of ITP

Supportive care involving the avoidance of aspirin and other NSAIDs as well as avoidance of intramuscular shots, contact sports, and diving is recommended.

Acute and persistent ITP: The risk of spontaneous bleeding is high at platelet counts of less than 10,000/mm^3. Most of the available treatments for ITP transiently increase the platelet count to a safer range but do not change the natural history of ITP. Patients with minimal bleeding may be watched closely. Patients with very low platelet count and/or mucocutaneous bleeding or active adolescents for whom restricted activity may not be a desirable option may be treated with intravenous immunoglobulin (IVIG) or steroids. For patients requiring therapy, IVIG at 0.8 to 1.0 g/kg per day IV for 1 to 2 doses generally raises the platelet levels in 80 to 90 percent of patients within 3 days of therapy (23). A short course of corticosteroids 1 to 2 mg/kg per day until the platelet count reaches a normal level and then tapered over 1 to 2 weeks can also be used as the first line of therapy. In nonsplenectomized Rh-positive patients with stable hemoglobin, a single dose of anti-D immunoglobin 50 to 75μg/kg, can be given intravenously. The response to these therapies lasts for 4 to 6 weeks. Most patients will require repeated treatment.

Anti-D and IVIG both are derived from human blood. Side effects of IVIG include headache, nausea, vomiting, fever, malaise, and a septic meningitis – like picture. The symptoms can occur up to 72 hours postinfusion. The side effect of anti-D may be a drop of 1 to 2 g/dL in hemoglobin as the coated RBCs are destroyed. Rarely patients may develop intravascular hemolysis and renal failure. Steroids cause fluid retention, weight gain, irritability, mood swings, hyperglycemia, hypertension, and acne (23).

In rare resistant cases immunosuppressive agents like azathioprine, cyclosporine A, cyclophosphamide, danazol, dapsone, mycophenolate mofetil, and vinca alkaloids have been tried. Rituximab (anti-CD 20 antibody) has been used for the treatment of patients who fail to respond to the above measures. It may also be considered as an alternative to splenectomy in adolescents with chronic ITP. High-dose dexamethasone may also be considered (23,24).

6.4.2 Disseminated Intravascular Coagulation (DIC)

Intravascular coagulation activation, fibrin deposition in the microvasculature, and platelet consumption is the hallmark of DIC. Bleeding is common and microthrombi lead to organ dysfunction. A variety of conditions such as sepsis, trauma, burns, abortions, and malignancies are associated with DIC. PT, APTT, and D-dimer are elevated and fibrinogen and platelets are low. Schistocytes are seen on peripheral smear. Successful treatment of the underlying condition corrects the platelet count and hemostatic abnormality. Platelet transfusion and cryoprecipitate can be used to control bleeding.

6.4.3 Thrombotic thrombocytopenic purpura (TTP)

Thrombotic thrombocytopenic purpura is rare disorder of hemostasis. The hallmarks of TTP are aggressive aggregation of platelets leading to occlusion of microvasculature, thrombocytopenia, and microangiopathic anemia. Schistocytes are seen on peripheral smear. These distinctive features are often accompanied by varying degrees of neurologic deficit, renal impairment, and fever. Decreased activity of a von Willebrand cleaving metalloprotease, ADAMTS 13, results in increased levels of very adhesive large von Willebrand multimers. The platelets adhere to these multimers and aggregate and form microthrombi. Decrease ADAMTS 13 activity can be either congenital or caused by an antibody that inhibits ADAMTS 13 activity. Most cases are idiopathic and occur abruptly in previously healthy individuals. Females and African Americans are at higher risk for TTP. Antibodies to ADAMTS 13 have been isolated in 44 to 84 percent of patients with TTP (25,26).

Diagnosis

The pentad of thrombocytopenia, microangiopathic hemolytic anemia, neurologic abnormalities, renal dysfunction, and fever is diagnostic of TTP (25,26). Decreased ADMTS 13 activity and presence of ADMTS antibody further supports the diagnosis.

Treatment

There is no pharmacologic treatment for TTP. Plasma-exchange (PE) therapy (40–60 mL/kg) is the primary treatment for idiopathic TTP. It replenishes ADAMTS 13 and removes the circulating long multimers of vWF. Supportive care is usually continued on a daily basis until clinical symptoms resolve and platelet count is restored to $150 \times 109/L$.

6.4.4 Disorders of hemostasis

Hemophilia A (factor VIII deficiency) and hemophilia B (factor IX deficiency) are the most common X-linked bleeding disorders. Von Willebrand Disease (VWD) is the most common autosomal bleeding disease, due to a deficiency or abnormality of the von Willebrand factor (VWF), a carrier protein for FVIII. The other rare autosomal bleeding disorders include deficiencies of factors II, VII, XI, XIII, and fibrinogen.

Epidemiology

The incidence of hemophilia is 1 in 5,000 males (27). It affects males almost exclusively; 80 to 85 percent have hemophilia A and 10 to 15 percent hemophilia B. The prevalence of VWD is 0.6 to 1.3 percent (28). Individuals with severe hemophilia and type 3 VWD bleed spontaneously and are diagnosed in early childhood. Patients with mild hemophilia and types 1 and 2 VWD often go undiagnosed until adolescence or adulthood and may experience bleeding with severe trauma or surgery. An adolescent with menorrhagia should be screened for a bleeding disorder, especially VWD, since approximately 11 to 33 percent could have an underlying bleeding disorder (29). Both adolescent boys and girls may present with prolonged bleeding following dental extraction. Occasionally the diagnosis is made on screening tests done prior to a surgical procedure.

Diagnosis

Hemophilias A and B are clinically indistinguishable and specific plasma factor assays are the only way to differentiate between them and confirm the diagnosis. Based on plasma levels of circulating FVIII or IX (normal levels are 50%–100% or 100 IU/dL), the hemophilias are classified as mild, moderate, and severe (▶Tab. 6.18).

VWD is characterized by either a quantitative (types 1 and 3) or a qualitative (type 2 and the subtypes) defect of the VWF. The diagnosis of VWD includes measurement of plasma VWF antigen (VWF: Ag), VWF ristocetin cofactor assay (VWF: RCo), and FVIII assay. Normal levels of VWF: Ag and VWF: RCo range from 50–150 IU/dL. Multimeric analysis of VWF to identify subtypes of VWD is done in specialized laboratories.

The classification of VWD is shown in ▶Tab. 6.19. The hallmark of hemophilia is bleeding in the joints; common sites of bleeding in hemophilia and VWD are shown in ▶Tab. 6.20. Patients with bleeding disorders are otherwise healthy. The differential

Tab. 6.18: Clinical Classification of Hemophilia.

Characteristics	Classification of hemophilia A and B		
	Severe	Moderate	Mild
Plasma factor VIII or IX levels (normal levels = 50%–150%)	<1%	1%–5%	6%–30%
Cause of bleeding episodes	Spontaneous	Minor trauma	Postsurgery or major trauma
Frequency of bleeding episodes	2–4 per month	4–6 per year	Rare

Tab. 6.19: Classification of von Willebrand Disease (VWD).

VWD Types	VWF:RCo* (IU/dL) Normal = 50–200	VWF:Ag† (IU/dL) Normal = 50–200	FVIII levels	Ratio of VWF:RCo/ VWF: Ag
Type 1	<30	<30	↓/ N	>0.5–0.7
Type 2 (A, B, M, N)	<30 30–200 (N type)	<30–200	↓/ N	Usually <0.5–0.7
Type 3	<3	<3	↓↓↓(<10 IU/dL)	Not applicable

*von Willebrand factor: ristocetin cofactor.
†von Willebrand factor: antigen.

Tab. 6.20: Bleeding sites in hemophilia and von Willebrand disease (VWD).

Hemophilia	VWD
Hemarthroses, soft tissue, muscle hematomas, intracranial hemorrhage, gastrointestinal hemorrhage	Epistaxis Reproductive tract bleeding (including menorrhagia), bleeding with dental procedures Type 3 may present with bleeding episodes similar to hemophilia

diagnoses of the inherited bleeding disorders includes trauma, drugs, thrombocytopenia both primary and secondary.

Management

The half-life of FVIII is 10 to 12 hours and that of FIX is 18 to 24 hours. Minimal hemostatic levels are 30 percent (30). The half-life of plasma VWF is 12 hours (9–15 hours) (28,30). The goal of treatment of bleeding episodes in hemophilia and VWD is to raise factor levels to approximately 30 percent or more for minor bleeds (such as hematomas or joint bleeds) and 100 percent for major bleeds (such as intracranial hemorrhage or surgery) (31). This is accomplished by administering appropriate factor (F VIII, F IX, or VWF) concentrates; 1 unit (U)/kg raises F VIII levels by 2 percent, F IX levels by 1.2 to 1.5 percent, and VWF (ristocetin cofactor activity) raises levels by 1.5 percent (28,30). ▶Tabs. 6.21 and 6.22 provide dosage guidelines for the treatment of specific bleeding episodes.

In the 1980s, transfusion-transmitted pathogens such as human immunodeficiency and hepatitis C viruses contaminating pooled plasma concentrates claimed the lives of many hemophiliacs. This eventually led to the development of recombinant and

Tab. 6.21: Dosage guidelines for treatment of specific bleeding episodes in hemophilia.

Type of bleeding	Hemophilia A (1 U/kg raises levels by 2%)		Hemophilia B (1 U/kg raises levels by 1.2%–1.5%)		Adjunctive therapy
	Desired level	Dose (U/kg)	Desired level	Dose (U/kg)	
Epistaxis	20%–30%	10–15	30%–45%	20–30	Nasal packing, Nosebleed QR, antifibrinolytics
Oral mucosal bleeds Dental procedures	30%–50%	15–25	45%–75%	30–50	Use 1 hour prior to procedure, antifibrinolytics, Desmopressin (DDAVP) for hemophilia A and VWD
Hemarthrosis	40%–100%	20–50	60%–100%	40–80	Non-weight bearing
Intramuscular bleed Iliopsoas bleed	40%–100%	20–50	75%–100%	50–80	Bed rest, non-weight bearing
Major bleeds Surgery Gastrointestinal bleed	Initial 80%–100% × 24 h, then 50%	40–50 × 24 h, then 25–30	Initial 80%–100% × 24 h, then 50%	80–100 × 24 h, then 25–50	Oral antifibrinolytics for GI bleed
Hematuria	30%–40%	15–20	45%–75%	30–50	Bed rest, increased oral or IV fluids
Intracranial hemorrhage	Initial 80%–100% × 24 h, then 50%	40–50 × 24 h, then 25–30	Initial 80–100% × 24 h, then 50%	80–100 × 24 h, then 25–50	Continue treatment for 14 days followed by prophylaxis

Tab. 6.22: Dosage guidelines for treatment of specific bleeding episodes in von Willebrand disease.

	Major surgery/bleeding	Minor surgery/bleeding
Loading dose (VWF: Rco* IU/dL)	40–60 U/kg	30–60 U/kg
Maintenance dose	20–40 U/kg every 8 to 24 hours	20–40 U/kg every 12 to 48 hours
Therapeutic goal	Trough VWF:RCo and FVIII >50 IU/dL for 7–14 days	Trough VWF:RCo and FVIII >50 IU/dL for 3–5 days

*von Willebrand factor: ristocetin cofactor.

Tab. 6.23: Adjunctive medications.

Types	Uses	Dose
DDAVP	Mild hemophilia A, VWD type 1	Intravenous: 0.3 µg/kg, over 30 minutes Subcutaneous: 0.3 µg/kg Intranasal spray: 150mcg in *one nostril* (<50 kg) or in *both nostrils* (>50 kg). May be repeated after 24 hours. Do not use in children under 2 years or in pregnant women.
Nosebleed QR*	Epistaxis	
Aminocaproic acid (antifibrinolytic)	Mucosal bleeds (epistaxis, dental extraction, oral bleeds etc.), menorrhagia	Loading dose: oral 4–5 g (adults) or 100–200 mg/kg (max 10 g in children) Maintenance: 4–6 g (adults) or until bleeding is controlled or 5–7 days after surgery; 50–100 mg/kg (max 5 g in children) every 6 hours
Tranexamic acid (antifibrinolytic)		Intravenous: 10 mg/kg every 6–8 hours Oral: 25 mg/kg every 6–8 hours, 1,300 mg every 8 hours for 5 days in menorrhagia

*Nosebleed QR is a commercial product to stop nosebleeds. It is a powder that interacts wtih the tissues to form a scab.

virally safe plasma-derived concentrates. A list of products licensed in the United States for the treatment of hemophilia, VWD, and rare bleeding disorders is available on the National Hemophilia Foundation (NHF) website (32).

Prophylactic administration of concentrates (F VIII 25–40 U/kg every other day, F IX 25–40 U/kg twice weekly because of the longer half-life of F IX) is aimed at preventing debilitating effects of joint disease and is often begun at 1 to 2 years of age and continued throughout the life of the patient. Longer-acting products are currently being developed. Tailored or escalating dose prophylaxis may be an option for adolescents (33). Adolescents should be encouraged to self-infuse regularly and prior to any planned strenuous activity. Because of the complications of central venous catheters (infections, thrombosis, and mechanical problems), use of a peripheral vein is encouraged.

Listed in ▶Tab. 6.23 are other adjunctive products that are helpful for minor bleeds in mild hemophilia and VWD. Inhibitory antibodies to F VIII and F IX should be suspected if a patient fails to respond to an appropriate dose of clotting factor concentrate. They further exacerbate bleeding episodes and hemophilic arthropathy (see chapter 13).

Issues in adolescents

Adolescents with hemophilia should be encouraged to participate in sports activities that promote not only "joint health" by muscle building and strengthening but also psychological well-being and acceptance by peers. Sport activities have been divided into three categories. Category 1 activities such as swimming, golf, and running are safe; category 2 activities include weight lifting, bowling, and bicycling, where the psychological, social, and physical benefits outweighs the risks; and category 3 comprises sports such as boxing, skateboarding, and football, which should be avoided.

Adolescents should be encouraged to wear MedicAlert tags (necklace or wrist or ankle bracelet) that may be lifesaving, allowing early and appropriate treatment in the event of an accident. They are also encouraged to join support groups such as the National Hemophilia Foundation (NHF). The goal of the NHF's national prevention program is to prevent or reduce complications of bleeding disorders by "doing the 5," namely (a) annual comprehensive checkups, (b) vaccination for hepatitis A and B, (c) early treatment of joint bleeds, (d) exercise for joint health, and (e) regular testing for bloodborne pathogens.

Travel for an adolescent reflects independence. For individuals with a bleeding disorder it is important to be educated about their disorder and have a letter that specifies the diagnosis and management in case of an emergency. Furthermore, they should be taught to self-infuse, travel with a supply of factor concentrate, wear a MedicAlert bracelet or necklace, and avoid risky behavior during their travels. Sexual activity may pose a risk not only for bleeding but also for the transmission of pathogens.

Compliance is an important issue in adolescents. It is vital to educate them on the long-term complications, such as joint damage. Adequate support from parents, health care providers, and support groups is very important. Transition to an adult provider may sometimes be anxiety provoking and a team approach may be helpful. Guidelines for transition at every stage, from infancy to adulthood, are available at the NHF (MASAC document #147, available at www.hemophilia.org)(32).

Hereditary deficiencies of the other clotting factors (i.e., fibrinogen; prothrombin; factors V, VII, X, XI, XII, and XIII; Fletcher factor; etc.) are rare and are mostly associated with milder forms of bleeding tendencies. Manifestations include umbilical cord bleeding (especially in afibrinogenemia); bleeding in the mucosa, skin, muscle, or joint; and menorrhagia and intracranial hemorrhage. Since the availability of fibrinogen concentrates, FXIII concentrates and recombinant FVIIa, the use of fresh frozen plasma or cryoprecipitate has become less popular.

6.4.5 Thrombotic disorders and thrombophilia

Thrombosis is the presence of coagulated blood (thrombus) either in an artery or in the deep venous system. The term *thrombophilia* indicates an inherited or acquired predisposition to clot formation. Thrombotic disorders in adolescents are being recognized with increased frequency and may be inherited or acquired as a result of a blood vessel or coagulation factor abnormality. They are frequently associated with risk factors such as infections, obesity, cancer, or pregnancy. Arterial thrombi are generally considered as platelet thrombi, though they may sometimes have a venous origin and enter the systemic circulation through a shunt or a defect in the cardiac septum.

Epidemiology

The incidence of symptomatic venous thromboembolism (VTE) in the Canadian Thrombophilia Registry is 0.07 per 10,000 children and 5.3 per 10,000 hospital admissions. The annual rate of VTE admissions increased by 50 percent from 2001 to 2007 and the proportion of patients with recurrent VTE also significantly increased to 37 percent among children between 13 to 18 years of age (34).

Diagnosis

A strong family history of thrombosis at a young age may suggest an inherited thrombophilia. Adolescents without an underlying medical condition who present with a thrombotic episode should be screened for thrombophilia. ▶Tab. 6.24 lists some of the risk factors for VTE in children and adolescents. The single most important risk factor in children is VTE related to central venous lines, seen in more than 50 percent of DVT in children (35). Laboratory workup could include a CBC, coagulation profile including fibrinogen, D-dimer, and investigation of risk factors depending on the site of thrombus and associated comorbidity. Radiologic imaging is vital in the diagnosis of thrombosis.

Although venography is the gold standard, it is seldom used in view of its invasiveness. Compression ultrasonography with Doppler remains the primary modality of choice in VTE involving the upper and lower limbs. Other imaging techniques include echocardiography and magnetic resonance (MR) angiography for the superior vena cava and atrium, diffusion MR for cerebral sinus venous thrombosis, spiral computed

Tab. 6.24: Risk factors for thromboembolism.

Thrombophilia
• Factor V Leiden deficiency (most prevalent in whites, 5%)
• Prothrombin G20210A, methylenetetrahydrofolate reductase (MTHFR) and plasminogen activator inhibitor polymorphism (PAI-1 4G/4G)
• Deficiency of proteins C & S and antithrombin III
• Elevation of lipoprotein (a) and homocysteine
• Abnormalities of fibrinogen and factors VIII, VII, FXII
• Antiphospholipid antibody syndrome (lupus anticoagulant, anticardiolipin, anti-β2 GP)

Acquired risk factors
Trauma, surgery, sepsis/systemic inflammatory response syndrome, inflammatory bowel disease, systemic lupus erythematosus, nephrotic syndrome, SCD, diabetes, hyperlipidemia, hypertension, malignancy, hormone therapy, oral contraceptives, obesity, smoking, pregnancy, prolonged travel/ immobility, indwelling venous catheters, etc.

tomography (CT), or a ventilation/perfusion scan for pulmonary embolism and CT or MR imaging for deep pelvic or abdominal veins.

Management

The therapeutic goals should be to prevent thrombus propagation and/or embolization, restore blood flow (rapidly when necessary), and minimize long-term sequelae. The duration of anticoagulant therapy for the first episode of VTE varies anywhere from 3 to 6 months in cases where the risk factor can be resolved to being indefinite in inherited thrombophilia. Postthrombotic syndrome (PTS) is a syndrome of chronic venous insufficiency following VTE with a calculated weighted mean frequency of 26 percent. Physical findings of PTS can include edema, pain, dilated superficial collateral veins, stasis dermatitis, and ulceration involving the affected limb (36). Compression stockings are recommended although compliance with their use in adolescents is problematic. Stasis ulcers are common in adolescents and are difficult to treat. Obesity is a risk factor for venous stasis ulcers, hence nutritional and exercise counseling should be a part of the standard care.

The current standard of treatment of VTE is low-molecular-weight heparin (LMWH), although unfractionated heparin (UFH) is used in situations where rapid reversal is needed. Subsequent follow up with oral vitamin K antagonists (VKA) such as warfarin, while feasible, is difficult in children and adolescents since it requires frequent monitoring. Risks of bleeding with therapeutic doses of oral anticoagulant are estimated to occur in 20 percent of all cases. With LMWH, the risk of bleeding is 17 percent. VTE itself has a recurrence rate of 17 to 22 percent as reported in literature (37).

▶Tab. 6.25 lists the anticoagulant therapy for VTE in children and adolescents. Thrombolysis should be considered in patients with completely occlusive proximal limb DVT in whom D-dimer is greater than 500 ng/mL and/or FVIII levels are greater than 150 U/dL. In such persons, the risk of PTS appears to be elevated with conventional care anticoagulation alone (38). Newer anticoagulants such as direct thrombin inhibitors (lepirudin, bivalirudin, and argatroban) and a synthetic antithrombin-dependent inhibitor of factor Xa (fondaparinux) are currently being investigated in children and adolescents. For arterial thrombosis the recommendation is either LMWH or UFH or aspirin (1–5 mg/kg per day) as initial therapy until dissection and embolic causes have been excluded (39).

6.5 Summary

The most common nonmalignant blood disorders in adolescents include the various forms of cytopenias, anemias, bleeding and clotting disorders, and hemoglobinopathies. The public health impact of these disorders is enormous and recognition is important not only for prevention of complications but also for treatments to improve quality of life. Early recognition also provides an opportunity to address preconception care during adolescence and education. Management often requires comprehensive care that includes plans for transition of care to adults, especially in those disorders that are inherited. This chapter reviews the common nonmalignant hematologic disorders and pharmacologic approaches for the treatment and prevention of complications (such as factor concentrate prophylaxis in hemophilia, use of hydroxyurea in sickle cell disease, and chelation therapy in hemoglobinopathies).

Tab. 6.25: Anticoagulant therapy in children and adolescents.

Unfractionated heparin

- Main advantages: short half-life, easy reversibility
- Main disadvantages: unreliable therapeutic levels, bleeding, HIT (1%)
  1. Loading dose: 50–75 U/kg, then continuous infusion at15–25 U/kg per hour
  2. Monitoring: anti-Xa activity (8 hours after initiation of infusion): 0.3–0.7 U/mL OR aPTT: 60–85 seconds or approximately 1.5–2 times the upper limit of age-appropriate values
  3. Usual duration: 5–10 days with overlap transitioning to low-molecular-weight heparin (LMWH) or warfarin
  4. For heparin resistance, may give antithrombin concentrates

LMWH (enoxaparin)

- Main advantages: more predictable, easy monitoring, longer half-life
- Main disadvantages: less of a HIT, no antidote
  1. Dosage: 1.25 mg/kg subcutaneously every 12 hours (no bolus needed)
  2. Monitoring: anti-Xa activity (4 hours after first few doses): 0.5–1.0 U/mL

Thrombolysis (tissue-type plasminogen activator [tPA])

- Uses: high-risk clots, limb-threatening VTE, or ischemic stroke
  1. Systemic bolus/infusion or local catheter-directed infusion
  2. Dose (continuous infusion): 0.03 mg/kg per hour; max 2 mg/h for 48–96 hours
  3. Monitoring: repeated imaging to assess clot lysis, D-dimer, PT, aPTT, fibrinogen

Vitamin K antagonist (warfarin)

- Uses: Primarily for extending anticoagulant therapy
- Main advantages: oral route, antidote in vitamin K
- Main disadvantages: risk of bleeding, affected by diet/antibiotics, no good liquid prep, compliance on daily taking, need for frequent laboratory monitoring
  1. Loading dose: 0.2 mg/kg per day and subsequent dose adjustments needed to maintain an INR of 2–3

HIT, heparin-induced thrombocytopenia; INR, international normalized ratio; PT, prothrombin time; aPTT, activated partial thromboplastin time; VTE, venous thromboembolism.

References

1. Brugnara C, Oski FA, Nathan DG. Diagnostic approach to the anemic patient: Hematology of infancy and childhood. Philadelphia, PA: Saunders, 2009:455–66.
2. Dallman PR, Barr GD, Allen CM, Shinefield HR. Hemoglobin concentration in white, black and oriental children: is there a need for separate criteria in screening for anemia? Am J Clin Nutr 1978;31:377–80.
3. Kulkarni R, Gera R, Scott-Emuakpor AB. Adolescent hematology. In: Greydanus DE, Patel DR, Pratt HD, eds. Essential adolescent medicine. New York: McGraw-Hill, 2006:371–90.

4. Merkel D, Huerta M, Grotto I, Blum D, Tal O, Rachmilewitz E, et al. Prevalence of iron deficiency and anemia among sternously trained adolescents. J Adolesc Health 2005;37:220–23.

5. Ganz T. Hepicidin a key regulator of iron metabolism and mediator of anemia of inflammation. Blood 2003;102:783–88.

6. Silverstein SB, Rogers GM. Parenteral iron therapy options. Am J Hematol 2004;76: 74–78.

7. Young NS, Calado T, Schinberg. Current concepts in to Pathophysiology and treatment of aplastic anemia. Blood 2006;108: 2509–19.

8. Conley CL. Sickle cell anemia; the first molecular disease; In Wintrobe MM, ed. Blood, pure and eloquent. New York; McGraw Hill, 1980:319–73.

9. National Institute of Health, National Heart Lung and Blood Institute. The management of sickle cell disease. Washington, DC: NIH publication 02-2117, 2002:59–71.

10. Charache S, Terrin ML, Moore RD, Dover GJ, Barton FB, Eckert SV, et al. Effect of hydroxyurea on the frequency of painful crises in sickle cell anemia. Investigators of the Multicenter Study of Hydroxyurea in Sickle Cell Anemia. N Engl J Med 1995;332(20): 1317–22.

11. Kinney TR, Helms RW, O'Branski EE, Ohene-Frempong K, Wang W, Daeschner C, et al. Safety of hydoyurea in children with sickle cell anemia: results of the HUG-KIDS study. A phase I/II trial. Blood 1999;94:1550–54.

12. Adams RJ, McKie VC, Hsu L, Files B, Vichinsky E, Pegelow C, et al. Prevention of first stroke by transfusion in children with sickle cell anemia and abnormal results on transcranial Doppler ultrasonography. N Engl J Med 1998;339(1):5–11.

13. Adams RJ, Brambilla D. Optimizing primary stroke prevention in sickle cell anemia (STOP 2) trial investigators. Discontinuing prophylactic transfusions used to prevent stroke in sickle cell disease. N Engl J Med 2005;353(26):2769–78.

14. Collins FS, Weismann SM. The molecular genetics of human hemoglobin. Prog Nucleic Acid Res Mol Biol 1984;31:315.

15. Piomelli S, Danoff SJ, Becker MH, Lipera MJ, Travis SF. Prevention of bone malformation and cardiomegaly in Cooley's anemia by early hypertransfusion regimen. Ann NY Acad Sci 1969;165(1):427–36.

16. Borgna-Pignatti C, Rugolotto S, De Stefano P, Zhao H, Cappellini MD, Del Vecchio GC, et al. Survival and complications in patients with thalassemia major treated with transfusion and deferoxamine. Haematologica 2004;89(10):1187–93.

17. Olivieri NF, Brittenham GM, McLaren CE, Templeton DM, Cameron RG, McClelland RA, et al. Long term safety and effectiveness of iron chelation therapy with deferiprone for thalasemia major. N Engl J Med 1998;339(7):417–23.

18. Cappellini MD, Cohen A, Piga A, Bejaoui M, Perrotta S, Agaoglu L, et al. A phase 3 study of deferasirox (ICL 670), a once daily-oral iron chelator in patients with ß-thalassemia. Blood 2006;107(9):3455–62.

19. Boxer LA. Neutrophil abnormalities. Pediatr Rev 2003;24(2):52–62.

20. Kyono W, Coates TD. A practical approach to neutrophil disorders. Pediatr Clin North Am 2002;49(5):929–71.

21. Rosenberg PS, Zeidler C, Bolyard AA, Alter BP, Bonilla MA, Boxer LA, et al. Stable long-term risk of leukaemia in patients with severe congenital neutropenia maintained on G-CSF therapy. Br J Haematol 2010;150(2):196–99.

22. Gera R, Pawar A, Saah EN, Scott-Emuakpor AB, Kulkarni R. Pediatric hematology and oncology. In: Greydanus DE, Patel DR, Reddy VN, Feinberg AN, Omar HA, eds. Handbook of clinical pediatrics. An update for the ambulatory pediatrician. Singapore: World Scientific, 2010:389–451.

23. Neunert C, Lim W, Crowther M, Cohen A, Solberg L Jr, Crowther MA. The American Society of Hematology 2011 evidence-based practice guideline for immune thrombocytopenia. Blood 2011;117(16):4190–207.
24. McCrae K. Immune thrombocytopenia: No longer idiopathic. Cleve Clin J Med 2011;78 (6):358–73.
25. Bouw MC, Dors N, van Ommen H, Ramakers-van Woerden NL. Thrombotic thrombocytopenic purpura in childhood. Pediatr Blood Cancer 2009;53(4):537–42.
26. Lowe EJ, Werner EJ. Thrombotic thrombocytopenic purpura and hemolytic uremic syndrome in children and adolescents. Semin Thromb Hemost 2005;31(6):717–30.
27. Soucie JM, Evatt B, Jackson D. Occurrence of hemophilia in the United States.The Hemophilia Surveillance System Project Investigators. Am J Hematol. 1998;59:288–94.
28. Nichols WL, ed. The diagnosis, evaluation and management of von Willebrand disease. Bethesda, MD: National Institutes Health, National Heart Blood Lung Institute, 08-5832, 2007.
29. Miller CH, Philipp CS, Stein SF, Kouides PA, Lukes AS, Heit JA, et al. The spectrum of haemostatic characteristics of women with unexplained menorrhagia. Haemophilia 2011;17:e223–29.
30. Montgomery RR, Gill JC, Paola JD. Hemophilia and von Willebrand disease. In: Orkin SH, Fisher DE, Look AT, Lux SE, Ginsburg D, Nathan DG, eds. Nathan and Oski's hematology of infancy and childhood. 7th ed. Philadelphia, PA: Saunders Elsevier, 2009: 1487–1524.
31. Kulkarni R, Chitlur M, Lusher J. Treatment of congenital coagulopathies. In: Mintz PD, ed. Transfusion therapy: Clinical principles and practice, 3rd edition. Bethesda, MD: AABB Press, 2011:167–208.
32. National Hemophilia Foundation. MASAC recommendations concerning products licensed for the treatment of hemophilia and other bleeding disorder. MASAC document 202, 2011. Accessed 2011 Jun 20. URL: http://www.hemophilia.org/NHFWeb/MainPgs/MainNHF.aspx?menuid=57&contentid=693
33. Blanchette VS. Prophylaxis in the haemophilia population. Haemophilia 2010;16: 181–88.
34. Raffini L, Huang YS, Witmer C, Feudtner C. Dramatic increase in venous thromboembolism in children's hospitals in the United States from 2001 to 2007. Pediatrics 200;124: 1001–8.
35. Male C, Julian JA, Massicotte P, Gent M, Mitchell L. PROTEKT Study Group. Significant association with location of central venous line placement and risk of venous thrombosis in children. Thromb Haemost 2005;94:516–21.
36. Goldenberg NA, Donadini MP, Kahn SR, Crowther M, Kenet G, Nowak-Göttl U, Manco-Johnson MJ. Post-thrombotic syndrome in children: a systematic review of frequency of occurrence, validity of outcome measures, and prognostic factors. Haematologica 2010;95:1952–59.
37. Bick RL, Haas S. Thromboprophylaxis and thrombosis in medical, surgical, trauma, and obstetric/gynecologic patients. Hematol Oncol Clin North Am 2003;17:217–58.
38. Goldenberg NA, Branchford B, Wang M, Ray C Jr, Durham JD, Manco-Johnson MJ. Percutaneous mechanical and pharmacomechanical thrombolysis for occlusive deep vein thrombosis of the proximal limb in adolescent subjects: findings from an institution-based prospective inception cohort study of pediatric venous thromboembolism. J Vasc Interv Radiol 2011;22(2):121–32.
39. Monagle P, Chalmers E, Chan A, DeVeber G, Kirkham F, Massicotte P, et al. American College of Chest Physicians. Antithrombotic therapy in neonates and children: American College of Chest Physicians evidence-based clinical practice guidelines, 8th ed. Chest 2008;133:887S–968S.

7 Pharmacotherapeutics of cancer in adolescents

Renuka Gera and Elna Z. Saah

Cancer is the leading cause of mortality in adolescence. Improved understanding of molecular biology, effective combination chemotherapy, and advances in supportive care have all contributed to significant improvement in the long-term survival of adolescents with cancer. However, improvement in the outcome of adolescents with cancer has lagged behind the success rates seen in children. Differences in the biology of the disease, access to care, and compliance with treatment regimens are some of the factors responsible for these differences. To improve the care of the adolescent with cancer, the National Cancer Institute and Children's Oncology Group both now have separate sections for the treatment of adolescents and young adults. Clinical trials focusing on disease biology, access to care, compliance, and supportive care are being developed for adolescents and young adults with cancer. The treatment of common cancers seen in adolescents is discussed in this chapter.

7.1 Introduction

Cancer is the leading cause of death in adolescents. In the United States and most developed countries, 2 percent of all invasive cancers are seen in ages 15 to 30 years. This number is 2.7 times higher than the number of cancers seen in children below 15 years of age. Although the long-term disease-free survival rates in children range between 70 and 90 percent, improvement in the outcome for this age group has lagged behind (1). Limited access to care, poor adherence to treatment, and a poor understanding of biology in this age group may be responsible for the poor outcomes (2).

Additionally limited emphasis on early detection, such as routine testicular examination and inadequate health care coverage, cause delays in diagnosis. This is further complicated by the inability of adolescents to remain compliant with treatments. With the recognition of these barriers to care for adolescent and young adults with cancer, the National Cancer Institute has formed a separate section called Adolescent and Young Adult (AYA) Cancer. The Children's Oncology Group has formed the Adolescent and Young Adult committee addressing the cancer-related needs of these patients.

The distribution of cancers in adolescents 15 to 19 years of age as reported by the National Cancer Institute's Surveillance Epidemiology and End Result (SEER) program, 1975–2000, is shown in ▶Tab. 7.1. Adolescent females are at higher risk for cancer than males, and non-Hispanic white populations have the highest incidence of cancer in this age group.

7.1.1 Etiology and risk factors

The causes of cancer in adolescent are not known. Cancers due to exposure to environmental carcinogens take a long time to develop and usually do not occur until later in life.

Tab. 7.1: Incidence and distribution of cancer in ages 15 to 19 from the SEER program, 1975–2000.

Type of cancer	Proportion of invasive cancers (%)
Hodgkin's lymphoma	19
Leukemia	11
Non-Hodgkin's lymphoma	8
Central nervous system neoplasm	10
Soft tissue sarcoma	8
Bone sarcoma	8
Testicular cancer	7
Melanoma	7
Female genital tract	6
Non-gonadal germ cell tumors	3
Others	7

In adolescents both genetics and environmental factors may play an important role. Melanoma after sun exposure is more common in Australian adolescents and points to a genetic predisposition. Clear cell carcinoma in adolescent girls is the result of exposure to diethylstilbestrol prenatally. A second malignant neoplasm may occur in adolescents after exposure to chemotherapy and/or radiation therapy in childhood.

7.1.2 Diagnosis and treatment

The clinical presentation of a cancer in adolescence is similar to the same cancer in another age group. Knowledge of the presentation and distribution of cancers in this age group helps the clinician perform an appropriate, thorough physical examination, develop an appropriate differential diagnosis, request appropriate tests and referrals, and follow patients after they have completed treatment. Surgery is the main modality for the diagnosis and treatment of solid tumors. Chemotherapy plays an important role in the treatment of lymphoma and leukemia and other cancers seen in adolescents. Cancer cells develop resistance against cytotoxic drugs when one of these is used as a single agent. Combination chemotherapy rather than a singleagent is used for the treatment of most cancers. Effective combination chemotherapy uses the following principles (3):

- Each drug in the combination has some activity against the cancer as a single agent and the dose-limiting toxicities of the agents used in the combination are different. For example, two nephrotoxic agents are seldom used together.
- The drugs with different mechanism of action as well as resistance are combined.
- Interaction of the drugs at the cellular level to provide the best synergy is taken into account in deciding on the sequence and timing of administration of various cytotoxic agents the combination. For example, drugs specific to the S-phase, such as methotrexate, are most effective during the periods of rebound DNA synthesis in the recovery phase.

With improved understanding of molecular defects and their association with a specific cancer potential, genetic targets have been identified and drugs are being developed to target the defect and induce apoptosis. For example, t(15;17) translocation in promyelocytic leukemia (PML) disrupts the function of the retinoic acid receptor a (RARa). This type of PML responds well to all trans-retinoic acid (ATRA). Imatinib mesylate (Gleevec) is a low-molecular-weight drug that inhibits aberrant tyrosine kinase function and now is the standard therapy for chronic myelogenous leukemia. Combination chemotherapy with tyrosine kinase inhibitors has also improved the outcome of patients with Philadelphia chromosome–positive B precursor acute lymphoblastic leukemia (ALL).

Recombinant human growth factors such as granulocyte colony stimulating factor (G-CSF), granulocyte macrophage colony-stimulating factor (GM-CSF), as well as newer broad-spectrum antifungals and antibiotics have significantly reduced the morbidity and mortality caused by chemotherapyrelated neutropenia and infection (refer to chapter 6 on neutropenia).

7.1.3 Chemotherapy-induced nausea and vomiting (CINV)

Last but not least, an important advancement in cancer care is the availability of a broad range of drugs to control chemotherapy-induced nausea and vomiting. Nausea and vomiting can be immediate (onset within 24 hours of chemotherapy administration) or delayed (onset 24 hours after chemotherapy administration). Delayed CINV may last as long as 5 to 7 days. Anticipatory nausea and vomiting is a complex problem. It is a conditioned response and occurs with increased frequency if nausea and vomiting is poorly controlled with first course of chemotherapy. Therefore effective control of CINV with the first course is essential for compliance with prescribed treatment. The mechanism of nausea and vomiting is complex. Peripheral as well as central receptors and neurotransmitter pathways are involved in the pathogenesis of CINV. The brain plays a major role as a recipient of noxious stimuli. Newer medications block these neurotransmitters to control CINV (see ▶Tab. 7.2).

Tab. 7.2: Antiemetic drugs.

Class	Indication	Dose (for an average adult-size adolescent)
Serotonin(5-HT3) receptor antagonists	Prophylaxis of low-to moderate-risk chemotherapy	
Ondansetron		32mg/day TID, PO, ODT, or IV
Granisetron		2 mg IV or PO once or 1 mg twice a day (max dose 3 mg/day)
Neurokinin-1(NK$_1$) receptor antagonist Aprepitant	Acute or delayed prophylaxis	125 mg PO on day 1, 80 mg PO on days 2 and 3
Dexamethasone	Acute or delayed	20mg* IV or PO on day 1, 8 mg on days 2–4

*Use 50 percent dose of dexamethasone with aprepitant.

Tab. 7.3: Emetogenicity of antineoplastic agents.

CINV >90%	CINV 60%–90%	CINV 30%–60%	CINV 10%–30%	CNIV <10%
Cisplatin	Carboplatin	Lower-dose cyclophosphamide	Etoposide	Vincristine
Cyclophosphamide >1,500 mg/m²	Procarbazine	Anthracyclines	Low-dose methotrexate	Vinblastine
Mechlorethamine	Cyclophosphamide 750–1,500 mg/m²	Methotrexate 250–1,000 g/m²	Paclitaxel	6-Thioguanine 6-Mercaptopurine
Dacarbazine	Cytarabine >1 g/m² High-dose methotrexate	Ifosfamide		Bleomycin

Antiemetics may be used as single agents or in combination with dexamethasone and aprepitant to control moderate to severe acute and delayed nausea and vomiting. The choice of antiemetic depends on the emetogenic potential of the antineoplastic agent. The severity of nausea and vomiting is drug- and dose-specific (4). The risk of CINV varies between less than 10 percent to over 90 percent (▶Tab. 7.3).

The American Society of Clinical Oncology (ASCO) recommends a combination of a 5-HT3 receptor antagonist, dexamethasone, and neurokinin-1 (NK$_1$) receptor antagonist for highly emetogenic chemotherapy and the combination of a 5-HT3 receptor antagonist and dexamethasone for chemotherapy with a moderate risk of vomiting (5). Metoclopramide, dronabinol, and prochlorperazine are used as rescue medications when the above combinations fail. Common adolescent cancers and their treatment are discussed in sections 7.2–7.7.

7.2 Lymphoma

Lymphoma is the most common malignancy seen in adolescents. Hodgkin's disease and non-Hodgkin's lymphoma together account for 27 percent malignancies seen in this age group.

7.2.1 Hodgkin's disease (HD)

Most cases of HD in pediatrics occur during adolescence. The incidence is higher in non-Hispanic whites. Thepresence of Reed-Sternberg or Hodgkin's cells is the hallmark of HD. The cause of HD is not known. The Epstein-Barr virus (EBV) genome has been identified in Reed-Sternberg cells in young children, but HD in adolescent is seldom associated with EBV (6). Siblings and children of patients with HD are at higher risk for developing HD. Other risk factors include immune deficiency, autoimmune disorders, and family history of cancer. There are two major subtypes of HD: nodular lymphocyte-predominant HD and classic HD. Classic HD has four subtypes: mixed cellularity, nodular sclerosis, lymphocyte-rich, and lymphocyte-depleted. Mediastinal involvement is common. Approximately 80 percent of cases in adolescents have a nodular sclerosis histology.

Painless enlargement of cervical, supraclavicular or mediastinal lymph nodes is seen at presentation. Mediastinal lymph node enlargement may also cause cough or dyspnea. Axillary or inguinal lymph nodes may also be involved. The disease usually spreads to adjacent lymph node regions. It may present in extralymphoid locations. Systemic symptoms, unexplained fever above 38°C for more than 3 days, weight loss greater than 10 percent over preceding 6 months, or drenching night sweats are called "B symptoms" and are seen in 30 percent cases. Diagnostic tests are listed in ▶Tab. 7.4.

Clinical staging: The Ann Arbor classification system is widely used. Stage 1 is localized to one lymph node region or extranodal organ; stage 2 involves two lymph node regions on the same side of the diaphragm or an extranodal region with one lymph node region on the same side of the diaphragm; stage 3 disease is on both side of the diaphragm; and stage 4 disease represents diffuse or disseminated involvement of one or more extralymphatic organs or tissues with or without associated lymph node involvement. Each stage is further subclassified as A if there are no constitutional symptoms or B if one of the following three is present:

- Weight loss greater than 10 percent over the previous 6 months
- Night sweats
- Fever 38°C or greater without any other source

Tab. 7.4: Hodgkin's disease diagnostic tests and expected results.

Tests	Rationale
ESR	N↑
Ferritin	N↑
Hemoglobin	N↓, Poor iron utilization or immune destruction DAT (direct antiglobulin test +)
WBC/ neutrophil	N↑/N↑
Imaging	
CT neck, chest, abdomen, pelvis PET scan Bone scan	For staging For staging and response If clinically indicated
Bone marrow evaluation	Involved in 3%
Surgery: biopsy of largest accessible node	To establish the diagnosis
ECG and ECHO	Baseline, during therapy and follow up to monitor toxicity
PFT with DLCO	Baseline, during therapy and follow up to monitor toxicity

CT, computed tomography; N, normal; WBC, white blood count; ECG, electrocardiogram; ECHO, echocardiogram; ESR, erythrocyte sedimentation rate; PET scan, positron emission tomography; PFT, pulmonary function testing; DLCO, diffusing capacity of the lungs for carbon monoxide.

Treatment/management

HD is curable in 70 to 95 percent of cases. The goal of the treatment is to maximize the recurrence-free survival and cause minimal immediate and late treatment-related toxicity. Stage 1 and 2 are stratified as early stage and stages 3 and 4 as advanced stage. Early-stage disease is treated with mantle radiation to the axillae, neck, and chest with doses of 40 to 44 Gy followed by "inverted Y" radiation to the spleen and paraaortic/pelvic lymph nodes. High-intensity radiation used as a single modality is associated with higher relapse rates, higher delayed side effects, and poor quality of life. Combination chemotherapy is used to treat advanced-stage disease. Combination chemotherapy consisting of mustard, oncovin, prednisone, procarbazine, doxorubicin (Adriamycin), bleomycin, vinblastine, and dactinomycin can be used to treat advanced-stage HD with excellent results. However, these combinations are associated with significant late organ toxicity, anthracycline-related cardiomyopathy, pulmonary fibrosis due to bleomycin, infertility, and a second malignancy resulting from the use of an alkylating agent (7).

High-dose mantle radiation used to treat early-stage HD has resulted in unacceptable delayed toxicity in children. Chemotherapy alone has been used to successfully treat early-stage disease in developing countries. Combined-modality treatment consisting of the reduced dose of an alkylating agent, anthracyclines, and reduced dose of radiation given to the involved field may lower the toxicity without reducing the efficacy. The "risk-adapted" approach – based on stage, symptoms, gender, and bulk of the tumor – has been used in pediatric trials and has resulted in excellent survival and a reduction in delayed toxicity. Response to therapy is also a significant marker and is being used in current treatment plans.

The results of recent risk-adapted therapy suggest that patients with early-stage disease who do not have bulky disease or B symptoms may be treated with chemotherapy alone (8). To reduce toxicity and increase efficacy, the combination chemotherapy has been modified in recent years. Two of the newer combinations are BEACOPP (bleomycin, etoposide, doxorubicin [Adriamycin], oncovin, prednisolone, procarbazine) and ABVPC (doxorubicin [Adriamycin], bleomycin, vinblastine, prednisone, and cytoxan).

Late effects

Adolescent treated for HD are at risk for delayed toxicity. Treatment with alkylating agents causes gonadal damage and decreased fertility in males. Exposure to anthracyclines may cause cardiomyopathy, and pulmonary fibrosis may develop after treatment with bleomycin. Thoracic radiation amplifies pulmonary and cardiac toxicity. Girls treated with thoracic radiation at age 10 to 16 years are at higher risk for breast cancer. Both boys and girls are also at risk for radiation-induced solid tumors. Myelodysplastic syndrome and/or treatment-related acute myeloblastic leukemia may be seen 5 to 10 years after treatment. Newer response and risk-adapted therapies hopefully will reduce these delayed treatment-related side effects.

7.2.2 Non-Hodgkin's lymphoma

The incidence of non-Hodgkin's lymphoma (NHL) also increases with age. Over the past several years there has been an increase in the number of new cases of NHL.

The incidence is higher in non-Hispanic whites. American Indians/Alaska Natives have the lowest incidence. NHL is also more common in males than females. Most cases of NHL present de novo. Patients with congenital or acquired immune deficiency either due to HIV infection or immunosuppressive therapy are at higher risk for NHL. EBV plays an important role in the pathogenesis of NHL seen in patients with organ or bone marrow transplant.

Clinical presentation

The clinical presentation depends on the site, extent, and histologic subtypes of NHL. Burkitt's lymphoma usually arises in the abdomen from the gastrointestinal tract as a large, rapidly growing mass with signs and symptoms of obstruction and ascites. Intussusception is occasionally the presenting sign. Lymphoblastic lymphoma usually presents as a large mediastinal mass with signs and symptoms of respiratory difficulty or superior vena cava syndrome. Anaplastic large cell lymphoma presents as a large, sometimes painful nodal mass or skin involvement.

Diagnosis

The complete blood count (CBC) is normal. Lactic dehydrogenase (LDH) is usually elevated. There is a good correlation between LDH and tumor load. A rapidly growing tumor may present with signs and symptoms of tumor lysis syndrome, consisting of hyperuricemia, hyperkalemia, and hyperphosphatemia. Bilateral bone marrow aspiration and biopsy and cerebrospinal fluid examination are done to establish the stage of disease.

Imaging studies – computed tomography (CT) scan, magnetic resonance imaging (MRI), or bone scan – are used to determine the extent and stage of disease. Biopsy is required in most cases to make the diagnosis. Diagnosis could also be made by cytology done on pleural, peritoneal, or pericardial fluid. Positron emission tomography is used for staging and to evaluate the response to therapy. St. Jude's staging system classifies NHL as stage 1 when only one lymphoid region or extranodal organ is involved. Involvement of two lymphoid organs or one extranodal region with one involved node on the same side of the diaphragm is stage 2. A gastrointestinal tumor with greater than 90 percent resection also falls into stage 2. Disease on both sides of the diaphragm or primary intra-abdominal or intrathoracic (pleural, mediastinal, or thymic) disease is stage 3. Involvement of bone marrow or the central nervous system (CNS) in addition to stages 1 to 3 is stage 4.

Treatment

NHL is a chemotherapy-sensitive cancer with an excellent response to combination chemotherapy. Treatment depends on histology (▶Tab. 7.5) biology, and clinical stage (9). With treatment, long-term disease-free survival for patients with localized disease is 90 to 100 percent; for advanced-stage disease with more aggressive therapy, the rate is 65 to 90 percent.

Combination chemotherapy to treat Burkitt's and large B-cell lymphoma includes cyclphosphamide, high-dose methotrexate, doxorubicin, and cytosine arabinoside.

Tab. 7.5: Histologic subtypes of NHL.

Type	Burkitt's	Lymphoblastic	Diffuse Large-B Cell	Anaplastic Large Cell
% of total number	40	30	20	10
Location	Abdomen, head, and neck	Mediastinum, bone, cutaneous	Abdomen, thymus, bone	Lymph nodes, skin
Immunophenotype	Mature B cell	T cell, precursor B cell	B cell	T or null cell, occasionally B
Molecular defect	Transcriptional deregulation of c-myc	Nonspecific	Transcriptional deregulation of bcl6	NPM/Alk fusion protein
Cytogenetics	t(8;14), t(2;8), t(8;22)	–	variable	t(2;5)
Treatment	Vincristine, Prednisone, cyclophosphamide, methotrexate, doxorubicin, cytosine arabinoside, rituximab	ALL-like therapy	Vincristine, prednisone cyclophosphamide, methotrexate, doxorubicin, cytosine arabinoside, rituximab	Doxorubicin, vincristine, prednisone, Cytosine arabinoside, etoposide

ALL, acute lymphocytic leukemia; t, translocation.

Anti-CD 20 antibody rituximab is used to treat lymphomas expressing CD20 antigen on their cell surfaces. With aggressive combination chemotherapy, 70 to 90 percent of these patients are expected to become long-term survivors of the cancer. Diffuse large B-cell lymphoma, like Burkitt's lymphoma, is treated according to initial resection and stage. The chemotherapy and long-term disease-free survival rates are similar.

Lymphoblastic lymphoma is treated with precursor B-ALL or T-cell ALL therapy respectively (10). Large cell anaplastic lymphoma localized to the skin is treated with surgery. Disease in any other location is treated with combination chemotherapy consisting of vincristine, , and prednisone. Some treatment regimens use etoposide and/or cytosine arabinoside. Patients with recurrent disease are candidates for autologous or allogeneic bone marrow transplant.

7.3 The leukemias

Leukemias are disorders of the hematopoietic progenitors. Molecular abnormalities in the leukemia cells give them a proliferative advantage; uncontrolled proliferation occurs at the expense of normal hematopoietic cells. Leukemias constitute about 6 percent of all cancers seen in 15- to 19-year-olds (11). The incidence of acute lymphoblastic leukemia

(ALL) decreases and that of acute myeloblastic leukemia (AML) gradually increases with age. Two-thirds of all acute leukemia in 10- to 19-year-olds are ALL. The incidence of chronic leukemia and myelodysplastic syndrome remains low.

The etiology of leukemia is not known. Patients with Down's syndrome, Fanconi's anemia, neurofibromatosis-1, Bloom's syndrome, ataxia telangiectasia, Klinefelter's syndrome, Turner's syndrome, severe combined immunodeficiency, and congenital neutropenia are at higher risk for developing leukemia. Exposure to ionizing radiation, alkylating agents, epipodophyllotoxins, nitrosourea, and benzene may increase the risk. Most patients with leukemia, however, do not have an underlying genetic disorder and the cause of leukemia remains elusive.

The clinical presentation of acute leukemia is nonspecific. The bone marrow's inability to make normal hematopoietic cells results in anemia, thrombocytopenia, and neutropenia. Expansion of the marrow by the abnormal cells causes bone pain. Leukemia cells can infiltrate almost every organ in the body and may cause hepatosplenomegaly, lymphadenopathy, testicular enlargement, gum swelling, joint swelling, eye involvement, cranial nerve involvement, meningeal involvement, periosteal elevation, and spinal cord involvement. As a result, ALL can mimic a variety of acute infectious or inflammatory illnesses such as rheumatoid arthritis, infectious mononucleosis, or osteomyelitis. The clinical presentations of AML and ALL are similar.

7.3.1 Acute lymphoblastic leukemia (ALL)

In the United States approximately 600 new cases (1) of ALL are diagnosed in individuals 10 to 19 years of age. According to the 2000 SEER data, the rates were highest in Hispanics, followed by non-Hispanic whites. The incidence is lowest in African Americans. More males than females are diagnosed with ALL.

Pathogenesis

Immunophenotyping and cytogenetics help differentiate ALL from AML. Precursor B ALL is the most common phenotype, followed by T-cell leukemia. The French American British (FAB) morphologic classification of ALL classifies ALL as L1, L2, and L3. There is no correlation between L1 and L2 subtypes and immunophenotype. L3 morphology is always seen with mature B-cell leukemia and is treated as mature B-cell lymphoma. Cytogenetics and ALL fluorescent in situ hybridization (FISH) of leukemia cells show chromosomal abnormalities of number, deletion, or translocation in most patients. These abnormalities are of prognostic significance and help tailor chemotherapy. Chromosomal abnormalities such as hyperdiploidy resulting in trisomies 4 and 10, or t(12;21) markers for good outcome, are less common in adolescents (12). Philadelphia chromosome t(9;22), a marker of poor outcome, is seen in 3 percent of adolescent ALL.

Diagnosis

A patient presenting with the symptoms listed in ▶Tab. 7.6 and an abnormal complete blood count (CBC) affecting more than one cell line or circulating leukemic blast cells

Tab. 7.6: Laboratory abnormalities seen at presentation in ALL.

Laboratory test	Abnormality
Hemoglobin	N, L
WBCs	N, L, H
Platelets	N, L
ANC	L
Circulating Blasts	Present in 90% of the cases
LDH	N, H
Uric acid	N, H

ANC, absolute neutrophic count; N, normal; L, low; H, high; LDH, lactate dehydrogenase; WBCs, white blood cells.

should be further evaluated for leukemia with bone marrow examination. The presence of more than 25 percent lymphoblasts in the bone marrow is consistent with the diagnosis of ALL.

Treatment

ALL without treatment is fatal. There has been a significant improvement in long-term disease-free survival rates over last 40 years. The most important prognostic factor for long-term survival is age at diagnosis. The outcome of a patient greater than 10 years of age is worse than that for younger children. With increasing age the outcome becomes progressively worse. This has to do mainly with the biology of the disease. It is interesting that adolescents treated on pediatric protocols have better outcomes than those treated on adult protocols (13). The current high-risk ALL protocols of the Children's Oncology Group are designed to enroll patients up to 30 years of age. Older adolescents have a higher incidence of T-cell ALL t(4;11) and minimal residual disease at the end of remission induction. Five years of 78 to 87.5 percent disease-free survival has been reported with risk-adjusted intensive chemotherapy (14,15)

The treatment consists of combination chemotherapy given over a period of 2 to 3 years. The intensity of the therapy is tailored to the biology of the disease and the patient's response to therapy as measured by minimal residual disease (MRD) at the end of the remission induction phase, lasting 4 to 6 weeks. Combination chemotherapy consisting of antineoplastic agents active against ALL is given in variety of combinations (▶Tab. 7.7), sequences, and durations; it has been used worldwide. The typical treatment regimen often used in the United States is a modified BFM regimen consists of five to six treatment phases as described below. The induction phase consists of vincrstine, asparginase, prednisone, and daunorubicin.

Approximately 95 to 98 percent of patients go into remission with this therapy. The risk of death in induction is higher in adolescents than in younger children. Induction is followed by consolidation and CNS prophylaxis. CNS prophylaxis consists of weekly intrathecal methotrexate for 4 weeks and either prophylactic brain radiation or subsequent ongoing intrathecal chemotherapy given at least once every 3 months for the entire duration of therapy. Without CNS prophylaxis the risk of CNS relapse followed by systemic relapse is very high.

Tab. 7.7: Treatment of ALL.

Drug	Mechanism of action	Route of administration	Side effects
Vincristine	Antimitotic, inhibits tubulin formation	IV	A, Peripheral neuropathy sensory, motor, autonomic, SIADH
Prednisone/ dexamethasone	lympholysis	Oral/IV	Weight gain, hyperglycemia, hypertension, osteonecrosis, mood changes, psychosis
Asparginase	Catalyzes asparagine, inhibits protein synthesis	IM/IV	Hypersensitivity, clotting defects (thrombosis and bleeding), pancreatitis, hyperglycemia
Cyclophosphamide	Alkylating	IV	A, B, C, CY, G, M, N, V
Anthracyclines Daunorubicin and doxorubicin	Free radical–mediated DNA break and DNA cross-linking	IV	A, B, C, N, V, M
Methotrexate	Antimetabolite: antifolate	PO, SC, IV, IM, IT	A, B, N, V, H, M, CNS
6-Mercaptopurine	Antimetabolite: blocks purine synthesis	PO	B, N, V, H,
Cytosine arabinoside	Antimetabolite: inhibits DNA polymerase	IV, SC, IT	A, B, D, N, V, fever, CNS

A, alopecia; B, myelosuppression; C, cardiac; CNS, central nervous system; Cy, cystitis; D, diarrhea; G, gonad; H, hepatic; IM, intramuscular; IT, intrathecal; IV, intravenous; M, mucositis; N, nausea; PO, oral; SC, subcutaneous; SIADH, syndrome of inappropriate antidiuretic hormone.

This phase is followed by interim maintenance for 8 weeks consisting of escalating doses of methotrexate. Reintesification with vincristine, asparginase, doxorubicin, cyclophosphamide, cytosine arabinoside, and 6-thioguanine given over 8 weeks follows this phase (▶Tab. 7.7). The maintenance therapy consists of oral 6-mercaptopurine daily and methotrexate once a week for 2 years. These patients also receive monthly vincrstine pulses with 5 days of prednisone/dexamethasone for 2 to 3 years. Thiopurine S-methyltransferase (TPMT) is an enzyme that converts 6-thioguanine and 6-mercaptopurine from a prodrug to an active metabolite. Patients with TPMT gene mutations do not metabolize these drugs effectively and need dose adjustment. Genetic testing for these mutations is available.

Prophylactic cranial radiation is used for poor responders; bone marrow transplant is reserved for patients who fail treatment and relapse. Treatment-related toxicity – including avascular necrosis, pancreatitis, and thrombosis – is higher in adolescents than in younger children (16). The risk of avascular necrosis (AVN) of the bone is high in children above 10 years of age, especially with a treatment regimen that uses dexamethasone (17).

Supportive care

Supportive care is based on these basic concepts:

- An indwelling central venous line (CVL) will ease the stress caused by repeated venipunctures and extravasation of chemotherapy. Patients need close monitoring for CVL-related infections and thrombosis.
- Infections, especially during neutropenia, are a major cause of morbidity. Patients with fever who are receiving chemotherapy should be promptly evaluated and treated with empiric broad-spectrum antibiotics (see discussion of neutropenia in chapter 6).
- Most centers in the Unite States give patients some form of prophylaxis against *Pneumocystis carinii*, now *Pneumocystis jirovecii* (PCP), consisting of trimethoprim/sulfamethoxazole two to three times per week for the duration of treatment and continued for 8 to12 weeks after chemotherapy is discontinued. Alternatives to trimethoprim/sulfamethoxazole are dapsone, inhaled pentamidine, or atovaquone.
- Once in the maintenance phase of therapy, patients may return to school full time.
- Influenza immunization is encouraged.
- Live virus vaccines are contraindicated.
- Ongoing long-term follow-up to monitor for relapse and delayed treatment-related toxicity is warranted.

7.3.2 Acute myelogenous leukemia (AML)

AML constitutes one third of the cases of acute leukemia in adolescence. There has been a slight increase in the incidence of AML in adolescents and young adults. However, the outcome of treatment has significantly improved over the last three decades. The 5-year disease-free survival rate with treatment is now 50 to 60 percent.

Pathogenesis

AML is a heterogeneous malignancy involving hematopoietic progenitors. The precursors of myeloid monocytes, erythroid cells, or cells of megakaryocytic lineage may be affected. The diagnosis is usually made by bone marrow aspiration and biopsy. The presence of greater than 20 percent myeloblasts in the bone marrow or increased blasts with cytogenetically abnormal AML clones is required to make the diagnosis of AML.

Morphologically there are eight FAB subtypes, M0 to M7 (▶Tab. 7.8). These subtypes have characteristic cytochemistry, immune, and cytogenetic profiles. t(8;21), inv(16), t(16;16) are usually seen with M1 or M2 AML and are associated with better outcomes. t(15;17) is seen with promyelocytic leukemia and is associated with good outcomes. Monosomy 5 o 7 or del(5), del(7) are associated poor outcomes. The new World Health Organization classification of AML is based on cytogenetic abnormalities and correlates better with outcome. Patient with no cytogenetic abnormality are classified using the FAB classification.

Clinical presentation

The clinical presentations of ALL and AML are similar and are discussed under acute leukemia, above. Findings specific to AML include granulocytic sarcoma or chloroma.

Tab. 7.8: FAB classification.

M0	Undifferentiated
M1	AML without maturation
M2	AML with maturation
M3	Promyelocytic leukemia
M4	Myelomonocytic leukemia
M5	Acute monoblastic leukemia
M6	Erythroleukemia
M7	Acute megakaryocytic leukemia

Chloroma is a mass consisting of leukemic blasts that has a greenish hue imparted by myeloperoxidase (MPO) present in myeloid cells. Although chloroma is usually seen in the orbital or periorbital area, it can involve any anatomic location. Occasionally the patient may present with isolated chloroma without evidence of leukemia in the bone marrow. Disseminated intravascular coagulation (DIC) may develop in patients with promyelocytic leukemia owing to the release of granules containing thromboplastin activity. Patients presenting with very high WBC counts (above 200,000/μL) may develop cell clumping in the small blood vessels of the lungs or brain, causing symptoms of respiratory failure, headache, somnolence, or stroke.

Laboratory

Initial laboratory features are similar to those of ALL (▶Tab. 7.4). Coagulation abnormalities such as elevated prothrombin time (PT), activated partial thromboplastin time test (aPTT), and low fibrinogen due to DIC are more common in AML and require close monitoring.

Treatment

Outcomes and survival have improved significantly over the last 30 to 40 years. This improvement is the result of intensified chemotherapy, improved supportive care as well as the use of hematopoietic stem cell transplantation (HSCT). Although FAB subtypes are distinct, the treatment of all subtypes with the exception of promyelocytic leukemia is the same. The drugs most active against AML are cytarabine and anthracyclines; these constitute the backbone of therapy. The mechanisms of action and side effects of these drugs are outlined in ▶Tab. 7.7. This combination causes significant mucositis and prolonged myelosuppression.

With intense chemotherapy, about 85 percent patients achieve remission. This phase is followed by consolidation therapy. Without postremission consolidation, most patients will relapse within a couple of years. In the United States so far, postremission therapy has consisted of allogeneic HSCT from haplo-identical sibling donors. Patients who do not have donors are treated with consolidation chemotherapy consisting of high-dose cytosine arabinoside. Autologous HSCT has failed to show major benefit (18) over chemotherapy.

Trials recently conducted by the Medical Research Council of Britain (MRC) show that a subset of patients with AML may be treated with chemotherapy alone (19). Clinical trials to evaluate the treatment of AML in children and adolescents with favorable cytogenetics and response to therapy with chemotherapy alone are currently being done. High-risk patients without a matched related donor for HSCT are candidates for HSCT from an unrelated donor.

Acute promyelocytic leukemia (M3) is a distinct subtype of acute myeloid leukemia. It is associated with t(15;17) and is responsive to All-trans retinoic acid (ATRA). Treatment with ATRA and anthracyclines during induction and consolidation followed by ATRA-based maintenance has resulted in long-term disease-free survival rates of 64 to 100 percent (20)

High-dose chemotherapy to treat AML is associated with life-threatening complications such as infections and bleeding. Infection is the number one cause of mortality during remission. Bacterial infections are responsible for 40 percent cases of neutropenia and fever, followed by fungal and viral infections.

The improvement in survival of the patients with AML is due to better supportive care and the treatment of infections. Febrile neutropenic patients are empirically treated with broad-spectrum intravenous antibiotics to cover both gram-negative and gram-positive bacteria. Patients with persistent fever after 4 to 7 days of broad-spectrum antibiotics should also receive an antifungal. They should also receive prophylactic antibiotics to prevent *P. jirovecii*. Trimethoprim/sulfamethoxazole is the drug of choice. Dapsone, atovaquone and inhaled pentamidine are other alternatives. To prevent cytomegalovirus (CMV) infection, these patients are given CMV-negative or leukoreduced blood products. Patients with recurrent mucocutaneous herpes simplex infection should receive acyclovir prophylaxis.

7.4 Osteogenic sarcoma (osteosarcoma)

Osteosarcoma is a primary malignant bone tumor derived from mesenchymal spindle cells that produces osteoid tissue or immature bone (21). Only about 50 percent of pediatric bone tumors are malignant, with osteosarcoma being the most common, accounting for about half. The peak incidence occurs in the second decade of life, during the growth spurt, suggesting an association with a period of rapid growth. It involves predominantly the long bones (femur, tibia, and humerus most commonly). This is clearly a very debilitating tumor to deal with, especially since management involves surgery.

As stated above, management is primarily surgical and chemotherapy has, over the years, been shown with multiple cooperative studies to have a role in both neoadjuvant timing and postoperative treatment. Neoadjuvant chemotherapy is given prior to surgery to decrease bulk and gain some biologic response. With this approach, limb-salvage surgical procedures have become standard when anatomically feasible, thereby decreasing the psychological catastrophe of major deformity in the majority of patients (22).

The same agents that have been found to be effective are used pre- and postoperatively and are called MAP – high-dose methotrexate, doxorubicin (Adriamycin), and cisplatin (▶Tab. 7.9). Other agents that have been shown to have activity are still being investigated and are outside the scope of this chapter.

Tab. 7.9: MAP (methotrexate, doxorubicin [Adriamycin], cisplatin).

Drug	Mechanism of action	Side effects
Methotrexate (Used at very high doses in this regimen)	Antifolate antimetabolite	Mucositis, alopecia, myelosuppression Transaminitis, renal impairment
Doxorubicin (Adriamycin)	Antitumor antibiotic DNA strand breaks and intercalation, free radical formation	Colors urine red CINV, alopecia, mucositis Cardiotoxicity
Cisplatin	Heavy metal (platinum) derivative Plastination and DNA cross-linking	CINV, alopecia, ototoxicity. myelosuppression Nephrotoxicity (Fanconi-like tubular damage)

CINV, chemotherapy-induced nausea and vomiting.

7.5 Ewing's sarcoma

Ewing's sarcoma is the second most common malignancy of bone. It is believed to arise from bone even though soft tissue (extraosseous) sites are encountered. It also occurs most commonly in the second decade of life. The primary sites of occurrence of Ewing's sarcoma are the extremities. It has, however, a higher predilection, (almost 50% of the time) than osteosarcoma for the central axis (flat bone in pelvis, and ribs), vertebral column, and skull (23).

Unlike osteosarcoma, Ewing's tumors are radiosensitive; therefore therapy involves a multimodality approach including neoadjuvant chemotherapy, surgery, and/or radiation. Once again, over years of cooperative studies, the first-line therapy for non-advanced Ewing's sarcoma should include vincristine, doxorubicin, and cyclophosphamide (VDC) plus or minus ifosfamide and etoposide (IE) (▶Tab. 7.10). Other agents and combinations are in use whereas some are still investigational and therefore not mentioned here.

7.6 Brain tumors

After the leukemias and lymphomas, tumors involving the CNS as a group form the second most common malignancies in childhood (24). Of note is that these constitute the greatest cause of mortality in pediatric malignancies. They include medulloblastoma, low- and high-grade astrocytoma, ependymoma, pontine glioma, craniopharyngioma, pineal tumors, and others.

The presentation depends on the anatomic site, with supratentorial tumors presenting more with headaches and infratentorial tumors more associated with cranial nerve deficits. MRI has become the diagnostic modality of choice in brain tumors. In addition to delineating the origin of the tumor, surrounding brain parenchyma and central nerve structures can be easily evaluated for appropriate surgical planning. Gross (complete) surgical resection impacts significantly on the outcome of these tumors, and the goal would be to achieve gross total resection with minimal sequelae.

Tab. 7.10: Combination chemotherapy for Ewing's sarcoma.

Drug	Mechanism of action	Side effects
Vincristine	Plant product Mitotic inhibitor	Vesicant, SIADH Neuropathy (motor and sensory)
Doxorubicin	Antitumor antibiotic DNA strand breaks and intercalation, free radical formation	Colors urine red CINV, mucositis, alopecia, mucositis Cardiotoxicity
Cyclophosphamide	Alkylating agent. DNA cross-linking	Nausea, vomiting, alopecia Hemorrhagic cystitis
Ifosfamide	Alkylating agent, DNA cross-linking	Nausea, vomiting, alopecia Renal tubular acidosis
Etoposide	Plant product, Topo II DNA strand breaks	Nausea, vomiting, alopecia Mucositis, allergic reaction Secondary leukemia

SIADH, syndrome of inappropriate antidiuretic hormone secretion; CINV, chemotherapy-induced nausea and vomiting.

The approach to therapy is once again a multimodality one, involving surgical resection, chemotherapy, and radiation. Some exceptions are as noted:

- Low-grade astrocytoma, craniopharyngioma, and choroid plexus papillomas where surgery alone might suffice.
- Diffuse intrinsic pontine glioma where resection is anatomically not feasible. Radiation therapy is the mainstay of palliative therapy for most gliomas.

The following chemotherapeutic agents are used in various chemotherapeutic regimens (24): vincristine, cisplatin, carboplatin, lomustine, and carmustine, temozolomide, cyclophosphamide, and etoposide (see ▶Tab. 7.11). Vincristine, cyclphosphamide, and cisplatin are specifically useful in the treatment of brain tumors.

7.7 Germ cell tumors

Malignant germ cell tumors are very infrequent in early childhood and are thought to be biologically different than adult germ cell tumors; they represent less than 1 percent of all pediatric malignancies in patients under age 15 years (25).The incidence of testicular tumors increases following the onset of puberty.

Histologically, malignant germ cell tumors show varied cell types and can be described as yolk sac tumors (endodermal sinus tumor), germinomas (dysgermino-mas), embryonal carcinomas, choriocarcinomas, and mixed (having different components). Such a tumor usually presents as a nontender testicular mass (in males), with abdominal distention and possibly menstrual irregularities in females. Endodermal tumors or those with an endodermal component have alpha-fetoprotein as a marker, whereas the dysgerminomas secrete beta-human chorionic gonadotropin. These markers are helpful in the diagnosis and monitoring of such tumors (26). Ovarian tumors,

Tab. 7.11: Chemotherapy for brain tumors.

Drug	Mechanism of action	Side effects
Carboplatin	Heavy metal (platinum derivative) plastination and DNA cross-linking	Nausea, vomiting, alopecia Mucositis, ototoxicity
Temozolomide	Alkylating agent, Methylation	Mucositis, nausea, vomiting Thrombocytopenia
Lomustine	Alkylation, DNA cross-linking	Mucositis, nausea, vomiting Renal and pulmonary toxicity
Carmustine	Alkylation, DNA cross-linking	Mucositis, nausea, vomiting Renal and pulmonary toxicity

Tab. 7.12: Cisplatin, etoposide, and bleomycin for germ cell tumors.

Drug	Mechanism of action	Side effects
Cisplatin	Heavy metal (platinum) derivative Plastination and DNA cross-linking	Nausea, vomiting, alopecia, ototoxicity, myelosuppression Nephrotoxicity (Fanconi-like tubular damage)
Etoposide	Plant product; Topo II DNA strand breaks	Nausea, vomiting, alopecia Mucositis. allergic reaction Secondary leukemia
Bleomycin	Antitumor antibiotic; DNA strand breaks	Nausea, vomiting, mucositis, pulmonary toxicity

on the other hand, both benign and malignant, can be composed of mature and immature teratomas.

Because these cancers are heterogenous as a group and vary in histologic subtype and site of origin, the approach to their treatment is individualized and employs multiple modalities. Surgical resection is all that is indicated for benign lesions and total excision is recommended for resectable tumors. Most of our regimens were gleaned off the adult experience and the addition of platinum based drugs improved the outcomes significantly (27). The combination of cisplatin, etoposide, and bleomycin is the standard first-line therapy for malignant nonseminomatous germ cell tumors (28). Multiple other agents and combinations are in use or under investigation for platinum-resistant disease (see ▶Tab. 7.12).

7.8 Late effects

As noted in the discussion of side effects, the main issues plaguing adolescents after initial disease-free survival are returning to normalcy as much as possible. Restrictions and follow-up requirements are more difficult to implement in late adolescence and early adulthood.

The Children's Oncology Group has a free website with guidelines for long-term follow-up care. There are both disease-and organ-specific recommendations; all patients and families should be referred there. Primary care physicians should encourage their patients to visit the site and thus be empowered to thrive after cancer (www.curesearch.org). A few pertinent issues are:

- Second malignant neoplasms: The risk of acute myelogenous leukemia after most alkylating agents and etoposide is present and can occur following any chemotherapeutic regimen.
- Cardiac toxicity: This is a dose-dependent toxicity causing decreased cardiac function and risk of heart failure. This is a main side effect of the anthracyclines (and exacerbated by the addition of radiation therapy to chest). Therefore these patients are restricted from heavy weight lifting for life and need cardiac monitoring by 2D echocardiography and electrocardiography. The frequency of monitoring depends on the total lifetime anthracycline dose and radiation exposure.
- Pulmonary toxicity: Interstitial fibrosis is a side effect of bleomycin, busulfan, and carmustine. These patients are monitored with pulmonary function tests and are generally limited from situations of high-pressure submersion such as scuba/deep sea diving.
- Fertility issues: Patients who present in late adolescence are usually offered sperm banking. However, in most cases that is not feasible. The majority of these patients still go on to lead full reproductive lives.
- Other possible endocrine issues are delayed growth and maturation and hypothyroidism. Patients treated for brain tumors in early adolescence may experience delayed puberty and growth. They are also at risk for hypothyroidism if radiation therapy was used in conjunction with chemotherapy.

7.9 Summary

Cancer is the leading cause of mortality in adolescence. Improved understanding of molecular biology, effective combination chemotherapy, and advances in supportive care have all contributed to significant improvements in the long-term survival of adolescents with cancer. However, improvements in the outcome of adolescents with cancer has lagged behind the success rates seen in children. This chapter reviews common causes of cancer in adolescence, including Hodgkin's disease, non-Hodgkin's disease, the leukemias (ALL, AML), osteosarcoma, Ewing's sarcoma, brain tumors, and germ cell tumors. Issues of management for the various types of oncology are presented. Research continues to provide improvements in access to care, compliance, and supportive care for adolescents and young adults with cancer.

References

1. Bleyer WA, OLeary M, Barr R, Ries LAG, eds. Cancer epidemiology in older adolescents and young adults 15–29 Years of age, including SEER incidence and survival, 1975–2000. Bethesda, MD: National Institute Cancer, NIH Pub. No. 06–5767, 2006.
2. Bleyer WA, Albritton KH, Ries LAG, Barr A. Introduction: Cancer in adolescent and young adults. Berlin: Springer, 2007:1–23.
3. Sparreboom A, Evans WE, Baker DB. Chemotherapy in the pediatric patient. In: Orkin SH, Nathan DG, Ginsburg D, Look AT, Fisher DE, Lux SE, eds. Nathan and Oski's hematology of infancy and childhood, 7th ed. Philadelphia, PA: Saunders, 2009:175–208.

4. Hesketh PJ, Kris MG, Grunberg SM, Beck T, Hainsworth JD, Harker G, et al. Proposal for classifying the acute emetogenecity of cancer chemotherapy. J Clin Oncol 1997; 15:103–9.
5. Kris MG, Hesketh PJ, Somerfield MR, Feyer P, Clark-Snow R, Koeller JM, et al. American Society of Clinical Oncology guidelines for antiemetics in oncology: Update 2006. J Clin Oncol 2006;24(18): 2932–47.
6. Hjalgrim H, Askling J, Rostgaard K, Hamilton-Dutoit S, Frisch M, Zhang JS, et al. Characteristics of Hodgkin lymphoma after infectious mononucleosis. N Engl J Med 2003; 349(14):1324–32.
7. Gobbi PG, Broglia C, Levis A, La Sala A, Valentino F, Chisesi T, et al. MOPPEEBVCAD chemotherapy with limited and conditioned radiotherapy in advanced Hodgkin's lymphoma: 10 tears results, late toxicity, and second tumors. Clin Cancer Res 2006;12(2): 529–35.
8. Nachman JB, Sposto R, Herzog P, Gilchrist GS, Wolden SL, Thomson J, et al. Randomized comparison of low-dose involved field radiotherapy and no radiotherapy for children with Hodgkin's disease who achieve a complete response to chemotherapy. J Clin Oncol 2002;20(18):3765–71.
9. Burkhardt B, Zimmermann M, Oschlies I, Niggli F, Mann G, Parwaresch R, et al. The impact of age and gender on biology, clinical features and treatment outcome of non-Hodgkin lymphoma in childhood and adolescence. Br J haematol 2005;131(1):39–49.
10. Burkhardt B, Oschlies I, Klapper W, Zimmermann M, Woessmann W, Meinhardt A, et al. Non-Hodgkin's lymphoma in adolescent: experience in 378 adolescent NHL patients treated according to pediatric NHL_BFM protocols. Leukemia 2011;25(1):153–60.
11. Mattano LJr, Nachman J, Ross J, Stock W. Leukemias. In: Bleyer A, O'Leary M, Barr R, Ries LAG, eds. Cancer epidemiology in older adolescents and young adults 15–29 years of age. Bethesda, MD: National Cancer Institute, NIH 06-5767, 2006:39–51.
12. Stock W. Adolescent and young adults with acute lymphoblastic leukemia. Hematology Am Soc Hematol Educ Program 2010;2010:21–29.
13. Boissel N, Auclerc MF, Lhéritier V, Perel Y, Thomas X, Leblanc T, et al. Should adolescent with acute lymphoblastic leukemia be as old children or young adults? Comparison of the Frech FRALLE-93 and LALA −94. J Clin Oncol 2003;21(5);774–80.
14. Barry E, Deangelo DJ, Neuberg D, Stevenson K, Loh ML, Asselin BL, et al. Favorable outcome for adolescents with acute lymphoblastic leukemia treated on Dana-Farber Cancer Institute. Acute Lymphoblastic Leukemia Consortium Protocols JCO 2007; 25:813–19.
15. Pui C, Pei D, Campana D, Bowman WP, Sandlund JT, Kaste SC, et al. Improved prognosis for older adolescents with acute lymphoblastic leukemia. J Clin Oncol 2011; 29:387–91.
16. Strauss AJ, Su JT, Dalton VM, Gelber RD, Sallan SE, Silverman LB. Bony morbidity in children treated for acute lymphoblastic leukemia. J Clin Oncol 2001;19(12):3066–72.
17. Mattano LA Jr, Sather HN, Trigg ME, Nachman JB. Osteonecrosis as a complication of treating acute lymphoblastic leukemia in children: a report from children's Cancer Group. J Clin Oncol 2000;18(18):3262–72.
18. Woods WG, Neudorf S, Gold S, Sanders J, Buckley JD, Barnard DR, et al. A comparison of allogeneic bone marrow transplantation, autologous bone marrow transplantation and aggressive chemotherapy in children with acute myeloid leukemia in remission. Blood 2001;97(1):56–62.
19. Stevens RF, Hann IM, Wheatley K, Gray RG. Marked improvement in outcome with chemotherapy alone in pediatric acute myeloid leukemia: results of the United Kingdom Medical research Council's 10th AML trial. MRC Childhood Leukemia Working party. Br J Haematol 1998;101:130–40.

20. Sanz MA. Treatment of acute promyelocytic leukemia. Hematology Am Soc Hematol Educ Program 2006:147–55.
21. Huvos A. Bone tumors: Diagnosis, treatment, and prognosis, 2nd ed. Philadelphia, PA: WB Saunders, 1991.
22. Meyers PA, Heller G, Healey J, Huvos A, Lane J, Marcove R, et al. Chemotherapy for non-metastatic osteogenic sarcoma: The Memorial Sloan-Kettering experience, Clin Oncol 1992;10(1):5–15.
23. Simon MA. Limb salvage for Osteosarcoma. J Bone Joint Surg Am 1988:70:307–10.
24. Craft AW, Pearson D, Bullimore J. The UKCCSG first Ewing's tumor study 9ET-1. Med Pediatr Oncol 1989;17:287.
25. Wexler LH, DeLaney TF, Tsokos M, Avila N, Steinberg SM, Weaver-McClure L, et al. Ifosfamide and etoposide plus vincristine, doxorubicin and cyclophosphamide for newly diagnosed Ewing's sarcoma family of tumors. Cancer 1996;78(4):901–11.
26. Smith M, Freidlin B, Ries LA, Simon R. Trends in reported incidence of primary malignant brain tumors in children in the United States. J Natl Cancer Inst 1998:90(17): 1269–77.
27. Ater JL, van Eys J,Woo SY, Moore B III, Copeland DR, Bruner J. MOPP chemotherapy without irradiation as primary post surgical therapy for brain tumors in infants and young children. J Meurooncol 1997; 32:243–52.
28. Rescorla FJ, Breitfield PP. Pediatric germ cell tumors. Curr Probl Cancer 1999;23: 257–303.
29. Hawkins E, Perlman EJ. Germ cell tumors in childhood, morphology and biology In: Parham DM, ed. Pediatric neoplasia: Morphology and biology. New York: Raven, 1996:297.
30. Einhorn LH, Williams SD. Chemotherapy of disseminated testicular cancer: a random prospective study. Cancer 1980;46:1339–44.
31. Giller R, Cushing B, Lauer S. Comparison of high dose or standard dose cisplatin with etoposide and bleomycin (HDPEB vs PEB) with children with stage III and IV malignant germ cell tumors (MGCT): a Pediatric Intergroup Trial (POG 9049/CCG 8882). PROC Am Soc Clin Oncol 1998:17:525a.
32. Pizzo PA, Poplack DG, ed. Principles and practice of pediatric oncology, 4th ed. Philadelphia, PA: Lippincott Williams Wilkins, 2002:246–47.

8 Sleep disorders in adolescents

Donald E. Greydanus and Cynthia L. Feucht

Healthy sleep-wake cycles are essential for normal physical and psychological health in humans. There are a number of sleep disorders in adolescents, including excessive daytime sleepiness, insomnia, narcolepsy, restless legs syndrome, parasomnias, nocturnal enuresis, and others. Behavioral management (including establishing proper sleep hygiene) is the key to many sleep problems in youth, although the judicious use of pharmacologic agents is helpful in some, as reviewed in this discussion. Sedative medications, particularly those with addictive qualities, should be prescribed only with great caution and restraint for patients with insomnia. There is no established role for the use of herbal products for insomnia except perhaps for melatonin. Research in sleep medicine is expanding and promises more treatment options for sleep concerns and disorders in youth.

8.1 Introduction

The three basic stages of human consciousness are identified as wake, non-REM (rapid eye movement) sleep, and REM sleep (see ▶Tab. 8.1) (1). High-quality sleep is important for all humans, allowing for proper health and good function during the waking hours (2,3,4,5,6,7,8,9,10,11,12). Individuals between 6 and 12 years of age generally need 10 of 11 hours of sleep per 24 hours and adolescents need an average of 9 hours per 24 hours, although there is some variation from individual to individual. Delta sleep (slow-wave or deep sleep) occurs in stages 3 and 4 of non-REM sleep and is the most restorative type of sleep as well as the sleep from which it is most difficult to arouse someone. REM sleep ("dream sleep") is characterized by generalized atonia of muscles, bursts of rapid eye movement, dreaming, and the inhibition of erections and diaphragmatic movements. In contrast to non-REM sleep, REM sleep involves increased cardiovascular and cerebrovascular activity along with irregular breathing.

Human beings need less total night sleep as they mature from infancy to late adolescence; also a later sleep onset hour (bedtime) is characteristic of many adolescents, along with a 40 percent reduction in REM sleep stage from ages 10 to 20 years. As the adolescent matures, the sleep ratio of non-REM to REM becomes 75 to 25 percent, with a normal pattern of four to six cycles of change (i.e., every 90 minutes) from non-REM to REM sleep with normal transient periods of arousal during night sleep. Daytime naps are not needed by adolescents unless night sleep is significantly interrupted.

A number of factors regulate and influence sleep-wake cycles, especially the endogenous circadian rhythm or internal biological clock mechanism. This internal clock mechanism is affected by light exposure, which turns off endogenous melatonin production, whereas absence of light (dark) turns on melatonin production. Research in sleep medicine has identified a number of "zeitgebers," or external stimuli, that affect the internal clock, such as meal timing, a ringing alarm clock, or other environmental cues. The circadian pacemaker is located in the suprachiasmatic nucleus of the brain. Puberty initiates a normal circadian sleep delay in most adolescents that results in a later desired bedtime than is noted in childhood.

Sleep disorders and abnormal sleep patterns are found in as many as half of adolescents, with a potentially very negative impact on their mental and/or physical health.

A number of sleep disorders have been classified as listed in ▶Tab. 8.2. Some adolescents are at increased risk for sleep problems, including those with chronic illnesses, psychiatric disorders, and developmental disorders, as noted in ▶Tab. 8.3.

Tab. 8.1: Stages of human consciousness.

1. Being awake
2. Non-REM sleep (rapid eye movement)
   a. Stage 1 sleep (transition of wake and sleep): light sleep
   b. Stage 2 sleep (starts true sleep state)
   c. Stage 3: first part of deep sleep (also called delta- or slow-wave sleep)
   d. Stage 4: second part of deep sleep
3. REM sleep (rapid eye movement with generalized muscle atonia)

Used with permission from Greydanus DE: Sleep disorders in children and adolescents. In: DE Greydanus, JL Calles Jr, DR Patel, eds. Pediatric and Adolescent Psychopharmacology. Cambridge, UK: Cambridge University Press; 2008:200.

Tab. 8.2: Sleep disorders.

1. Excessive daytime sleepiness
2. Insomnia
   a. Delayed-sleep-phase disorder (delayed sleep phase type)
   b. Limit-setting sleep disorder
   c. adjustment sleep disorder
   d. Psychophysiologic insomnia
   e. Altitude insomnia
3. Posttraumatic hypersomnolence
4. Narcolepsy
5. Klein-Levin syndrome
6. Sleep-disordered breathing: OSAHS (obstructive sleep apnea/hypopnea syndrome)
7. Parasomnias
   a. Sleep talking
   b. Nightmares
   c. Sleep terrors (*pavor nocturnes*)
   d. Nocturnal enuresis
   e. Others seen in childhood (bruxism; rhythm movement disorders [head banging, head rolling, body rocking])
8. Restless legs syndrome (periodic limb movement disorder)

Tab. 8.3: Disorders with increased incidence of sleep disorders.

1. Chronic medical disorders
    a. Asthma
    b. Cystic fibrosis
    c. Hyperthyroidism
    d. Organ failure (i.e., liver, kidney)
    e. Gastroesophageal reflux
2. Psychiatric disorders
    a. Attention deficit/hyperactivity disorder (ADHD)
    b. Mood disorders
    c. Anxiety disorders
    d. Conduct disorder
    e. Oppositional defiant disorder
    f. Schizophrenia
    g. Others
3. Developmental disorders
    a. Autistic spectrum disorders
    b. Severe mental retardation
    c. Angelman's syndrome
    d. Rett's syndrome
    e. Smith-Magenis syndrome
    f. Down's syndrome
    g. Prader-Willi syndrome
    h. Others
4. Fatal familial insomnia (noted in adults)
5. Neuromuscular disorders
    a. Myotonic dystrophy
    b. Duchenne's muscular dystrophy
6. Medications (prescription and over-the-counter)

Used with permission from Greydanus DE: Sleep disorders in children and adolescents. In: DF Greydanus, JL Calles Jr, DR Patel, eds. Pediatric and Adolescent Psychopharmacology. Cambridge, UK: Cambridge University Press; 2008:202.

Youths with chronic medical conditions may develop abnormal sleeping patterns due to the impact of pain, intermittent hospitalizations (with frequent awakings at night from staff), family dynamics issues, mental health problems (anxiety, depression, others), and consumption of various medications (over-the-counter and prescription) that can cause sleep disruption (see ▶Tab. 8.4). Clinicians should always be cognizant the side effects of medications they recommend, including those that can lead to nocturnal arousals, daytime sleepiness, worsened obstructive sleep apnea, or restless legs syndrome (see ▶Tab. 8.4).

Tab. 8.4: Medications interfering with normal sleep patterns.

Drug	Sleep effect
Alcohol	Insomnia due to delayed sleep onset
Anticonvulsants	Sedation during the day
Antihistamines (first-generation) • diphenhydramine • hydroxyzine • chlorpheniramine	Daytime sleepiness; lowered efficiency
Antidepressants • SSRIs • TCAs • Bupropion • Duloxetine (SNRI)	Activating effects with sleep interruption Sleepiness in the day due to slow wave sleep blunting
Caffeine	Insomnia due to delayed sleep onset
Corticosteroids	Stimulating effects leading to insomnia
Opioids	Daytime sleepiness, insomnia, nightmares, worsening of obstructive sleep apnea
Nicotine (tobacco)	Insomnia due to delayed sleep onset
Stimulants • Methylphenidate • Dextroamphetamine	Stimulant effects with insomnia (delayed sleep onset)
Theophylline	Delayed sleep onset, increased arousals during sleep

SNRI, serotonin noradrenaline reuptake inhibitor; SSRIs, selective serotonin reuptake inhibitors; TCAs, tricyclic antidepressants.
Used with permission from Greydanus DE: Sleep disorders in children and adolescents. In: DE Greydanus, JL Calles Jr, DR Patel, eds. Pediatric and Adolescent Psychopharmacology. Cambridge, UK: Cambridge University Press; 2008:203.

Perhaps half of adolescents with attention deficit/hyperactivity disorder (ADHD) develop sleep problems that include insomnia, frequent night awakenings, and incomplete sleep caused or complicated by the stimulant effects of anti-ADHD medications and other ADHD comorbidities, such as anxiety, depression, oppositional defiant disorder, and others. A variety of sedating medications are often used to improve insomnia in ADHD patients, include alpha agonists, antihistamines, and antidepressants given at bedtime: clonidine (0.1–0.3 mg), imipramine (50–75 mg), trazodone (25–50 mg), exogenous melatonin (3–6 mg), paroxetine (20–mg), mirtazapine (7.5–15 mg), and others, as noted in section 8.2, on insomnia.

8.1.1 Sleep evaluation

A careful medical history and physical examination are crucial to identifying the specific sleep abnormality of an adolescent (13,14,15,16). One should inquire about the regular time of sleep onset and waking up, nocturnal sleep duration, sleep awakening frequencies, and the presence of such issues as excessive snoring, daytime sleepiness, sleepwalking, sleep talking, nightmares, and others. The examination may document the presence of enlarged tonsils; fatigue during the physical examination, suggesting excessive daytime sleepiness; and others. It is very helpful to have the these patients keep a sleep diary to record their sleep habits, which can later be used to diagnose various abnormal sleep-wake cycles.

Those with complicated sleep problems and/or those resistant to therapy should be referred to a local sleep center, which can use such tools as actigraphy and a sleep lab studies. Actigraphy involves use of a wrist or ankle device to record sleep-wake cycles, while a sleep lab study provides a detailed recording of the youth while sleeping. This procedure includes electrocardiography and electroencephalography as well as the study of chin and tibial movements, oronasal flow, movements of the chest and abdomen, oxyhemoglobin saturations, end-tidal carbon dioxide levels, and others. A careful evaluation of the youth's sleep problems allows for a more accurate diagnosis, thus facilitating the development of an effective management plan. Various sleep disorders are considered in the following sections, with emphasis on pharmacologic management.

8.2 Insomnia

Insomnia is a term – not a specific diagnosis – referring to an acute or chronic difficulty in falling asleep; it can be due to many factors, such as chronic poor sleep hygiene, obstructive sleep apnea, effects of medications (prescription, over-the-counter, or illicit), and others (5). Sleep onset–associated disorder is described in infants or young children who normally awaken frequently; it is complicated by the frequent intervention of parents with rocking or feeding, so that the infants learns to fall asleep only with some type of parental intervention.

Limit-setting sleep disorder is described in those 3 years of age and older who refuse to go to bed because of various issues, such as parents who do not insist on a regular bedtime hour, effects of medications, the development of primary sleep disorders, concomitant anxiety, and others. Adjustment-setting sleep disorder may arise in a child who does not want to go to bed or wakes up frequently from normal nightmares, often due to a traumatic event; the parents become worried and then the child becomes excessively worried, leading to a chronic pattern of sleep dysfunction. Behavioral management that identifies and corrects the underlying mechanism is usually sufficient treatment for these three sleep disorders.

Sleep dysfunction may arise from exposure to high altitude (altitude insomnia), with abnormal, intermittent breathing (Cheyne-Stokes) occurring in non-REM sleep, probably because of the combined effects of hypoxia and hypocapnia. Fortunately this usually clears rapidly over a few days with acclimatization to the higher attitude. Acetazolamide has been used for severe and/or persistent situations.

An older child or adolescent may develop psychophysiologic insomnia, in which he or she is unable to fall asleep or remain asleep normally owing to a wide variety of factors such as an erratic bedtime schedule, medication effects (i.e., caffeine, ADHD stimulants, illicit drugs, others), underlying disorders (medical and/or psychiatric), development of anxiety about sleep, and others. As noted, puberty alters the circadium rhythm for young people, so that many prefer to stay up later yet need to get up early for school while still in a deep sleep stage.

This sleep dysfunction can evolve into an overt delayed sleep phase disorder (DSPD) complicated by daytime sleepiness, the development of a school-avoidant or refusal pattern, and/or anxiety or depression about school. This is a common problem for many adolescents that can range from mild to severe. A significant sleep debt may develop with the frequent emergence of transient, unconscious "microsleeps" that may be misdiagnosed as ADHD. Placing such an individual on an stimulant ADHD medication only makes the situation worse.

8.2.1 Management

The management of psychophysiologic insomnia or overt DSPD is based on the under-lying causative factors. The differential diagnosis includes psychiatric disorders, circadian preference, primary insomnia, and inadequate sleep hygiene. Youths with underlying psychiatric disorders can present with insomnia but usually not with a delay in the sleep-wake pattern. Those with circadian preference can conform to a normal sleep-wake pattern if they are motivated to do so. Many sleep well when allowed to choose their sleep-wake patterns, thus distinguishing them from those with primary insomnia who have problems with falling asleep and staying asleep even when allowed to choose their own sleep-wake patterns.

Management of such cases of delayed sleep onset or DSPD involves the correction of the underlying factors with behavioral management where possible. If there is poor sleep hygiene, education is required to correct the underlying disruptors. Thus the clinician can seek to recommend a strict sleep schedule for going to bed and waking up 7 days a week (including weekends!), avoidance of daytime napping, and avoidance of drugs interfering with sleep (i.e., nicotine, caffeine, others). Chronotherapy is part of a behavioral therapy program that seeks to adjust the sleep-wake schedule until the desired times are achieved. Bright-light therapy utilizes light boxes that provide 10,000 lux of blue light (or exposure to bright sunlight) to take advantage of a major zeitgeber – light.

Melatonin

Melatonin (N-acetyl-5-methoxytryptamine) is a pineal gland hormone that is regulated by the suprachiasmatic nucleus and can be given 30 to 120 minutes before the attempted bedtime. Since melatonin is considered an herbal supplement, its production is unregulated by the U.S. Food and Drug Administration (FDA); thus there may be a lack of standardization and risk of impurities in the melatonin as well. Dosages range from 0.3 to 6 mg at a time given orally. If these treatments are not beneficial or if there are concomitant problems (sleep, psychiatric, or medical), consultation is recommended. See ▶Tab. 8.5.

Alpha-2-agonist

Clonidine is a centrally acting alpha-2 agonist used for its hypnotic effects, especially to combat the stimulant effects of anti-ADHD stimulant medications. It has not been approved as a sedative drug. See ▶Tab. 8.5.

Tab. 8.5: Medications for insomnia.

Drug class	Examples	Adult dosages and comments	Side effects
Alpha-2 agonists	Clonidine (Catapres)	Dosing typically starts at 0.05 mg at night with increases of 0.05 mg every 3–7 days to a maximum of 0.4 mg at bedtime. Its onset of action is 45–60 minutes, the half-life is 8–12 hours, and its sedative effect peaks in 2–4 hours. Gradual tapering is recommended when stopping to avoid rebound hypertension. Effects include lowered latency to sleep and suppression of REM sleep. Clonidine is not FDA-approved as a hypnotic drug. It is not a Drug Enforcement Administration (DEA) controlled-schedule drug.	Hypotension, dyphoria, dry mouth, irritability, bradycardia, dizziness, fatigue, tolerance
Antidepressants	Tricyclic antidepressants (TCAs)		TCAs: anticholinergic effects; agitation, arrhythmias, overdose with TCAs; tachycardia, arrhythmias, hypotension (orthostatic), death
	Amitriptyline (Elavil)	Amitriptyline (25–100 mg).	Trazodone: hangover effect, dry mouth, constipation, priapism (rare)
	Doxepin (Silenor)	Doxepin (3–6 mg).	Mirtazapine: dry mouth, constipation, abnormal dreams, increased appetite, dizziness
	Nortriptyline (Pamelor) Other antidepressants	Nortriptyline (25–100 mg).	
	Mirtazapine (Remeron)	Mirtazapine (7.5–45 mg).	
	Trazodone (Desyrel)	Trazodone (25–100 mg).	

(Continued)

Tab. 8.5: Medications for insomnia. (*Continued*)

Drug class	Examples	Adult dosages and comments	Side effects
		These are sedating antidepressants; except Silenor they are not FDA-approved as sedative-hypnotic drugs. They are not DEA controlled-schedule drugs.	
		TCAs: acetylcholine antagonist, H1 antagonist.	
		Mirtazapine/trazodone: H1 antagonists.	
Antihistamines	Diphenhydramine (Benadryl)	Diphenhydramine: commonly used in children as a hypnotic agent despite a lack of confirmatory research; pediatric dose: 1 mg/kg up to 50 mg at night; sedation peaks at 1–3 hours and may last 4–7 hours; may lower latency to sleep onset and increase total sleep time; crosses blood-brain barrier and blocks histamine (H1) receptors; FDA-approved for insomnia age ≥12 years.	Anticholinergic side effects: dry mouth, tachycardia, hypotension, irritability, urinary retention, daytime sedation; tolerance; paradoxic excitation in children may be seen; overdose: respiratory depression, seizures, hypotension, rhabdomyolysis
	Doxylamine (Unisom)		
Benzodiazepines (BZDs)	Clonazepam (Klonopin)	BZDs are used for the treatment of anxiety, insomnia, and other conditions. These are DEA-controlled schedule IV drugs; except for clonazepam and lorazepam they are FDA-approved for adults with insomnia. They bind to several gamma-aminobutyric acid (GABA) type A receptor subtypes, with aresultant decreased sleep latency and delta sleep and increased total sleep time, increased stage N2 sleep, and REM latency; arousals (awakenings) between sleep-stage changesare reduced. These drugs also have anxiolytic and anticonvulsant effects.	Dependence with chronic use; common cause of addiction; daytime sleepiness, memory impairment, depression, behavioral disinhibition, anterograde amnesia, rebound insomnia, withdrawal, tolerance, many others. Abuse of prescription medications has become a public health dilemma as seen in the current abuse and misuse of BZDs.

	Estazolam (Prosom) (initial adult dose: 1 mg)	To be used with great caution in adolescents owing to many side effects including dependence. Clonazepam is used in adolescents with disorders of severe partial arousal at doses of 0.25–0.5 mg at bedtime. All agents except lorazepam and temazepam are hepatically metabolized and have active metabolites with a potential for CYP 450 drug interactions.
	Flurazepam (Dalmane) (initial adult dose: 15 mg)	
	Lorazepam (Ativan) (initial adult dose: 1 mg)	
	Quazepam (Doral) (initial adult dose: 7.5 mg)	
	Temazepam (Restoril) (initial adult dose: 7.5–15 mg)	
	Triazolam (Halcion) (initial adult dose: 0.125–0.25 mg)	
Herbal supplements	Melatonin	Melatonin: see text. Half-life is 30–50 minutes and onset of action is ½ to 1 hour; widely used; formulation not standardized. Wide range of dosages: 0.3–10 mg; may lower latency for	Melatonin: common side effects include fatigue, dizziness, headache, and irritability. Long-term side effects unknown; may reduce seizure threshold; to be used with caution in patients with vascular disorders; avoided in those with

(Continued)

Tab. 8.5: Medications for insomnia. (*Continued*)

Drug class	Examples	Adult dosages and comments	Side effects
	Chamomile	sleep onset and increase sleep maintenance and total sleep time. Other dietary supplements: only anecdotal reports of benefit; no overt research and not FDA-approved.	immune disorders or on immunosuppressants or corticosteroids; not FDA-approved or regulated. Melatonin from animal sources is to be avoided owing to risk for contamination.
	Lavender Kava-kava Valerian		
Melatonin agonist	Ramelteon (Rozerem)	Half-life up to 5 hours; 8 mg given 1/2 hour before bedtime; onset within 30 minutes. Binds to melatonin receptors MT1 and MT2 in the suprachiasmatic nucleus; FDA-approved in adults for insomnia; metabolized by cytochrome (CYP) 1A2 and used with caution if combined with other such drugs; fatty meal to be avoided before taking. Not a scheduled drug and is not limited to short-term use. See text.	Side effects include sedation, dizziness, fatigue, and headaches. Reports of overt dependence, tolerance, addiction, or rebound effects are not found in the literature.
Nonbarbiturate hypnotic	Chloral hydrate (Somnote)	Formerly popular as a hypnotic agent in children but no longer owing to side-effect profile; pediatric dosage: 25–50 mg/kg every 24 hours (maximum 1 g); peaks at 1/2 to 1 hour and lasts 4–8 hours; lowering of latency to sleep onset seen as well as increased total sleep time; not FDA-approved. Should not be used long-term for sedation. Can lead to tolerance,	Nausea, emesis, malaise, disorientation, ataxia, hangover effect (due to long half-life), paradoxical excitement, drowsiness, gastric distress; avoided or used very cautiously in for those with severe organ dysfunction (cardiac, liver), renal insufficiency (CrCl <50 mL/min), gastritis/esophagitis, porphyria.

			dependence (if used over 2 weeks); withdrawal symptoms (delirium and seizures) can be seen if stopped suddenly after chronic use. Classified as a controlled substance, schedule IV.
Nonbenzodiazepines	Eszopiclone (Lunesta)	Zolpidem has a half-life of 2.5 hours and an adult dosage of 5–10 mg (immediate release [IR]) and 6.25–12.5 mg (controlled release [CR] formulation). Potential CYP 3A4 interactions. In adults, IR used for sleep initiation concerns and CR for sleep onset as well as sleep maintenance.	Controlled substance, schedule IV. Dizziness, amnesia (dose-dependent), excess sedation, fatigue, hyperexcitability, ataxia. Not to be combined with CNS depressants. Can cause sleepwalking, sleep-related eating disorders, sleep-driving, parasomnias; untreated sleep-disordered breathing problems can worsen; to be used with caution in hepatic impairment. Overdose leads to respiratory depression.
	Zalepon (Sonata)	Zalepon has a half-life of 1 hour; the adult dose is 10–20 mg. Used in adults for sleep onset problems or to maintain sleep in cases of midsleep awakenings (up to 4 hours before wake time).	Also with eszopiclone: headache, nervousness, unpleasant taste, dry mouth.
	Zolpidem (Ambien)	Eszopiclone has a half-life of 6 hours. The adult dose is 2–3 mg, reduced to 1 mg with potent CYP 3A4 inhibitors. Used for adults to initiate sleep and maintain sleep. FDA-approved for chronic insomnia in adults. Minimal risk for rebound insomnia, withdrawal symptoms, and development of tolerance or dependence.	

Melatonin agonist

The use of melatonin receptor agonists such as ramelteon is controversial since it is best to utilize nonpharmacologic approaches for adolescents with DSPD. Ramelteon is FDA-approved for adults with insomnia, and pharmaceutical companies are marketing their sleep-inducing products directly to the general public as well as to clinicians. One advantage is it is the only nonscheduled (U.S. DEA), prescription drug that is FDA-approved as a sedative-hypnotic and is not limited to short-term use.

Ramelteon is a melatonin 1 and 2 receptor agonist and is called a chronohypnotic; it is available as an 8-mg tablet. There is no dose-response relationship and effective daily doses range from 4 to 8 mg orally. The introduction of such medications to adolescents, with their changing central nervous systems (CNSs) and when other measures can be beneficial, are issues clinicians should consider before prescribing such medications. Mechanisms of action include aiding sleep onset, improvement of circadian rhythm dysfunction, and increase in the total sleep duration. Patients should be counseled to avoid mixing such medications with illict drugs. Other medications used for adults with insomnia are listed in ▶Tab. 8.5.

Benzodiazepines

Several benzodiazepines are indicated for the short-term treatment of insomnia. They are associated with a decrease in sleep latency and an increase in total sleep time; they alter sleep architecture by increasing stage 2 sleep and decreasing stage 4 or delta sleep. Benzodiazepines should be used very cautiously to correct insomnia in adolescents because of their side effects, which include tolerance and dependence. (See Tab. 8.5 and chapter 10 in Greydanus DE, Patel DR, Omar HA, Feucht C, Merrick J: Adolescent Medicine – Pharmacotherapeutics in General, Mental and Sexual Health. Berlin: de Gruyter; 2012.)

Nonbenzodiazepine hypnotics

These include eszopiclone (Lunesta), zaleplon (Sonata), and zolpidem (Ambien). They are usually well accepted in adults for insomnia, as reviewed in ▶Tab. 8.5. Nonbenzo-diazepine hypnotics are associated with a decrease in sleep latency, increase in total sleep time (expect possibly zaleplon due to its short half-life), and maintenance of sleep architecture. Zolpidem immediate release is beneficial for the short-term treat-ment of sleep-onset insomnia compared with zolpidem extended release, which is effective for both sleep-onset and sleep-maintenance insomnia and may be used for longer time periods. Zaleplon is beneficial for sleep onset and for situations such as jet lag, where short sleep duration is the goal; it is FDA-approved for short-term use in adult insomnia. Eszopiclone is FDA-approved for adult insomnia and is beneficial for sleep onset and sleep maintenance with less nighttime awakening. It can be used for the long-term treatment of insomnia. Nonbenzodiazepine hypnotics have been associated with minimal risk for rebound insomnia, withdrawal symptoms, or the development of tolerance and dependence. See ▶Tab. 8.5.

8.2.2 Excessive daytime sleepiness

As noted with insomnia, excessive daytime sleepiness is a symptom and not a specific diagnosis (17). Potential causes are noted in ▶Tab. 8.6. Chronic daytime sleepiness can lead to many consequences, including irritability, impulsivity, ADHD-like features, depression, academic problems, and even death and/or injury from motor vehicle accidents. As noted, puberty can stimulate alteration in circadian rhythm, with adolescents delaying bedtime, staying up later, and sleeping in until late morning or even afternoon; if they get up early for school or other activities, a sleep debt develops.

Many adolescents develop poor sleep hygiene with trouble falling asleep owing to many distractions even in their bedrooms, such as watching television, playing video games (or other Internet activities such as Facebook), and/or listening to music (CD players, MP3 players, radio, others); this can lead to DSPD, as noted earlier, which is also complicated by having too much light in the bedroom, having a room that is too cold or hot, eating within a few hours of planned bedtime, consumption of caffeinated beverages, and others.

Management is based on correction of the issues preventing the adolescent from getting to sleep on time, improving sleep hygiene, and using behavioral management to

Tab. 8.6: Causes of excessive daytime sleepiness.

Poor sleep hygiene (see text)

Delayed sleep phase disorder (DSPD; see text)

Drug effects (due to caffeine in caffeinated beverages, alcohol, others; see Tab. 8.4)

Psychiatric disorders (see Tab. 8.3)

Medical disorders
- Hypothyroidism
- Anemia
- Infectious mononucleosis
- Lyme disease
- Substance abuse disorder
- Epilepsy
- Central nervous system (CNS) tumor
- Trauma to the paramedian thalamic areas of the CNS

Narcolepsy

Klein-Levin syndrome

Restless legs syndrome

Parasomnias

Obstructive sleep apnea/ hypopnea syndrome (OSAHS)

Jet lag (rapid time-zone change) syndrome

Others

Used with permission from Greydanus DE: Sleep disorders in children and adolescents. In: DE Greydanus, JL Calles Jr, DR Patel, eds. Pediatric and Adolescent Psychopharmacology. Cambridge, UK: Cambridge University Press; 2008:206.

establish regular, healthy sleep-wake cycles. Use of medication to correct this form of "insomnia" is discussed in the previous section. As noted, medication in these situations should be used with great caution and only for a short time in connection with behavioral management. Medications used to manage excessive daytime sleepiness, as noted in narcolepsy, include modafinil, methylphenidate, and amphetamines; these are reviewed in the next section.

8.3 Narcolepsy

Narcolepsy is a chronic neurologic disorder with REM sleep dysfunction; it has an incidence of approximately 0.1 percent (range of 0.02%–0.18%) with a positive family history in about 25 percent of patients; the prevalence increases 40-fold if there are first-degree relatives with narcolepsy (5,18,19). In some situations there is a history of CNS trauma. Those with narcolepsy usually have some but not all of the classic narcolepsy characteristics: excessive daytime sleepiness, cataplexy, hypnagogic hallucinations, and sleep paralysis. There can be frequent night awakenings, interrupted sleep, problems with initiating or maintaining sleep, and nightmares. Children with narcolepsy may be misdiagnosed as having ADHD.

A deficiency of hypocretin from the hypothalamus is found in some patients with narcolepsy; hypocretin is a neuropeptide transmitter that is part of the process in both being awake and inhibiting REM sleep. Thus narcolepsy is a process of sleep intruding into wakefulness and wakefulness interrupting sleep. Narcolepsy has an association with two HLA class II antigens: DR2 and DQ1. DQA*0102 is found in narcolepsy as well, whereas HLA DQB1*0602 is the most closely associated marker for narcolepsy, particularly for cataplexy.

8.3.1 Excessive daytime sleepiness

This is associated with REM-onset sleep and usually occurs while the youth is not in motion, such as when sitting down; however, it can be seen in other situations, as while standing or even eating. There are many causes for excessive daytime sleepiness, as noted in ▶Tab. 8.6, often leading to a delay in the diagnosis of narcolepsy. That diagnosis may therefore not be made until adulthood, although this condition may actually peak in incidence in adolescence.

Management of narcolepsy-based excessive daytime treatment includes behavioral treatment as reviewed earlier (i.e., improve sleep hygiene, allow two 20-minute naps in the daytime, others), with the use of medications to help keep the patient awake (see ▶Tab. 8.7). Such medications include modafinil and psychostimulants (i.e., methylphenidate [MPH] or dextroamphetamine). Medication is used for a lifetime to control symptoms, and it is important that patients (as well as parents, guardians, and schoolteachers) be educated regarding this disorder. Repeated counseling is needed, especially regarding the importance of having good sleep hygiene and sleep-wake patterns.

Modafinil is a nonamphetamine medication that is FDA-approved for patients with narcolepsy who are over 16 years of age; it is a wakefulness-promoting drug and is the first-line medication for excessive daytime sleepiness for adults with narcolepsy. Its mechanism of action is linked to its effects on dopaminergic signaling. It is not FDA-approved as a pediatric drug for ADHD management.

Tab. 8.7: Medications used to manage narcolepsy: daytime sleepiness.

Class	Agent	Dose	Side effects
Psychostimulants	Methylphenidate (MPH)	10–60 mg/day; started at 5–10 mg twice daily; no more than 20 mg in a single dose or 60 mg/day; dosing can be a single AM dose (long-acting products) or three times a day (immediate-release products).	Both MPH and amphetamines: insomnia, reduced appetite, loss of weight. Nausea, elevated blood pressure, headache, depression, rebound symptoms, FDA black box warning for potential of drug dependence (avoid abrupt discontinuation); tolerance; controlled schedule II substance with abuse risk; others.
	Mixed amphetamines; dextroamphetamine	Dose similar to MPH dose.	
Wakefulness promoting agent (long-acting)	Modafinil	Started at 100–200 mg once a day in the morning; some need a morning and noon dose; maximum dosage is 400 mg/day in divided doses. Avoid using after 2 PM (1400 hours) to avoid interference with night sleep; it has a long half-life (15 hours).	Controlled substance (schedule IV) owing to potential for abuse; FDA-approved for narcolepsy. In those above 16 years of age; headache, nervousness, hypertension, rhinitis, diarrhea, back pain, dry mouth, nausea, insomnia, dizziness, dyspepsia. Substrate for CYP 3A4; potential for drug interactions. Associated with life-threatening skin reactions and psychiatric symptoms (anxiety, mania, hallucinations).

Used with permission from Greydanus DE: Sleep disorders in children and adolescents. In: DE Greydanus, JL Calles Jr, DR Patel, eds. Pediatric and Adolescent Psychopharmacology. Cambridge, UK: Cambridge University Press; 2008:208.

MPH (methylphenidate) (see ▶Tab. 8.7) is a CNS stimulant used to treat ADHD but also excessive daytime sleepiness in narcolepsy. (See chapter 11 in Greydanus DE, Patel DR, Omar HA, Feucht C, Merrick J: Adolescent Medicine – Pharmacotherapeutics in General, Mental and Sexual Health. Berlin: de Gruyter, 2012.) Its sympathomimetic effects and DEA schedule II status makes it a second-line drug after modafinil, at least for those over 16 years of age. Amphetamine (dextroamphetamine) is another CNS stimulant that is an alternative to MPH for the treatment of excessive daytime sleepiness; it is also used to treat ADHD. Patients on psychostimulants should have certain parameters periodically checked, such as the blood pressure, pulse, and weight. Owing to cardiovascular side effects, its use should be avoided in patients with serious cardiovascular disease, including structural and rhythm abnormalities. A baseline ECG may be considered as part of a cardiovascular assessment prior to the initiation of medication. These medications also have a potential for dependency and should be used with caution in individuals with a history of dependence. Avoid abrupt discontinuation after prolonged administration in order to prevent withdrawal.

8.3.2 Other features of narcolepsy

Cataplexy is more a feature of adults with narcolepsy and involves a transient loss of tone in striated muscles of the face and extremitieswithout the development of unconsciousness; it may be precipitated by the individual becoming suddenly fearful, angry, or even laughing. The patient is conscious during such an episode, which can last from seconds to minutes. Patients with cataplexy may be misdiagnosed as having epilepsy.

Hypnagogic hallucinations are dream-like states that are very real to the patient, involve various senses in these states, and occur either while falling asleep or waking up. The other classic feature of some patients with narcolepsy is sleep paralysis, which is typically transient (lasting less than 1 minute) but can be frightening in that the patient cannot move during the time of waking up or falling asleep.

▶Tab. 8.8 reviews medications used to manage cataplexy, sleep paralysis, and hypnagogic hallucinations; these drugs suppress both REM sleep and deep delta sleep and lower inter-sleep-cycle arousals. These medications include antidepressants (i.e., SSRIs, [fluoxetine], venlafaxine, tricyclic antidepressants [imipramine, protriptyline, clomipramine], benzodiazepines [clonazepam], and sodium oxybate). The clinician should use these drugs very cautiously, keeping in mind their various side effects and the fact that they do not directly treat the underlying sleep disorder. The issues of overdose (as with tricyclic antidepressants and benzodiazepines) as well as tolerance and addiction (with benzodiazepines) must be considered at all times. (See chapter 10 in Greydanus DE, Patel DR, Omar HA, Feucht C, Merrick J: Adolescent Medicine – Pharmacotherapeutics in General, Mental and Sexual Health. Berlin: de Gruyter; 2012.) Tolerance and rebound may occur when these drugs are stopped. It is not known what the exact effect of chronic suppression of deep sleep waves has on adolescents with maturing CNSs.

Gamma-hydroxybutyric acid (sodium oxybate) is a GABA metabolite and binds to GABA-B and gamma-hydroxybutyric acid (GHB) receptors. It is approved for the treatment of adults with narcolepsy with cataplexy and can improve both cataplexy and daytime sleepiness, although it may take up to 6 to 12 weeks for the latter. Its half-life is 30 to 60 minutes and it is given in two doses – one at bedtime (after patient is in bed) and then 3 (range 2.5–4) hours later. Sodium oxybate is a DEA schedule III agent when used for narcolepsy and physicians must enroll in the Xyrem Patient Success Program in order to prescribe it. Potential side effects can be severe, including death from an overdose; there is also a high risk for abuse. It should not be combined with other CNS depressants including alcohol.

Tab. 8.8: medications used to manage narcolepsy: cataplexy, sleep paralysis, hypnagogic hallucinations.

Class	Agent	Oral Dose	Side effects
SSRIs	Fluoxetine	10–20 mg/day (up to 60 mg/day)	Insomnia, headache, nausea. See chapter 5.
SNRI	Venlafaxine ER	37.5–150 mg/day	Sedation, dry mouth, dizziness, headache, nausea, dose-dependent hypertension. See chapter 5.
Tricyclic antidepressants	Imipramine Protriptyline Clomipramine	25–200 mg/day 10–40 mg/day 25–150 mg/day	Confusion, constipation, dizziness, sedation, dry mouth, tremor, urinary retention, weight gain; see chapter 5.
Benzodiazepines	Clonazepam	0.25–2 mg orally at night	Adverse effects: sedation, ataxia, confusion; if stopped too soon, rebound reactions. Schedule IV controlled substance.
Miscellaneous	Sodium oxybate (gamma-hydroxy butyrate)	Age ≥16: 4.5 g in two divided doses, maximum 9 g/day; formulation is liquid.	FDA-approved for cataplexy; to prescribe, must enroll in Xyrem Patient Success Program; sedation, headache, nausea, dizziness, disorientation, death from overdose, high abuse potential. Schedule III controlled drug when used for narcolepsy; see text.

Used with permission from Greydanus DE: Sleep disorders in children and adolescents. In: DE Greydanus, JL Calles Jr, DR Patel, eds. Pediatric and Adolescent Psychopharmacology. Cambridge, UK: Cambridge University Press; 2008:209.

8.4 Restless legs syndrome (RLS)

RLS is a neurologic sensorimotor disorder that is better identified in adults versus children or teenagers; it is often not diagnosed until the adult years (5,20,21,22,23,24). RLS causes discomfort in an extremity (lower more often than upper) that can be described as an aching sensation or "crawling-creeping." RLS is also associated with abnormal sleep patterns. It may present with "growing pains in childhood" and sleep dysfunction. Movement of the affected extremities typically relieves the uncomfortable feeling until the next wave occurs. Any extremity can be affected and the unpleasant feeling may delay or interrupt sleep. A formal sleep study (polysomnography) may corroborate the history and find nocturnal intermittent foot dorsiflexion, first-toe extensions, and periodic limb movements of five or more per hour. RLS implies that the symptoms occur while the patient is awake; if they occur during sleep, this condition is called periodic limb movement disorder (PLMD). At least 80 percent of people with RLS have PLMD, but the reverse is not necessarily true. An individual may experience RLS while awake or while asleep and the movements can be voluntary or involuntary.

The mnemonic URGE can be used to identify RLS: U, urge to move legs due to unpleasant feelings or sensations; R, worsens during periods of rest; G, gets better with activity; and E, is worse in the evenings. RLS is associated with ADHD, depression, anxiety, and parasomnias. A 2 percent prevalence is noted in adolescents and a higher prevalence in those with epilepsy and diabetes mellitus; a prevalence of 5 percent is noted in adults. One third of adults with RLS have a positive family history in a partial autosomal dominant pattern.

Complicating this association is that those with RLS also have a disturbed quality of sleep (i.e., prolonged sleep latency with disturbed night sleep), which can induce or worsen such associations, as anxiety, depression, ADHD, and others. It is also noted that RLS can be worse during the following conditions: pregnancy, increasing sleep debt, iron deficiency anemia, diabetic neuropathy, malignancy, amyloidosis, renal failure, and under the influence of caffeine.

The management of RLS includes nonpharmacologic measures, as noted in ▶Tab. 8.9. Proposed underlying mechanisms include iron deficiency and hypofunction of the dopaminergic system. Thus management strategies for RLS include iron supplementation (3 mg/kg per day of elemental iron) to maintain serum ferritin levels over 50 ng/mL as well as the use of dopaminergic drugs (▶Tab. 8.10). Iron absorption is enhanced if the iron is combined with vitamin C. Serum ferritin levels should be assessed periodically, the iron dose adjusted to the laboratory data, and an iron overload avoided. Calcium decreases iron absorption and should be avoided 1 to 2 hours before and 4 to 6 hours after the iron supplement is given.

Only ropinirole and pramipexole are FDA-approved for the treatment of adults with moderate to severe RLS (23). Ropinirole (Requip, Ropark, Adartrel) is a nonergot dopamine agonist approved by the FDA for use in adults with RLS; its initial adult dose is 0.25 mg 1 to 3 hours before bedtime; the daily dose is titrated over the next 7 to

Tab. 8.9: Nonpharmacologic measures to manage restless legs syndrome (RLS).

1. Avoid or reduce issues that make RLS worse:
    a. Nicotine
    b. Caffeine
    c. Alcohol
    d. Dopamine antagonists
    e. SSRIs
    f. Antihistamines
2. Establish a good sleep hygiene pattern and avoid a sleep debt
3. Massage the areas of unpleasant sensations
4. Apply hot or cold packs to areas of unpleasant sensations
5. Exercise
6. RLS support groups (www.RLS.org)

Tab. 8.10: Medications used to treat adults with restless legs syndrome (RLS).

1. Dopamine agonists
   a. Ropinirole (FDA-approved in adults; see text)
   b. Pramipexole (FDA-approved in adults; see text)
   c. Levodopa-carbidopa (not FDA-approved)
   d. Bromocriptine (limited use due to rare side effect of pleuropulmonary fibrosisand cardiac valvulopathy)
2. Opioids (narcotics)
   a. Codeine
   b. Oxycodone
   c. Tramadol
3. Anticonvulsants
   a. Gabapentin
   b. Carbamazepine
4. Benzodiazepine
   a. Clonazepam
   b. Diazepam
5. Oral iron replacement

8 weeks and should not be more than 4 mg/day. Side effects may include nausea, emesis, hallucinations, sedation, dizziness, fainting, peripheral edema, and postural hypotension. It can also induce sleepiness during daytime activities; this may occur without any warning symptoms of drowsiness or somnolence. This may, for example, occur during driving a motor vehicle even after chronic use. Dopamine agonists have also been associated with compulsive behaviors or loss of impulse control (e.g., gambling, binge-eating, and hypersexuality). Symptoms may improve with dose reduction or discontinuation of therapy.

Rebound of the RLS symptoms may occur usually in the early morning, as determined by the drug's half-life. Augmentation can be can be treated by giving the medication earlier in the day, lowering the dose, or using a different dopaminergic drug, such as pramipexole (a nonergot dopamine agonist also known as Mirapex, Mirapexin, and Sifrol), which is also FDA-approved for adults with RLS. The initial dose of pramipexole is 0.125 mg 2 to 3 hours before bedtime; the a maximum dosage is 0.5 mg/day based on manufacturer recommendations. Pramipexole has a similar side-effect profile as ropinirole.

Another dopaminergic agent that, although not FDA-approved, is carbidopa/levodopa (Sinemet), a medication used primarily to treat Parkinson's disease and dopa-responsive dystonia in adults (24). Its initial adult dose is 25/100 mg of the immediate-release formulation ½ to 1 hour before bedtime. Carbidopa/levodopa has a higher augmentation and rebound profile than ropinirole and pramipexole. Adverse effects are similar to those of the dopamine agonists described above; they include dry mouth, nasal congestion, nausea, emesis, constipation, anorexia, hypotension, dizziness, headache, daytime sedation, peripheral edema, abnormal dreams, and compulsive behaviors. Other medications used in RLS (not FDA-approved) include benzodiazepines, anticonvulsants, and opioids (▶Tab. 8.10).

8.5 Klein-Levin syndrome

The Klein-Levin syndrome is a combination of hypersomnia (as much as 20 hours in a 24-hour period) with episodes of behavior characterized by hyperactive (augmented) sexuality and confusion (5). The increased sleeping can be followed by bulimic episodes with compulsive overeating in combination with hypersexuality (i.e., excessive masturbation), irritability, and sometimes hallucinations. This unique syndrome is typically noted in males in late adolescence and may be precipitated by stress-induced hypothalamic dysfunction, major CNS trauma, or even a viral illness. There may be three to four episodes of this cycle in a year and polysomnography may show short REM latency with heightened REM and non-REM sleep patterns.

During the workup the clinician should consider a number of conditions in the differential diagnosis, including encephalitis, bipolar disorder, and temporal lobe epilepsy. There are no specific proven pharmacologic management protocols, although some clinicians have tried tricyclic antidepressants and anticonvulsant medications for severe situations. Some have also tried psychostimulants, but without proven efficacy. The history in most cases is that there is gradual improvement and no further episodes are recorded in the adult years.

Posttraumatic hypersomnolence is a variation of this pattern in which there is excessive daytime lethargy or sleepiness and prolonged nighttime sleeping within a few weeks of a history of major CNS trauma. The differential diagnosis includes depression, epilepsy, secondary narcolepsy, and encephalopathy. There is usually full resolution within 6 to 18 months.

8.6 Sleep-disordered breathing

Sleep-disordered breathing (SDB) may develop in adolescents because of upper airway obstruction; four basic types of SDB are noted: snoring (with no gas-exchange dysfunction), upper airway resistance syndrome (UARS), obstructive hypoventilation (OH), and obstructive sleep apnea syndrome (OSAS). There is a 10 percent incidence of snoring in adolescents versus a 2 to 5 percent incidence of OSAS and OH, with an equal female-to-male ratio.

▶Tab. 8.11 notes risk factors for OSAS. The underlying pathophysiology consists of increased upper airway resistance due to abnormal anatomy or abnormal upper airway neuromuscular control (25). In childhood the peak incidence is between ages 2 and 6 years in association with peak years for adenotonsillar hypertrophy. Nocturnal airflow obstruction leads to hypoxemia, hypercarbia with negative intrathoracic pressure, and paradoxical movements of the chest/abdomen.

Sleep is marked by snoring, sweating, enuresis, frequent arousals with choking and gasping, and severe sleep dysfunction. Severe obstruction leads to a number of problems, as listed in ▶Tab. 8.12. The correct diagnosis is based on a careful history and physical examination aided by a sleep diary and nocturnal polysomnogram (one or

Tab. 8.11: Risk factors for obstructive sleep apnea syndrome (OSAS).

Adenotonsillar hypertrophy

Allergic rhinitis

Arnold-Chiari malformation

Asthma

African American race

Cerebral palsy

Chronic sinus disease

Craniofacial syndromes

Down's syndrome

Gastroesophageal reflux disease (GERD)

Laryngeal masses

Laryngeal web

Laryngomalacia

Micrognathia

Mucopolysaccharidoses

Obesity

Positive family history

Prader-Willi syndrome

Prematurity

Smoke exposure

Ventilatory muscle weakness (due to neuromuscular disorders)

more respiratory events per hour). The clinicians should rule out allergic rhinitis and an antihistamine trial can be useful to eliminate allergy as a cause (primary or secondary).

Principles of management are noted in ▶Tab. 8.13. Pharmacologic agents have a limited role in OSAS management at this time. Adenotonsillectomy is the major treatment for those with OSAS due to adenotonsillar hypertrophy. Nasal CPAP is recommended for patients with postsurgical sleep apnea, those who cannot have or refuse surgery, or as a choice of management selected by the patient. Oxygen is a limited option as the only treatment and does not affect the apneic or arousal episodes. In addition, oxygen does not improve excessive daytime sedation and can lead to hypercapnea as well as higher oxygen saturations.

However, oxygen can be helpful to some patients, such as those unable to use nasal CPAP, who continue to have major residual sleep apnea after surgery (e.g., adenotonsillectomy), and/or are not willing to have a recommended tracheostomy. Intranasal steroids and leukotriene modifiers cannot be used as the sole treatment for OSAS since they do not lead to full resolution of apnea and hypopnea; they may be useful as adjuvant treatment in mild to moderate situations waiting for nasal CPAP and/or adenotonsillectomy. More research is needed to more clearly establish the role of these medications in OSAS.

Tab. 8.12: Potential consequences of OSAS.

1. Excessive daytime sleepiness
2. Snoring, restlessness, perspiration, and apneic episodes during sleep
3. Diaphoresis, neck hyperextension during sleep
4. Inward (paradoxical) rib-cage movement during inspiration
5. Unusual sleeping positions
6. Morning headaches
7. Growth delay
8. Ventricular hypertrophy
9. Cor pulmonale
10. Aspiration
11. Secondary enuresis
12. Gastroesophageal reflux disease (GERD)
13. Hypertension
14. Increased intracranial pressure
15. Parasomnias
16. Academic dysfunction (limited attention span, poor memory skills, cognitive dysfunction, and lowered reaction time)
17. Misdiagnosis of ADHD
18. Misdiagnosis of learning disorders
19. Others

Tab. 8.13: Principles of OSAS management.

1. Disorders noted in Tab. 8.11 first ruled out
2. Trial of antihistamine medication
3. Trial of protriptyline (REM-suppressant antidepressant)
4. Adenotonsillectomy for enlarged adenoids and tonsils (OSAS, UARS, OH, and select primary snorers)
5. Weight loss measures to treat obesity if present
6. Positive airway pressure to keep airways open during sleep
   a. Continuous positive airway pressure (CPAP)
   b. Bilevel positive airway pressure (B-PAP)
7. Uvulopalatopharyngoplasty (UPPP)
8. Tracheostomy
9. Rapid palatal expansion
10. Supplemental oxygen
11. Medication
    a. Fluticasone nasal spray: reduces the number of obstructions in mild disease
    b. Montelukast for those with obstruction with mild OSA and no allergic rhinitis/atopy

Used with permission from Greydanus DE: Sleep disorders in children and adolescents. In: DE Greydanus, JL Calles Jr, DR Patel, eds. Pediatric and Adolescent Psychopharmacology. Cambridge, UK: Cambridge University Press; 2008:218.

8.7 Enuresis

Primary nocturnal enuresis is often considered a parasomnia (see section 8.8) and refers to bedwetting at night after an age at which nocturnal bladder control is expected, such as 5 to 7 years of age; it can occur at any sleep stage. The incidence falls precipitously from 3 to 4 percent at age 12 to less than 1 percent in 19-year-old males. Factors associated with nocturnal enuresis are noted in ▶Tab. 8.14; ▶Tab. 8.15 notes causes of secondary enuresis (26,27,28).

Many cases of primary nocturnal enuresis can be managed with behavioral modification therapy, such using operant conditioning devices (wetting alarms), hypnosis, acupuncture, diet changes, and scheduled voiding programs. A number of medications are beneficial for primary nocturnal enuresis; they are reviewed in ▶Tab. 8.16.

8.8 Parasomnias

Parasomnias (▶Tab. 8.3) are arousal disorders (partial or full) along with dysfunction of sleep-wake transitioning involving CNS dysfunction and skeletal as well as autonomic muscular disturbances (2,5). Some are more common in children than in adolescents. For example, rhythmic movement disorders (i.e., head banging, head rolling, body rocking) are irregular movements that start during the first year of life at the sleep-wake transition in both normal and developmentally delayed infants. Parents can be reassured that this is a transient phenomenon that usually resolves before age 4, although bed padding may be necessary. Severe and refractory situations are usually associated with neuropsychiatric disorders and may be improved with the use of benzodiazepines or tricyclic antidepressants.

Bruxism is frequent teeth grinding at night and found in half of infants as teeth begin to erupt. Approximately 20 percent of older children may have bruxism as well, which can lead to excessive wear on the dental surfaces and temporomandibular joint pain. Children with persistent teeth grinding can be fitted for a mouth guard for night use in addition to analgesics and biofeedback therapy. Severe cases may improve with judicious use of benzodiazepines.

Sleep talking is a benign parasomnia characterized by talking while sleeping; the talking is purposeless to other hearing it and reassurance of its normal nature is usually all that is needed. Nightmares occur during the last phase of the night's sleep during REM sleep; they may be triggered by a number of issues, such as psychological factors (including sexual abuse, anxiety, depression, others) and withdrawal from alcohol as well as other illicit drugs. The youth can be reassured of the benign nature of nightmares and offered behavioral management for underlying psychological factors.

Tab. 8.14: Factors associated with primary nocturnal bedwetting.

Genetics (75% increased if both parents had childhood NB; 45% increase with one parent)
Being male
Small bladder
"Heavy sleeper"
Deficiency of nocturnal antidiuretic hormone surge
Chronic illness
Institutionalization
Poverty
Unstable bladder

Used with permission from Greydanus DE: Sleep disorders in children and adolescents. In: DE Greydanus, JL Calles Jr, DR Patel, eds. Pediatric and Adolescent Psychopharmacology. Cambridge, UK: Cambridge University Press; 2008:213.

Tab. 8.15: Causes of secondary enuresis.

Diabetes mellitus or insipidus
Posterior water intoxication
Mental subnormality
Hinman-Allen syndrome (nonneurogenic neurogenic bladder)
Unstable bladder
Intake of too much fluid
Consumption of caffeinated beverages
Urinary tract infection
Urethral or bladder obstruction
Lumbosacral abnormality (spinal cord tumor, tethered spinal cord)
Sickle cell disorder (anemia or trait)
Obstructive sleep apnea syndrome (OSAS)
Renal disorders (as tubulointerstitial disease)
Constipation
Anterior labial frenulum displacement
Food allergies

Used with permission from Greydanus DE: Sleep disorders in children and adolescents. In: DE Greydanus, JL Calles Jr, DR Patel, eds. Pediatric and Adolescent Psychopharmacology. Cambridge, UK: Cambridge University Press; 2008:213.

Sleepwalking (somnambulism) is a partial arousal parasomnia characterized by the person arising from sleep and walking, typically during the first part of sleeping, when there is a transition from slow-wave stage 4 sleep. There may be a positive family history of others with sleepwalking. The patient and parents can be reassured of the benign nature of this parasomnia, although injury can occur during sleepwalking. The youth's living space should be safeguarded with alarms set to tell others in the house that sleepwalking is occurring. Keeping the sleepwalker safe is the key to management.

Night terrors (pavor nocturnus, sleep terrors) is a partial arousal parasomnia that usually occurs in non-REM sleep in a child between 4 and 12 years of age; it can continue into the adolescent years in up to one third; persistence into adulthood is uncommon. It begins with vivid vocalizations (i.e., loud crying, screaming) with tachycardia, tachpnea, and sweating. The night terror does not usually exceed 30 minutes, usually recurs at the same time each night, and the child does not have any recall for the event. There may be a positive family history of others with this phenomenon. There may be underlying issues leading to prolonged slow-wave sleep induced by sleep deprivation and leading to an increase in pavor nocturnus. In the workup, clinicians should also consider temporal lobe epilepsy, complex partial seizure, confusional arousal, and nocturnal pain attack.

Sleep terrors usually resolve within a year and reassurance is all that is needed in this situation. Some individuals are helped if woken up ½ hour after falling asleep. If there is sleep deprivation, the underlying factors for this, such as medication effect or obstructive sleep apnea, should be corrected. Pharmacologic intervention for sleep terrors is usually not needed. If the situation is severe and/or persistent, clinicians can prescribe medications that suppress slow-wave sleep or change them to non-REM to REM sleep transition. A tricyclic antidepressant, such as imipramine; SSRI, such as sertraline; or benzodiazepine (e.g., clonazepam, 0.25–2 mg at night) may be tried. Medication

Tab. 8.16: Pharmacologic agents for primary nocturnal enuresis.

Agent	Dose	Adverse effects	Comments
Imipramine	25–75 mg orally at night. Age <12: maximum 50 mg/day Age ≥12: maximum 75 mg/day	Anticholinergic and other tricyclic antidepressant effects: sedation, restlessness, poor concentration, weight gain, syncope, dry mouth (decreased salivary flow and increased tooth decay), blurring of vision (including cycloplegia and mydriasis), confusion, dizziness, constipation, anxiety; urinary retention; drug interactions with SSRIs and MAOIs; electrocardiograph (ECG) changes (sinus tachycardia, AV blocks, prolonged PR interval, increased QTc interval); overdose can be fatal with arrhythmias and respiratory depression.	Start with 25 mg with gradual increase if necessary; 50% will respond; taken 60 minutes before bedtime. If helpful, may be used for 3–6 months. Avoid abrupt discontinuation.
Oxybutynin	5 mg orally at night; up to 5 mg thrice daily. Extended-release form available for treatment of overactive bladder and also detrussor overactivity due to neurologic disorders.	Anticholinergic adverse effects including dry mouth, constipation, sedation, blurred vision, dizziness and flushing; patient should avoid overheating on hot days.	Started at a low dose; may be used for 3–6 months if beneficial before gradual weaning; helps to suppress uninhibited bladder activity.
Desmopressin acetate (synthetic analogue of antidiuretic hormone [ADH])	0.2–0.6 mg orally	Anecdotal reports of hyponatremia in those with underlying liver and kidney disease; increased LFTs with oral formulation	First agent of choice for many clinicians. Started at a low dose 20–30 minutes before bedtime; increased after 2–3 weeks to max of 0.6 mg. The pills can be chewed if necessary. Best used at the most efficacious dose for 3–6 months before any attempt to wean off.

(Continued)

Tab. 8.16: Pharmacologic agents for primary nocturnal enuresis. (*Continued*)

Agent	Dose	Adverse effects	Comments
			Fluid intake restricted 1 hour prior to dose until the next morning or for at least 8 hours after dose; avoided in patients with hyponatremia, history of hyponatremia, or renal insufficiency.

Used with permission from Greydanus DE: Sleep disorders in children and adolescents. In: DE Greydanus, JL Calles Jr, DR Patel, eds. Pediatric and Adolescent Psychopharmacology. Cambridge, UK: Cambridge University Press; 2008:214–15.

can be used for 3 to 6 months and then stopped to see whether the sleep terrors return. Side effects for clonazepam, as noted before, include confusion, ataxia, rebound, and sedation.

8.9 Summary

Healthy sleep-wake cycles are essential for normal physical and psychological health in humans (5). There are a number of sleep disorders in adolescents as noted in this chapter. The most common issue with youth is excessive daytime sleepiness due to various factors (▶Tab. 8.6). A careful history and physical examination (including an otolaryngologic exam) are necessary to identify the nature of the sleep problem. Many medications can induce sedation, and sleep problems can worsen existing medical and psychiatric disorders. Youths who are sleepy in the daytime may be misdiagnosed as having learning problems, ADHD, laziness, or depression. A sleep diary may be helpful and a polysomnogram is also useful in selective situations to identify such disorders as narcolepsy, restless legs syndrome (periodic limb movement disorder), sleep apnea, and others.

Behavioral management (including establishing proper sleep hygiene) is the key to many sleep problems in youth, although the judicious use of pharmacologic agents is helpful in some, as reviewed in this chapter. For example, modafinil and psychostimulants are useful for daytime sleepiness of narcolepsy and a number of medications (imipramine, oxybutynin, and DDAVP) are useful for nocturnal enuresis. The prescription of sedative medications (▶Tab. 8.5), particularly those with addictive qualities, should be used only with great caution and restraint by clinicians in patients with insomnia. (See chapter 11 in Greydanus DE, Patel DR, Omar HA, Feucht C, Merrick J: Adolescent Medicine – Pharmacotherapeutics in General, Mental and Sexual Health. Berlin: de Gruyter: 2012.)

Abuse of these medications, such as the benzodiazepines, has reach epidemic proportions in the United States and many parts of the world. There is no established role for the use of herbal products for insomnia except perhaps for melatonin, although this and other popular agents (such as alpha-2 agonists in youths with ADHD) are not FDA-approved for insomnia (▶Tab. 8.5).

References

1. American Academy of Sleep Medicine. The international classification of sleep disorders, 2nd ed. New York: Westchester American Academy Sleep Medicine, 2005:125–29.
2. Chhangani B, Greydanus DE, Patel DR, Feucht C. Pharmacology of sleep disorders in children and adolescents. Pediatr Clin North Am 2011;58(1):273–91.
3. Colrain IM. Sleep and the brain. Neuropsychol Rev 2011;21:1–4.
4. Gradisar M, Gardner G, Dohnt H. Recent worldwide sleep patterns and problems during adolescence: a review and meta-analysis of age, region, and sleep. Sleep Med 2011;12:110–18.
5. Greydanus DE. Sleep disorders in children and adolescents. In: Greydanus DE, Dilip DR, CallesJr JL, eds. Pediatric and adolescent psychopharmacology. Cambridge, UK: Cambridge University Press, 2008:199–222.
6. Harvey AG. Sleep and circadian functioning: critical mechanisms in the mood disorders? Annu Rev Clin Psychol 2011;7:297–319.
7. Lewandowski AS, Ward TM, Palermo TM. Sleep problems in children and adolescents with common medical conditions. Pediatr Clin North Am 2011;58:699–713.
8. Owens JA. Sleep disorders in children and adolescents. In: Greydanus DE, Patel DR, Pratt HD, eds. Behavioral pediatrics, 2nd ed. New York: iUniverse Publishers, 2006:236–64.
9. Pandi-Perumal SR, Kramer M, eds. Sleep and mental illness. Cambridge: Cambridge University Press, 2010.
10. Brand S, Kirov R. Sleep and its importance in adolescence and common adolescent somatic psychiatric conditions. Int J Gen Med 2011;4:4235–42.
11. Gregory AM, Sadeh A. Sleep, emotional and behavioral difficulties in children and adolescents. Sleep Med Rev 2011;13:23–30.
12. Schuen JN.Sleep disorders in the adolescent. In: Greydanus DE, Patel DR, Pratt HD, eds. . Essential adolescent medicine. New York: McGraw-Hill, 2006:281–97.
13. Babcock DA. evaluating sleep and sleep disorders in the pediatric primary care setting. Pediatr Clin North Am 2011;58:543–54.
14. Owens JA. Etiologies and evaluation of sleep disturbances in adolescence. Adolesc Med State Art Rev 2010;21:430–45.
15. Roberts RE, Roberts CR, Xing Y. Restricted sleep among adolescents: prevalence, incidence, persistence, and associated factors. Behav Sleep Med 2011;9:18–30.
16. Weiss SK, Garbutt A. Pharmacotherapy in pediatric sleep disorders. Adolesc Med State Art Rev 2010;21:508–21.
17. Carrot B, Lecendreux M. Evaluation of excessive daytime sleepiness in child and adolescent psychopathology. Arch Pediatr 2011 Jun 14 [EPub ahead of print]
18. Kanbayashi T, Sagawa Y, Takemura F, Ito SU, Tsutsui K, Hishikawa Y, et al. The pathophysiologic basis of secondary narcolepsy and hypersomnia. Curr Neurol Neurosci Rep 2011;11:235–41.
19. Sullivan SS. Narcolepsy in adolescents. Adolesc Med State Art Rev 2010;21:542–55.
20. Durmer JS, Quraishi GH. Restless legs syndrome, periodic leg movements, and periodic limb movement disorder in children. Pediatr Clin North Am 2011;58:591–620.
21. Mitchell UH. Nondrug-related aspect of treating Ekbom disease, formerly known as restless legs syndrome. Neuropsychiatr Dis Treat 2011;7:251–57.

22. Picchietti DL, Stevens HE. Early manifestations of restless legs syndrome in children and adolescence. Sleep Med 2008;9(7): 770–81.
23. Scholz H, Trenkwalder C, Kohnen R, Riemann D, Kriston L, Hornyak M. Dopamine agonists for restless legs syndrome. Cochrane Database Syst Rev 2011;3:CD006009.
24. Scholz H, Trenkwalder C, Kohnen R, Riemann D, Kriston L, Hornyak M. Levodopa for restless legs syndrome. Cochrane Database Syst Rev 2011;2:CD005504.
25. Burg CJ, Friedman NR. Diagnosis and treatment of sleep apnea in adolescents. Adolesc Med State Art Rev 2010;21:457–79.
26. Greydanus DE, Torres AD, Wan JH. Genitourinary and renal disorders. In: Greydanus DE, Patel DR, Pratt HD, eds. Essential adolescent medicine. New York: McGraw-Hill, 2006:355–59.
27. Kiddoo D. Nocturnal enuresis. Clin Evid (Online) 2011 Jan 31; pii:0305.
28. Neveus T. Nocturnal enuresis-theoretic background and practical guidelines. Pediatr Nephrol 2011;26:1207-14.

9 Concepts of hypertension

Alfonso D. Torres and Donald E. Greydanus

Hypertension is a major disorder in adolescents; it has potentially severe consequences in adult life, with increased morbidity and mortality. This chapter considers important concepts in high blood pressure, including its definition, proper measurement, classification, etiology, evaluation, and pharmacologic management. Proper recognition and management of hypertension in youth will yield enormous dividends for health during the adolescent and adult years.

9.1 Introduction

The consensus recommendations of the Fourth Report of the U.S. National Heart, Lung and Blood Institute define normal blood pressure in children and adolescents as systolic and diastolic blood pressure (BP) below the 90th percentile for age, gender, and height; hypertension is defined as systolic and/or diastolic BP that is equal or above the 95th percentile for age, gender, and height (1). High-normal blood pressure or "prehypertension" is defined as BP between the 90th and 95th percentile (see ▶Tab. 9.1).

9.2 Measurement of blood pressure in children and adolescents

The measurement of BP in children and adolescents should be performed in a standardized manner by an experienced individual who utilizes the proper technique to prevent errors that could result in the misdiagnosis of hypertension. The most accurate results are obtained with mercury sphygmomanometers, but these are no longer available because of concerns regarding environmental toxicity. Currently accepted methods include auscultation with standard aneroid sphygmomanometers; these instruments require frequent calibration to ensure the accuracy of measurements. Automated oscillometric BP measurement devices are coming into more common use in the medical office, in the home to monitor very young infants and children, and in the intensive care units of hospitals.

Finally, ambulatory BP monitoring is being more widely utilized in outpatient clinics. Specific applications include circumstances when there is variability in BP values, in the evaluation of "white coat" hypertension, for the diagnosis of masked hypertension, for the measurement BP at night to determine the presence of non-"night BP dipping" (or, lowering of blood pressure), BP load, assessment of the effect of medication on BP, and other factors important in assessing the risk of chronic cardiovascular disease (2,3).

Accurate BP measurements require the appropriated BP cuff size for the specific patient, with a cuff that is appropriated for the child-size upper arm. In order to measure BP in children 3 years of age through adolescence, BP cuffs of different sizes are

Tab. 9.1: Classification of casual BP in adolescents (1).

HTN classification	2004 Working Group
Normotensive	<90th percentile
Prehypertensive	90th to <95th percentile or if BP ≥120/80 mm Hg even if <90th percentile at three separate visits
Stage 1 HTN	95th to 99th percentile + 5 mm Hg at three separated visits
Stage 2 HTN	>99th percentile + 5 mm Hg at three separated visits

required, including an adult cuff. For obese adolescents and the measurement of leg BP, an oversize BP cuff may be necessary (4).

Elevated BP in adolescents must be confirmed by at least three different visits before the adolescent can be categorized as hypertensive. In the measurement of BP, attention to details is important. The proper conditions include posture, equipment, technique, and measurement performance. Measurement of BP in the lower extremities is part of the evaluation of children and adolescents to exclude the possibility of coarctation of the aorta or midaortic syndrome. Symptomatic hypertensive patients require a rapid evaluation of target-organ involvement and prompt pharmacologic treatment even before the cause of the hypertension is definitively known.

The development of hypertension in the adult is closely associated with risk factors for cardiovascular disease and associated complications, including cerebrovascular disease, retinopathy, heart failure, renal failure, and compromised cognition. Hypertension is one of the leading causes of end-stage renal disease. It is increasingly recognized that many of these factors begin early in life; many are genetically determined and can result from intrauterine hypertension programming, as is seen with intrauterine growth retardation and preterm delivery, predisposing to hypertension and obesity. After birth, in childhood and adolescence, there is a mismatch between the conditions for which the fetus was programmed and the extrauterine conditions actually encountered (5,6).

The progression from normotensive males and females at 17 years of age to hypertensive young adults at 42 years of age (reaching a hazard ratio of 2.5 [95% CI: 1.75 to 3.57] for boys and 2.3 [95% CI: 0.71 to 7.60] for girls in the group with BP at 130 to 139/85 to 89 mmHg) correlates with body mass index (BMI) at 17 years of age and sex hormones. Longitudinal studies in young adolescent males from different ethnic groups in the United Kingdom indicate no difference in systolic BP at 12 years of age but greater differences with increased systolic BP in the adolescent years; this is also noted in African American males at 16 years of age as compared with Caucasians (9 + 2.9 mm Hg). The BP differences in girls were not significantly different at any age. The diastolic BP differences in girls were more significant, with socioeconomic disadvantages having a greater effect in girls in minority groups (7).

Primary hypertension (PH), or essential hypertension, has been considered to result from accelerated maturation in children and adolescents. The degree of maturation can objectively be assessed by determining of bone age using dual-energy x-ray absorptiometry (DEXA). Recently these observations have been validated by researchers in a group of newly diagnosed untreated adolescent patients (8).

9.3 Causes of hypertension in children and adolescents

Essential hypertension in adolescents has dramatically increased in the last 20 years from 2.7 percent to 5 percent of schoolchildren as defined by an average of systolic or diastolic BP greater than than the 95th percentile and corrected for age, gender, and height. This increase in BP correlates with an increase in overweight and obesity, hyperlipidemia, and insulin resistance; these factors are particularly evident in certain ethnic groups, where hypertension and obesity are observed in up to 50 percent the population (9,10).

Essential hypertension has become the most common cause of hypertension in adolescents. Criteria for the diagnosis of essential hypertension in adolescents include inability to identify a known secondary cause of hypertension, a positive family history of hypertension, heightened response to emotional stress, and stage 1 hypertension at presentation in most cases. Determination of plasma renin activity may not be useful for the diagnosis of essential hypertension. However, very low plasma renin activity may indicate other rare causes (monogenic causes) of hypertension (11).

Essential hypertension is considered to be a multifactorial and polygenic condition involving environmental, developmental, and genetic factors. Currently in the United States, the diagnosis of hypertension in children and adolescents is based on recent research (1). As noted, hypertension is defined as an average systolic BP (SBP) and/or diastolic BP (DBP) equal to the 95th percentile for gender, age, and height on three separate occasions. Prehypertension in children is defined as average SBP or DBP levels that are equal to the 90th percentile but below the 95th percentile.

Adolescents with BP levels of 120/80 mm Hg should be considered prehypertensive and preventive life style modifications should be recommended. A patient who is hypertensive at the physician's office or clinic but normotensive outside a clinical setting has "white-coat hypertension," Masked hypertension is diagnosed when the BP measured in the office is normal but is elevated in other settings. Masked hypertension is not a benign condition, since it may be associated with left ventricular hypertrophy.

Ambulatory BP monitoring (ABPM) is often necessary for the diagnosis of these conditions and is also useful for evaluation of adolescents with stage 2 hypertension. Left ventricular hypertrophy is found in 5.7 percent of normotensive adolescents, 9.4 percent of adolescents with white-coat hypertension, 22.2 percent of those with masked hypertension, 18 percent of individuals with stage 1 hypertension, and 32.4 percent of those with stage 2 hypertension (12,13). Other markers for cardiovascular risk that have been demonstrated in adolescents include carotid intima–media thickness. Obese hypertensive patients have higher cholesterol and higher insulin levels.

Secondary causes of hypertension continue to be the most frequent form of hypertension observed in children less than 12 years of age and can be characterized by the acuity and duration of the hypertension. Acute and transient forms of hypertension are seen with renal parenchymal diseases, vasculitis, tumoral diseases, trauma, neurologic disorders, and other causes (see ▶Tab. 9.2). These forms of acute transient hypertension usually respond well to treatment with antihypertensive medication with complete or partial resolution after an acute kidney injury. ▶Tab. 9.3 lists causes of secondary chronic hypertension.

As noted in the research on adults, there is a correlation between the severity of hypertension and evidence of target-organ damage if appropriate markers are utilized, such as left ventricular hypertrophy (LVH), retinopathy, microalbuminuria, and others.

Tab. 9.2: Acute and transients forms of secondary hypertension (4).

Renal parenchymal diseases:	Vascular:
Acute postinfectious glomerulonephritis	Renal vein and renal artery thrombosis
Interstitial nephritis	Embolic diseases
Hemolytic uremic syndrome	Vasculitis: Henoch-Schönlein purpura
Acute renal failure of any cause	Renal tumor, renal compression
Acute urinary tract obstruction	Renal trauma/surgery
Iatrogenic	
Fluid overload in acute renal failure	
Hormone treatment: corticosteroids	
Neurologic:	**Drugs:**
Increased intracranial pressure	Oral contraceptives
Guillain-Barre syndrome	Sympathomimetic drugs
Poliomyelitis	Erythropoietin
Dysautonomia	Stimulants
	Nonsteroidal anti-inflammatory drugs
Illicit drugs:	**Diet-mediated:**
Cocaine	Alcohol
Amphetamines	Licorice

The existence of comorbidity issues – such as diabetes mellitus, renal disease, cardiovascular disease, and positive family history – is an important consideration in the decision to intervene therapeutically. Common causes of hypertension in adolescents are indicated in ▶Tabs. 9.2 and 9.3.

9.4 Evaluation of the hypertensive adolescent

The evaluation of the hypertensive adolescent requires the confirmation that hypertension exist, utilizing objective measurements at the office, at home or school and if possible with the use of ABPM. A complete personal history provides important clues about the use of medications and other substances able to cause hypertension; such drugs include those used to treat ADHD, antidepressants, medications used to treat asthma, nonsteroidal anti-inflammatory drugs (NSAIDs), and others. Use of substances of abuse – such as alcohol, tobacco, and illicit drugs – is also associated with hypertension. The family history is important, given the observation that predisposing factors for hypertension (such as cardiovascular disease, diabetes mellitus, and obesity) accumulate in families. Adolescents with mild to moderate hypertension and a positive family history of primary hypertension will, as a general rule, have the diagnosis of primary hypertension.

The physical examination provides information regarding the growth and development of the individual patient; this can be affected by chronic diseases of the renal, cardiovascular, endocrine, and other systems, resulting in hypertension. Ophthalmoscopic examination may provide clues as to the chronicity and/or severity of the hypertension. The existence of a bruit in the flanks may point to renovascular hypertension. BP measurement of the four extremities is the most important finding for the diagnosis of aortic coarctation or midaortic syndrome.

Tab. 9.3: Secondary causes of chronic hypertension (4,11).

Renal disease:	Renovascular disease
Congenital abnormalities of the kidneys	Renal artery stenosis
and urinary tract (CAKUT)	Fibromuscular dysplasia
Hydronephrosis	Midaortic syndrome
Hypoplastic/dysplastic kidney	Coarctation of the aorta
Chronic glomerulonephritis	Takayasu's arteritis
Polycystic kidney disease	
Medullary cystic disease	
Interstitial nephritis	
Other parenchymal kidney diseases	
After an acute kidney injury	
Reflux nephropathy	
Chronic kidney disease with worsening	Endocrine causes
renal failure of multiple causes	Hyperthyroidism
	Catecholamine excess:
	Pheochromocytomas
	Paragangliomas
	Corticosteroid excess:
	Iatrogenic causes
	Cushing's disease
	Conn's syndrome
Tumors: Wilms' tumor	Monogenic forms of hypertension
Neuroblastoma	
Drugs:	Syndromes:
Corticosteroids	Alport's syndrome
Alcohol, nicotine	Williams syndrome
Appetite suppressants	Turner's syndrome
Anabolic steroids	Neurofibromatosis
Oral contraceptives	

Basic laboratory screening required for all hypertensive patients includes a complete blood count (CBC), electrolytes (sodium, potassium, chloride, and bicarbonate), glucose, blood urea nitrogen (BUN), creatinine, uric acid, and urinalysis. Serum uric acid elevation is a frequent finding in patients with primary hypertension; this should be measured, and a fasting lipid profile should be obtained. Echocardiographic examination is also indicated.

ABPM is now considered the preferred method of diagnosing and providing therapeutic monitoring of arterial hypertension in children and adults. It allows the determination of several BP patterns that are difficult to assess in the clinical setting, such as mean BP, diurnal BP rhythm (including dipping, morning surges, and variability), as well response to and duration of drug effects. Recommendations for the use of ABPM in clinical practice include white-coat hypertension, labile hypertension, resistant hypertension, hypotensive episodes, masked hypertension, postural hypertension, and in order to monitor response to treatment (2).

An effort should be made to obtain important laboratory tests of parameters that may be altered by the administration of certain medications, such as plasma catecholamines after the administration of labetalol or plasma renin levels after the administration of angiotensin converting enzyme (ACE) inhibitors, angiotensin receptor blockers (ARBs), or diuretics. The history, physical examination, basic laboratory data, and renal ultrasound results guide the clinical decision as to whether more specific testing is needed to evaluate secondary forms of hypertension.

The types of imaging studies for the identification of anatomic abnormalities will be dictated by the information obtained from the history, physical examination, and basic laboratory results. Given the predominance of renal disease among the secondary causes of hypertension, a bilateral retroperitoneal renal ultrasound with Doppler is indicated. When there is a history of recurrent febrile urinary tract infections, a voiding cystourethrogram (VCUG) will be useful to confirm or exclude reflux nephropathy. A dimercaptosuccinic acid (DMSA) scan is a valuable nuclear medicine study to identify the presence of the renal scars that are frequently associated with hypertension. Magnetic resonanace angiography (MRA) may be indicated when there is a significant difference in renal size, possibly suggesting renal artery stenosis (RAS), or when the captopril scan is suggestive of RAS.

9.5 Management of hypertension in adolescents

Patients with symptomatic severe hypertension, regardless of age, must be treated rapidly in order to bring their BP down to safer levels and thus prevent further target-organ damage; this should be done even before a definitive diagnosis is established. However, pharmacologic intervention is not the first step in the management of adolescents with prehypertension and stage 1 hypertension. The recommended approach is therapeutic life changes. This implies a lifelong commitment to changes lifestyle including modifications in diet, and exercise; the avoidance and treatment of obesity; and smoking avoidance or cessation (14).

Adolescents with mild to moderate hypertension will benefit from regular, moderate aerobic exercise. An increased intake of fruits and vegetables, as part of normal nutrition, is associated with a demonstrable decrease in systolic and diastolic BP; also a reduction in salt intake to less than 100 mmol (less than 3 g of sodium) a day causes a reduction in BP (15,16). Weight reduction in obese individuals decreases systolic and diastolic BP (17). Aerobic exercise of moderate intensity three to five times a week is associated with moderated reduction in BP. The effect of resistance exercise in BP is less clear.

These changes in lifestyle are the foundation that can reduce the risk for hypertension-related cardiovascular events later in life. Those individuals with more severe stage 2 hypertension and those who are symptomatic or with evidence of target-organ damage require prompt evaluation and pharmacologic treatment.

9.6 Pharmacologic treatment of hypertension in adolescents

BP is determined by the interrelationship of two independent variables: cardiac output and peripheral vascular resistance. The pharmacologic treatment of hypertension is based on the ability of a medication to modify either cardiac output and/or peripheral vascular resistance. Currently many therapeutic agents are available to the clinician for the management of hypertension, particularly in adults (see ▶Tabs. 9.4–9.8).

Tab. 9.4: Nondiuretic antihypertensive drugs.

Drug class	Mechanism of action	Side effects
Angiotensin converting enzyme (ACE) inhibitors; some class members: benazepril, captopril, enalapril, fosinopril, lisinopril	Decreases angiotensin II–induced vasoconstriction.	Cough, dizziness, hyperkalemia, rash, acute renal failure (particularly in patients with bilateral renal artery stenosis or hypovolemia). Contraindicated in pregnancy.
Angiotensin II type 1 receptor antagonists; some class members: candesartan, eprosartan, irbesartan, losartan, olmesartan, telmilsartan, valsartan	Decreases angiotensin II–induced vasoconstriction by blocking angiotensin II type 1 receptors.	Cough (less than ACE inhibitors), dizziness, angioedema (rare), hyperkalemia, acute renal failure (particularly in patients with bilateral renal artery stenosis or hypovolemia). Contraindicated in pregnancy.
Renin inhibitors: class member: aliskiren.	Decreases vasoconstriction by inhibiting renin formation necessary for transformation of angiotensinogen into angiotensin I. the precursor of angiotensin-II. High doses cause diarrhea.	Cough (less than ACE inhibitors), dizziness, angioedema (rare), hyperkalemia, acute renal failure (particularly in patients with bilateral renal artery stenosis or hypovolemia). Contraindicated in pregnancy.
Calcium antagonists; some class members (dihydropyridines): amlodipine, felodipine, isradipine, nifedipine ER, and others.	Attenuate cellular calcium uptake or its mobilization from intracellular stores. Direct-acting vasodilators; lower peripheral vascular resistance in all patients.	Dizziness, headache, peripheral edema, tachycardia, flushing, nausea.
Beta-adrenergic antagonists; there are many members of this class of antihypertensive agents.	Competitively inhibit catecholamines at the beta-adrenergic receptor. Reduce cardiac contractility and peripheral vascular resistance. Labetalol, carvedilol and celiprolol also inhibit alpha-adrenergic receptors. Pindolol, acebutolol,	Bradycardia, fatigue, dizziness, depression, insomnia, erectile dysfunction, decreased exercise tolerance, may mask symptoms of hypoglycemia, worsen peripheral arterial insufficiency, may worsen

(Continued)

Tab. 9.4: Nondiuretic antihypertensive drugs. (*Continued*)

Drug class	Mechanism of action	Side effects
	penbutolol, and carteolol have intrinsic sympathomimetic activity.	allergic reactions, bronchospasm (caution in patients with bronchospastic disease), increased serum triglycerides, decreased high-density lipoprotein. Avoid abrupt withdrawal; taper over 1–2 weeks.
Central adrenergic alpha-2 agonist and I_1 imidazoline receptors; class members: clonidine, alpha methyldopa. Rimenidine and moxomidine act on I_1 >alpha-2 receptors (not FDA-approved).	These cross the blood-brain barrier and have a direct agonist effect on alpha-agonist receptors in the midbrain and the brainstem and/or the I_1-imidazoline receptors by decreasing total sympathetic outflow, resulting in vasodilatation of the resistance vessels.	Sedation, dizziness, dry mouth, fatigue, orthostatic hypotension, rash (clonidine patch), rebound hypertension with abrupt withdrawal (clonidine), urine discoloration (methyldopa). Methyldopa (rare reactions): Coombs-positive hemolytic anemia, hepatitis, hepatic necrosis, lupus-like syndrome.
Central and peripheral adrenergic neuronal blocking agents; class member: reserpine.	Reduces BP by depleting catecholamines in the CNS and organ tissues, reduces cardiac output, heart rate, and peripheral vascular resistance.	Dizziness, headache, depression, nightmares, sedation, GI upset, bradycardia, nasal congestion. Use with caution in patients with a history of depression and discontinue if depression occurs.
Direct-acting vasodilators; class members: hydralazine and minoxidil.	Reduce systolic and diastolic BP by decreasing peripheral vascular resistance, acting directly in vascular smooth muscle cells. They have no significant effect on the venous capacitance vessels.	Tachycardia, headache, dizziness, aggravate angina, peripheral edema. Hydralazine: lupus-like syndrome(dose-related), hepatitis. Minoxidil: hair growth on face and body, pericardial effusion (may progress to tamponade).
Moderately selective peripheral alpha-1 adrenergic antagonists; class member: phenoxybenzamine.	Antihypertensive effect results from irreversible binding to the alpha-1 receptors; long-acting. Used only for the treatment of pheochromocytoma.	Orthostatic hypotension, tachycardia, sedation, fatigue, GI irritation, nasal congestion.

(*Continued*)

Tab. 9.4: Nondiuretic antihypertensive drugs. (*Continued*)

Drug class	Mechanism of action	Side effects
Peripheral alpha-1 adrenergic antagonists; some class members: doxazosin, prazosin, terazosin.	Selective competitive inhibitors of the postsynaptic alpha-1 receptor, blunting the increased vessel tone mediated by the release of norepinephrine, thus causing vasodilation and decreasing BP.	Headache, dizziness, vertigo, fatigue, orthostatic hypotension, syncope (especially with first dose), tachycardia, fluid retention, sedation.

Tab. 9.5: Diuretics class and site of action in the nephron.

Distal convoluted tubule diuretics, hydrochlorothiazide, chlorthalidone

Loop diuretics: furosemide, bumetanide, torsemide

Distal potassium-sparing diuretics
• Epithelial sodium channel blockers: amiloride, triamterene
• Aldosterone antagonists: spironolactone, eplerenone

Fortunately there is new information regarding the indications for the use of new pharmacologic agents for the treatment of hypertension in children and adolescents (3,18,19,20,21,22).

It is important for the clinician assuming the responsibility of prescribing these antihypertensive medications and to be certain that the selected medications have been found to be safe and effective in studies of children and adolescents. If this is not possible, it is important at least to make sure that there is abundant experience of their use in this population. The use of ACE inhibitors and ARBs in women of reproductive age requires special attention for the association of the teratogenic effects with these medications, as they are clearly contraindicated in any stage of pregnancy. In sexually active female adolescents, these medications should be avoided unless the adolescent is using an effective method of contraception. In order to improve compliance, the doses should number only once or twice a day in an easy-to-take regimen. Another consideration of increasing importance for families and clinicians is the cost factor, since in many instances patients and families are not able to afford the new and more expensive medications.

Beneficial changes with regard to target-organ damage can be seen within a few months of pharmacologic treatment. For example, left ventricular hypertrophy may regress within 6 months with effective treatment of hypertension. Normalization of BP seems to be more important than the type of medication used in decreasing the risks of development of cardiovascular events and strokes, particularly in adults, as demonstrated in a meta-analysis involving a large number of patients (23). This meta-analysis indicated that beta blockers are protective from recurrence of coronary events by 30 percent when initiated immediately after a myocardial infarction; this effect lasts for a few years as compared with other antihypertensive drugs (23). Only calcium channel blockers provide a slight benefit in the prevention of strokes as compared with other antihypertensive drugs. The study also indicates that BP-lowering drugs should be

Tab. 9.6: Dosing of antihypertensive medication in children adolescents and adults.

Drug	Pediatric dose/adolescent dose	Adult dose	Formulation
ACE inhibitors			
Benazepril	Start: 0.2 mg/kg per day Max: 0.6 mg/kg per day or 40 mg/day	Initial: 10 mg/day Max: 80 mg/day	T: 5/10/20/40 mg Extemp: 2 mg/mL
Captopril	Start: 0.2–0.5 mg/kg per dose every 12 hours or 12.5–25 mg dose 2–3 times a day Max: 6 mg/kg per day	Initial: 12.5 mg 2–3x/day Max: 450 mg/day	T: 12.5/25/50/100 mg Extemp: 1mg/mL
Enalapril	Start: 0.08 mg/kg per day, up to 5 mg Max: 0.6 mg/kg per day, up to 40mg/day	Initial: 2.5–5 mg daily Max: 40 mg/day	T: 2.5/5/10/20 mg Extemp1: mg/mL
Fosinopril	Start (≥6 years and 50 kg): 5–10 mg/day Max: 40 mg/day	Initial: 10 mg/day Max: 80 mg/day	T: 10/20/40 mg
Lisinopril	Start (≥6 years): 0.07 mg/kg per day, up to 5mg/day Max: 0.6 mg/kg per day or 40 mg/day	Initial: 10 mg/day Max 40 mg/day	T: 2.5/5/10/20/30/40 mg Extemp: 1 mg/mL
Quinapril	Start: 0.1–0.2 mg/kg per day	Initial: 10 mg/day Max: 80 mg/day	T: 5/10/20/40 mg
AT II receptor-1 antagonists			
Candesartan	Start: 0.13 mg/kg	Initial 8 mg/day Max: 32 mg/day	T: 4/8/16/32 mg
Irbesartan	Start (≥6–12 years): 75 mg/day Max: 150 mg/day	Initial: 150 mg/day Max: 300 mg/day	T: 75/150/300 mg
Losartan	Start (6–16 years): 0.7 mg/kg per day Max: 50 mg/day	Initial: 25–50 mg/day Max: 100 mg/day	T: 25/50/100 mg
Valsartan	Start (6–16 years): 1.3 mg/kg per day, up to 40 mg/day Max: 2.7 mg/kg per day, up to 160 mg/day	Initial: 80 mg/day Max: 320 mg/day	T: 40/80/160/320 mg Extemp: 4 mg/mL
Calcium channel blockers			
Amlodipine	Start (6–17 years): 0.1–0.2 mg/kg per day, up to 2.5–5 mg/day Max: 0.6 mg/kg per day, up to 10 mg/day	Initial: 5 mg/day Max: 10 mg/day	T: 2.5/5/10 mg Extemp: 1 mg/mL

(Continued)

Tab. 9.6: Dosing of antihypertensive medication in children adolescents and adults. (*Continued*)

Drug	Pediatric dose/adolescent dose	Adult dose	Formulation
Isradipine	Start: 0.15–0.2 mg/kg per day divided into 2–3 doses (CR in 1–2 doses) Max: 0.8 mg/kg per day, up to 20 mg/day	Initial: C: 2.5 mg 2x/day CR: 5 mg/day Max: 20 mg/ day	C: 2.5/5 mg CR: 5/10 mg Extemp: 1 mg/ mL
Atenolol	Start: 0.5–1 mg kg/day Max: 2 mg/kg per day, up to 100 mg/day	Initial: 25–50 mg/ day Max: 100 mg/day	T: 25/50/100 mg Extemp: 2 mg/ mL
Metoprolol	Start (≥6 years): 1mg/kg per day up to 50 mg/day (ER) Max: 2 mg/kg per day, up to 200 mg/day (ER)	Initial: 25–50 mg/ day (ER) Max: 400 mg/day	T: (ER): 25/50/ 100/200 mg Extemp: 10 mg/ mL
Propranolol	Start: 0.5–1 mg/kg per day in 2–3 divided doses Max: 16 mg kg/day	Initial: 40 mg twice a day; LA: 80 mg/day Max: 640 mg/day	T:10/20/40/60/ 80 mg C (ER): 60/80/ 120/160 mg Solution: 4– 8 mg/mL
Labetalol (alpha, beta-1, and beta- 2 adrenergic receptor site blocker)	Start : 1–3 mg/kg per day in 2 divided doses Max: 10–20 mg/kg per day, up to 1200 mg/day	Initial: 100 mg twice a day Max: 2,400 mg/ day	T: 100/200/300 mg Extemp: 40 mg/ mL
Central alpha-2 adrenergic agonists			
Clonidine	Start: (<12 years): 5 to 10 mcg/kg per day in 2–3 divided doses Start (≥12 years): 0.2 mg/day in 2 divided doses Max: (<12 years): 25 mcg/kg per day up to 0.9 mg/day Max: (≥12 years): 2.4 mg/day	Initial: 0.1 mg twice a day Max (oral): 2.4 mg/day Max (patch): 0.3 mg/week	T: 0.1/0.2/0.3 mg Transderm: 0.1/ 0.2/0.3 mg
Alpha-adrenergic antagonists			
Doxazosin	Start: 1mg/day Max: 4 mg/day	Initial: 1 mg/day Max: 16 mg/day	T: 1/2/4/8 mg
Prazosin	Start: 0.05–0.1mg/kg per day in 3 divided doses Max: 0.5 mg/kg per day	Initial: 1 mg two to three times a day Max: 20 mg/day	C: 1/2/5 mg
Terazosin	No data	Initial: 1 mg/day Max: 20 mg/day	C: 1/2/5/10 mg
Vasodilators			

Tab. 9.6: Dosing of antihypertensive medication in children adolescents and adults. (*Continued*)

Drug	Pediatric dose/adolescent dose	Adult dose	Formulation
Hydralazine	Start: 0.75–1mg/kg per day in 2–4 divided doses Max: 7.5 mg/kg per day, up to 200 mg/day	Initial: 10mg four times a day Max: 300 mg/day	T: 10/25/50/100 mg Extemp: 20 mg/5 mL
Minoxidil	Start (<12 years): 0.1–0.2 mg/kg per day divided in 1–2 doses, up to 5 mg/day Max: 50 mg/day	Initial: 2.5–5 mg/day Max: 100 mg/day	T: 2.5/10 mg Extemp: 2 mg/mL

CR, controled release; C, regular release; ER, extended release; LA, long-acting; Transderm, transdermal formulation (patch); T, tablets; Extemp, extemporaneously prepared.

Tab. 9.7: Diuretics used in the treatment of hypertension: suggested dosing of antihypertensive medications in children, adolescents, and adults (4,18,19,23).

Diuretics	Pediatric dosing	Adult dosing	Formulation	Comments / side effects
Amiloride	Start: 0.4–0.0625 mg/kg/day Max: 20 mg/day	Initial: 5–10 mg/day Max: 20 mg/day	T: 5 mg	Specific epithelial channel blocker and a potassium-sparing diuretic; potassium levels to be monitored. Side effects: hyperkalemia, GI upset, rash, headache.
Chlorothiazide	Start: 10–20 mg/kg per day in 1–2 divided doses Max: <2 years: 375 mg/day; 2–12 years: 1,000 mg/day	Initial: 125–500 mg/day in 1–2 divided doses Max: 2 g/day	T: 250/500 mg Susp: 250 mg/5 mL	Side effects: electrolytes disturbances: hypokalemia, hyponatremia, hypercalcemia and metabolic alkalosis. Long-term use associated with increased uric acid levels. May cause hypoglycemia, elevated cholesterol and triglycerides, rash, and photosensitivity reactions. To be avoided in renal insufficiency.
Chlorthalidone	Start: 0.3 mg/kg per day Max: 2 mg/kg per day, up to 50 mg/day	Initial: 25 mg/day Max: 100 mg/day	T: 25/50/100 g	
Hydrochlorothiazide	Start (2–17 years): 1 mg/kg per day in 1–2 divided doses Max: 3 mg/kg per day, up to 50 mg/day	Initial: 12.5–25 mg/day Max: 50 mg/day	C: 12.5 mg T: 25/50 mg	

(Continued)

Tab. 9.7: Diuretics used in the treatment of hypertension: suggested dosing of antihypertensive medications in children, adolescents, and adults (4,18,19,23). *(Continued)*

Diuretics	Pediatric dosing	Adult dosing	Formulation	Comments / side effects
Spironolactone	Start: 1mg/kg per day in 1–2 divided doses Max: 3 mg/kg per day, up to 100 mg/day	Initial: 25 mg 1–2 times a day Max: 100 mg/day	T: 25/50/ 100 mg Extemp: 25 mg/ml	Spironolactone, an aldosterone antagonist, is a potassium-spearing diuretic having antifibrotic effects. Spironolactone side effects: hyperkalemia, hyponatremia, gynecomastia, menstrual irregularities, GI upset, rash. Triamterene is an epithelial sodium channel blocker and a potassium-sparing diuretic. Triamterene side effects: hyperkalemia, GI upset, nephrolithiasis. To be avoided in renal insufficiency.
Triamterene	Start: 1–2 mg/kg per day in 2 divided doses Max: 3–4 mg/kg per day, up to 300 mg/day	Initial: 50– 100 mg/day in 1–2 divided doses Max: 300 mg/day	C: 50/100 mg	

C, regular release; Susp, suspension; GI, gastrointestinal; Max, maximum; T, tablet.

provided to all patients at high risk of cardiovascular events (23). Long-term studies of hypertensive children and adolescents are clearly necessary.

It is now accepted that for diabetic hypertensive patients, particularly those with albuminuria, ACEs and/or ARBs offer advantages over other antihypertensive drugs. Similar observations have been made in hypertensive patients with chronic kidney diseases and proteinuria. During randomized therapy, the beneficial effects of antihypertensive medications in decreasing the frequency and severity of cardiovascular diseases and death have been observed as compare with the control group. These beneficial effects persist in the actively treated group even after discontinuation of blinded therapy, when all the study patients were advised to continue with the same therapy. This observation indicates a legacy effect of early intervention that can result in improved outcomes for patients whose BP is controlled earlier (24).

The clinician prescribing antihypertensive medications must become familiar with the indications, contraindications, and side effects of these therapeutic agents. The different antihypertensive medications are listed in ▶Tabs. 9.4 to 9.7. Antihypertensive medications are divided into two groups: nondiuretics and diuretics; the most common nondiuretic and diuretics are listed in ▶Tabs. 9.4 and 9.5. Pharmacologic treatment of hypertension is indicated in adolescents with primary hypertension and evidence of target-organ damage, with BP consistently over the 99th percentile, in those that do

Tab. 9.8: Fixed combinations of antihypertensive drugs (23).

Fixed-dose combination therapy	
Class	Combination
Beta-adrenergic blockers and diuretics	Atenolol 50–100 mg/chlorthalidone 25 mg
	Bisoprolol 2.5, 5, and 10 mg /HCTZ 6.25
	Metoprolol 50–100 mg/HCTZ 25–50 mg
	Propranolol 40–80 mg/HCTZ 25 mg
	Nadolol 40–80 mg/bendroflumethiazide 5 mg
ACEIs and diuretics	Benazepril 5–20 mg/HCTZ 6.25 mg–25 mg
	Captopril 25–50 mg/HCTZ 15–25 mg
	Enalapril 5–10 mg/HCTZ 12.5–25 mg
	Lisinopril 10–20 mg/HCTZ 12.5–25 mg
Angiotensin II receptor blocker and diruetic	Losartan 50–100 mg/HCTZ 12.5–25 mg
	Valsartan 80–320 mg/HCTZ 12.5–25 mg
	Eprosartan 600 mg/HCTZ 12.5–25 mg
	Irbesartan 150–300 mg/HCTZ 12.5–25 mg
	Telmisartan 40–80 mg/HCTZ 12.5–25 mg
	Candesartan 16–32 mg/HCTZ 12.5–25 mg
	Olmesartan 20–40 mg/HCTZ 12.5–25 mg
Renin inhibitor and diuretic	Aliskiren 150–300 mg/HCTZ 12.5–25 mg
Calcium antagonists and ACEIs	Amlodipine 2.5–10 mg/benazepril 10–40 mg
	Verapamil ER 180–240 mg/trandolapril 1–4 mg
Calcium antagonists and angiotensin II receptor blockers	Amlodipine 5–10 mg/valsartan 160–320 mg
	Amlodipine 5–10 mg/olmesartan 20–40 mg

ACEI, angiotensin converting enzyme inhibitor; ER, extended release; HCT, HCTZ; hydrochlorothiazide; LA, long-acting.

not respond to or are unable to comply with lifestyle modifications, and in patients with secondary forms of hypertension.

Pharmacologic treatment must be individualized (25). Some of the factors to keep in mind include the effects of medication on electrolytes disturbances, glucose and lipid metabolism, and renal as well as cardiovascular function. Medication can also interfere with physical and intellectual activities and interact with other medications. Additional factors to consider include preexisting conditions, patient compliance with taking medications, and medication costs. Adolescents with hypertension requiring pharmacologic intervention should be under the supervision of consultants in nephrology or cardiology who are familiar with hypertension in adolescents. ▶Tab. 9.6 lists the most commonly used drugs for the management of hypertension in children, adolescents, and adults. ▶Tab. 9.7 reviews diuretic medications, and ▶Tab. 9.8 lists fixed-dose combinations.

9.7 Pregnancy

Pregnancy in adolescents deserves special consideration in view of the high risk for the development of hypertension in pregnant teens. The potential for complications in such pregnancies threatens the well-being of both mother and infant. Severe hypertension in the mother increases the risk of hypertensive encephalopathy, intracranial bleeding, and renal insufficiency in her child (26,27), as well as the risk of premature delivery with all its consequences. Preterm and small-for-gestational-age infants are born with a decreased number of nephrons and are at risk for developing hypertension.

Evaluation of the hypertensive mother is complicated. Common radiologic or nuclear scans are contraindicated. Angiotensin converting enzyme inhibitors and angiotensin II receptor antagonists are teratogenic; therefore their use is contraindicated in pregnancy. These patients are better served when followed by a team that includes an obstetrician, perinatologist, and nephrologist.

9.8 Summary

Hypertension is a major disorder in adolescents; it has potentially severe consequences in adult life, with increased morbidity and mortality. This chapter considers important concepts in high BP including its definition, proper measurement, classification, etiology, evaluation, and pharmacologic management (28). Proper recognition and management of hypertension in youth will yield enormous dividends for health during the adolescent and adult years.

References

1. National High Blood Pressure Education Program Working Group on High Blood Pressure in Children and Adolescents. The fourth report on the diagnosis evaluation and treatment in children and adolescents. National Heart, Lung and Blood Institute, Bethesda, Maryland. Pediatrics 2004;114:555–76.
2. Wühl E. Ambulatory blood pressure monitoring methodology and norms in children. In: Flynn JT, Ingelfinger JR, Portman RJ, eds. Pediatric hypertension, Second ed. New York: Humana Press, 2011:161–78.
3. De Moraes AC, de Carvalho HB. Evaluating risk factors in hypertension screening in children and adolescents. Hyperten Res 2011 Jun 9. [Epub ahead of print]
4. Falkner B. Hypertension in children. In: Oparril S, Weber MA, eds. Hypertension companion of Brenner and Rector's The Kidney, Second ed. Philadelphia, PA: Elsevier Saunders, 2005:603–15.
5. Lurbe E, Carvajal E, Torro I, Aguilar F, Alvarez J, Redon J. Influence of concurrent obesity and low birth weight on blood pressure phenotype in youth. Hypertension 2009;53: 912–17.
6. Dionne JM, Abitbol CL, Flynn JT. Hypertension in infancy: diagnosis, management and outcome. Pediatr Nephrol 2001 Jan 22. Epub ahead of print]
7. Harding S, Whitrow M, Lenguerrand E, Maynard M, Teyhan A, Cruickshank JK, et al. Emergence of ethnic differences in blood pressure in adolescence. The determinants of adolescent social well-being and health study. Hypertension 2010;55:1063–69.
8. Pludoski P, Litwin MK, Niemirska A, Jaworski M, Sladowska J, Kryskiewicz E, et al. Accelerated skeletal maturation in children with primary hypertension. Hypertension 2009;54:1234–39.
9. Feber J, Ahmed M. Hypertension in children: new trends and challenges. Clin Sci (Lond) 2010;119(4):151–61.

10. Kamboj M, Torres A, Patel D. Endocrine causes of systemic hypertension in children and adolescents: a clinical review. Pediatr Health Med Ther 2011:239–47.
11. McNiece KL, Gupta-Malhotra M, Samuels J, Bell C, Garcia K, Poffenbarger T, et al. Left ventricular hypertension in hypertensive adolescent analysis of risk by 2004 National High Blood Pressure Education Program Working Group Staging Criteria. Hypertension 2007;50:392–95.
12. Brady TM, Fivus B, Flynn FT, Parekh R. Lability of blood pressure adolescents Pediatr 2008;152:73–78.
13. Sorof JM, Alexandrov AV, Garami Z, Turmner JL, Grafe AE, Lai D, et al. Carotid ultrasonography for detection of vascular abnormalities in hypertensive children Pediatr Nephrol 2003;18:1020–102.
14. Siklar Z, Berberoglu M, Erdeve SS, Hacihamdioglu B, Ocal G, Egin Y, et al. Contribution of clinical, metabolic, and genetic factors on hypertension in obese children and adolescents. J Pediatr Endocrinol Metabol 2011;24:21–24.
15. Stabouli S, Papakatsika S, Kotsis V. The role of obesity, salt and exercise on blood pressure in children and adolescents. Expert Rev Cardiovasc Ther 2011;9:753–61.
16. Centers for Disease Control and Prevention. Vital signs: prevalence, treatment, and control of hypertension. United States, 1999–2002 and 2005–2008. MMWR 2011;60:103–8.
17. Flynn JT, Falkner BE. Obesity hypertension in adolescents: epidemiology, evaluation, and management. J Clin Hypertension 2011;13:323–31.
18. Flynn JT. Successes and shortcomings of the Drug and Food Modernization Act. Am J Hypertension 2003;16910:889–91.
19. Blowey DL. Pharmacotherapy of pediatric hypertension. In: Flynn JT, Ingelfinger JR, Portman RJ, eds. Pediatric hypertension, Second ed. New York: Humana Press, 2011:537–58.
20. Listernick R. A 15-year girl with hypertension. Pediatr Ann 2011;40:235–38.
21. Yoon SS, Ostchega Y, Louis T. Recent trends in the prevention of high blood pressure and its treatment and control, 1999–2008. NCHS Data Brief 2010;48:1–8.
22. Tocci G, Volpe M. Olmesartan medoxomil for the treatment of hypertension in children and adolescents. Vasc Health Risk Manag 2011;7:177–81.
23. Weir MR, Hanes DS, Klassen DK. Antihypertensive drugs. In: Brenner BM, ed. Brenner and Rector's The Kidney, eight ed. Philadelphia, PA: Saunders Elsevier, 2008:222–34.
24. Law MR, Morris JK, Wald NJ. Use of blood pressure lowering drugs in the prevention of cardiovascular disease: meta-analysis of 147 randomized trials in the context of expectations from prospective epidemiological studies BMJ 2009;338:1665.
25. Drugs for Hypertension. Treatment guidelines. Med Letter 2009;7(77):1–10.
26. Duley L. Pre-eclampsia, eclampsia, and hypertension. Clin Evid (Online) 2011;2011. pii:1402.
27. Cifkova R. Why is the treatment of hypertension in pregnancy still so difficult? Expert Rev Cardiovasc Ther 2011;9:647–49.
28. Kostis WJ, Thijs L, Richart T, Kostis JB, Staessen JA. Persistence of mortality reduction after the end of randomized therapy in clinical trials of blood pressure-lowering medications. Hypertension 2010;56:1060–68.

10 Pediatric cardiology

James Loker

This discussion provides information regarding the dyslipidemias; it includes concepts of lipid metabolism, familial hypercholesterolemias, and secondary hyperlipidemias. Management of dyslipidemias is considered, focusing on the role of statins as the mainstay of drug treatment for these disorders. Also reviewed are anticoagulants (i.e., warfarin, ximelagatran, rivaroxaban, others) and then medication used for syncope. Finally, this discussion considers the potential impact of stimulant medications on the cardiac system in those with heart disease and attention deficit hyperactivity disorder (ADHD). Medications have an important role in the management of youths with cardiac disorders. The application of these pharmacologic agents will improve the lives of these youths and the adults they will become.

10.1 Introduction

Pediatric cardiology can claim many recent advances. New surgical techniques and improvements in both perfusion and postoperative care have dramatically increased the survival rates for congenital heart surgery. Progress in catheter interventions, stents, and occluding devices has significantly improved outcomes for many patients who require surgery. Genetic analysis has not only helped to confirm suspected diagnoses but can also screen other family members and help to determine prognosis and treatment. (See chapter 6 in Greydanus DE, Patel DR, Omar HA, Feucht C, Merrick J: Adolescent Medicine – Pharmacotherapeutics in General, Mental and Sexual Health. Berlin: de Gruyter; 2012.) New medications capitalize on a better understanding of the pathophysiology of cardiac diseases. All of these factors have improved survival, so that currently there are more adults than children living with congenital heart disease. Adolescents with heart disease struggle to understand their condition while starting the transition from the pediatric caregivers they have trusted for many years to adult specialists and specialty clinics.

Almost all of the cardiac medications used in pediatrics today are administered off label (1). This increases the risk associated with treatment, as dosages are extrapolated for pediatric use. Unique features of the very young include a higher water- to-weight ratio and reduced intravascular space, which can dramatically affect pharmacokinetics. In addition, many medications do not come in liquid form. Dosing errors are the most common mistakes made in prescribing medication, particularly in infants less than 1 year old (2). Cutting or crushing tablets or making suspensions may increase the risk of dosage error and alter the bioavailability of the medication. Formulated suspensions frequently have a short shelf life. Even in adolescents, the smallest available dosage is not always low enough.

Caution is therefore urged in using any medications, especially cardiovascular medications. This discussion has derived dosages from several sources, and readers are encouraged to evaluate these and become acquainted with any medication that is prescribed. This article addresses only the medications suitable for outpatient use. Intravenous medications and those requiring inpatient monitoring during initiation are not discussed.

10.2 Dyslipidemias

Dyslipidemia can be broadly classified as primary, due to an underlying genetic abnormality with lipid metabolism, or secondary, due to obesity, diabetes, kidney or liver disease, hypothyroidism, or other conditions. The primary dyslipidemias are associated with overproduction and/or impaired removal of lipoprotein (see ▶Tab. 10.1). Impaired removal can result from an abnormality in either the lipoprotein itself or in the lipoprotein receptor. Secondary dyslipidemias are associated with dysregulation of key enzymes in the metabolic pathway, particularly lipoprotein lipase (LPL).

Numerous studies have documented the atherosclerotic changes that can occur in childhood and have been the driving force behind increased efforts to screen and treat pediatric hyperlipidemias. Autopsy studies have shown that antemortem low-density lipoprotein (LDL) and total cholesterol are highly associated with aortic fatty streaks in people 7 to 24 years old (3). Berenson et al reported that serum concentrations of total cholesterol, triglycerides, LDL, and high-density lipoprotein (HDL) were strongly associated with the extent of lesions in the aorta and coronary arteries at

Tab. 10.1: Lipoproteins.

Lipoprotein particle	Size	Origin and function	Composition	Predominant protein in shell
Chylomicrons	Large lipids, low density, will float on plasma	Small intestine	Triglycerides Cholesterol (2%–4%)	Apolipoprotein B (Apo B)
Very low density lipoprotein (VLDL)	Smaller than chylomicron but may also float	Liver, from triglycerides	Triglycerides Cholesterol (10%–15%)	Apo B 100
Intermediate-density lipoprotein (IDL)		Intermediate in metabolism from VLDL to LDL	Cholesterol 20%–35% Protein shell 5%–40%	Apo B 100
Low-density lipoprotein (LDL)	Derived from metabolism of VLDL as it shrinks	Functions to transport cholesterol	Cholesterol 35%–45% Surface protein 20%–30%	Apo B 100
High-density lipoprotein (HDL)	Synthesized in liver and small intestine with complex metabolism	Functions in reverse cholesterol transport and is antiatherogenic	Cholesterol 10%–20%	Apo A-l and Apo A-ll

autopsy in young persons who died of trauma (4). The Pathobiological Determinants of Atherosclerosis in Youth (PDAY) study demonstrated raised fatty streaks and accumulation of lipid-filled macrophages within the intima of the artery in 10 percent of coronary arteries and 30 percent of aortas in individuals 15 to 34 years of age (5).

10.3 Lipid metabolism

A brief introduction to lipid metabolism will help explain the mechanisms of atherosclerosis and how interventions can help. Lipoprotein particles are classified by their density on ultracentrifugation or their electrophoretic patterns (6). Triglycerides are the storage form of lipids, found mostly in adipose tissue but also in liver, heart, and muscle. Triglycerides originate from the dietary ingestion of fat and are secreted into lymph as chylomicrons. They can also be synthesized from carbohydrate and fatty acids in the liver and secreted as very low density lipoprotein (VLDL), an end-product that can be hydrolyzed by LDL. Once the hydrolyzed particles enter the cell, they can be reesterified into triglycerides. Lipolysis and free fatty acid (FFA) oxidation remove triglycerides from tissue. In the liver, VLDL secretion is increased by insulin, glucocorticoids, and ethanol and decreased by glucagon.

Cholesterol is a key component of cell membranes, steroidogenesis, and bile acid formation. Cholesterol can be absorbed in the diet or synthesized in most tissues. The rate-limiting step is the conversion of hydroxy-methylglutaryl coenzyme A (HMG-CoA) to mevalonate by HMG-CoA reductase. This enzymatic step is targeted by the statins. Internalized cholesterol inhibits cholesterol synthesis by decreasing HMG-CoA and also limits further cholesterol uptake by downregulating the LDL receptor. Esterification by lecithin cholesterol acyl transferase (LCAT), and shuttling of cholesterol esters by cholesterol esterase transfer protein (CETP) moves cholesterol from HDL to VLDL to the LDL molecule.

10.3.1 Enzymes and cellular receptors associated with lipid metabolism

Lipoprotein lipase is present on the endothelium of vessels, mostly in fat and muscle, where it hydrolyzes triglycerides in chylomicrons and VLDL to release FFAs. The activity of this enzyme is regulated by insulin and is diminished in poorly controlled diabetes, causing elevation of LDL levels. Hepatic lipase (HLA) facilitates the lipolysis of VLDL and intermediate-density lipoprotein (IDL) in hepatic endothelial cells, and hydrolyzes phospholipids and triglycerides in HDL. Its activity is modulated by sex steroid, the activity of which is increased by androgens and decreasedby estrogens.

The LDL receptor (LDLR) is the key mediator of entry of cholesterol as well as VLDL/LDL particles into cells. The gene for this receptor is coded on chromosome 19, and defects in this receptor are responsible for familial hypercholesterolemia. The dyslipidemias are broadly grouped phenotypically by the lipid abnormality in the Fredrickson classification (see ▶Tab. 10.2). Research continues into the genetic basis of protein and receptor abnormalities. Genetic research has opened up new ways to treat the underlying disorder and may help establish more accurate prognoses (6).

Tab. 10.2: Fredrickson classification of dyslipidemias.

Phenotype	Major lipid increased	Frequency
I	Triglyceride	Very rare
IIA	LDL	Common
IIB	LDL triglyceride	Common
III	Total cholesterol, triglyceride	Rare
IV	Triglyceride	Common
V	Triglyceride	Uncommon

10.4 Familial hypercholesterolemias

Familial chylomicronemia (type I) is characterized by chylomicrons and high triglycerides due to congenital deficiency of LPL or Apo C-II, which is required to remove triglycerides from chylomicrons. Symptoms include pancreatitis in children or young adults, eruptive xanthomas, and an enlarged liver and spleen but no coronary artery disease (CAD). The condition is very rare, occurring in 1 of 1 million individuals. Triglyceride levels are generally over 2,000 mg/dL. Secondary hypertriglyceridemia can be seen in patients with severe diabetic ketoacidosis and in those taking estrogen therapy.

Familial hypercholesterolemia FH (type IIA) occurs in 1 of 500 individuals as an autosomal dominant condition. It is due to abnormal LDL receptors, with over 150 mutations known. Type IIA FH includes a triad of hyperlipidemia, xanthoma, and premature CAD. Individuals heterozygous for this condition typically have LDL levels greater than 250 mg/dL. Diagnosis is based on LDL higher than 250 mg/dL, with a family history of premature CAD. Average life expectancy of heterozygous males with familial hypercholesterolemia is 45 years. Individuals homozygous for FH have total cholesterol levels exceeding 600 mg/dL and can have a myocardial infarction by 3 years of age. Fortunately this form of FH is very rare, occurring in only 1 of 1 million individuals.

Familial combined hyperlipidemia (type IIB) is also autosomal dominant trait, with several genetic loci being implicated. It is seen in 1 in 300 individuals, although there may be significant overlap with secondary dyslipidemias, including metabolic syndrome. Type IIB FH appears to be more complex than FH and consensus diagnostic criteria are lacking, which makes diagnosis more difficult. Individuals with type IIB FH do not have the xanthomas seen in FH.

Broad beta disease (type III) is caused by a defect in the metabolism of VLDL remnants, due to abnormal Apo E or hypothyroidism. Affected people may have palmar xanthomas and develop premature CAD. Both total cholesterol and triglycerides are elevated. This is noted in 1 of 10,000 individuals.

Familial hypertriglyceridemia (type IV) is characterized by elevated triglycerides and VLDL and is associated with obesity but not CAD. Triglyceride levels are greater than 1,000, with normal LDL levels. Type IV FH can sometimes be mistaken for type I disease, but since that is very rare, isolated elevations of triglycerides are usually felt to be type IV. Type IV FH occurs in 16 percent of adults.

Primary mixed hyperlipidemia (type V) is characterized by marked increases in triglycerides, chylomicrons, and VLDL. Pancreatitis, xanthomas, and hepatosplenomegaly can occur. Onset is in midlife; children or adolescents are apparently not affected. They do, however, have a higher risk of atherosclerosis. Both type IV and type V FH may exist secondary to uncontrolled diabetes mellitus, excessive ethanol intake, and use of glucocorticoids as well as estrogens. This condition is noted 1 in 1,000 individuals.

10.5 Secondary hyperlipidemia

Most secondary causes of hyperlipidemia are phenotypically similar to type IIA or IIB FH. In hypothyroidism, hepatic LDL receptors are decreased, causing an elevation in LDL cholesterol. Hypothyroidism can increase triglycerides by lowering LPL activity. In diabetes, glycosylation of apoprotein B causes increased VLDL synthesis with a concomitant rise in LDL levels. Insulin regulates LPL such that a deficiency (type 1 diabetes) or relative deficiency due to increased resistance (non–insulin dependent diabetes mellitus, renal disease, liver disease, Cushing disease, etc.) can cause hypertriglyceridemia. Treatment of secondary hyperlipidemia should be primarily directed at treating the underlying condition, although lipid-lowering medication can be used in the interim.

The National Cholesterol Education Program (NCEP) and the American Academy of Pediatrics (AAP) have published guidelines for cholesterol screening (7,8). Both groups recommend a targeted approach to individuals at higher risk rather than broad population screening. Children and adolescents whose parents have cholesterol measurements above 250 mg/dL or unknown family history should be screened with nonfasting total cholesterol testing. Children with a family history of dyslipidemia or who are at risk for secondary dyslipidemia should have a fasting lipid profile performed. If hyperlipidemia is noted, repeat testing is warranted and the two cholesterol values should be averaged. In addition, with the second lipid profile, thyroid studies, liver and renal function tests, and glucose or fasting insulin levels should be tested to evaluate for secondary causes of elevated cholesterol.

10.5.1 Management

Treatment of hyperlipidemias should start with dietary modifications for 6 to 12 months, especially for obese individuals. In adolescents with FH, nonpharmacologic measures usually are not sufficient and most specialists will prescribe statins along with dietary management. The American Heart Association (AHA) has abandoned the step 1 and step 2 diets in favor of a more uniform recommendation (9). Dietary reductions in cholesterol to less than 200 mg/day, less than 30 percent total fat, and less than 7 percent saturated fat are recommended by the NCEP (7). Calories should be 55 percent from carbohydrates, 20 percent from protein, and 25 percent from fat in a developing child. Consultation with a nutritionist is helpful, especially if caloric restriction is also indicated.

The goal of treatment is to reduce total cholesterol to less than 200 mg/dL, LDL to less than 130 mg/dL, and triglycerides to less than 125 mg/dL. Patients with dyslipidemias, such as FH, have stricter guidelines. The NCEP and AAP still recommend cholesterol-binding agents as the initial medication; however, problems with palatability and side effects usually limit compliance in most adolescents (7,8).

Statins have rapidly become the mainstay of pharmacologic treatment of dyslipidemia in both adults and children (see ▶Tab. 10.3). Numerous studies have shown statins to be both safe and efficacious in children older than 10 years (10). According to the 2007 AHA and 2008 AAP guidelines, treatment with statins can be recommended in boys older than 10 years and girls who have started their menses and have regular periods. Female patients should be counseled regarding the potential teratogenic effects of statin therapy and the need for appropriate contraception if warranted. Statins can be started in patients as young as 8 years old who have severe dyslipidemia (e.g, FH or type 1 diabetes mellitus) who have failed nonpharmacologic therapy (8). Recent studies suggest that statins may also upregulate endothelial nitric oxide (NO) synthase, thereby increasing the availability of endothelial nitrous oxide, which may have beneficial effects on endothelial vasomotor function (11).

In the adolescent, statins are indicated if the LDL is greater than 190 mg/dL without other risk factors or if the LDL is greater than 160 mg/dL but less than 190 mg/dL and one of the following conditions applies: (a) a family history of premature cardiovascular disease (CVD), (b) two or more other CVD risk factors after vigorous attempts to control

Tab. 10.3: Statins.

Statin	Adult dose	Pediatric dose
Lovastatin (Mevacor)	Initially: 20 mg/d orally at bedtime. Followed by: 10–80 mg/day orally at bedtime or divided twice daily.	10–17 years: 10–20 mg/day orally at bedtimeinitially; maintenance dosage ranges from 10–40 mg/day.
Simvastatin (Zocor)	Initially: 5–10 mg/day orally at bedtime. Followed by: 5–40 mg/day orally at bedtime or divided twice daily Simvastatin dosages of 80 mg have been associated with a higher risk of rhabdomyolysis.	10–17 years: 10 mg/day orally at bedtime initially; maintenance dosage ranges from 10–40 mg/day.
Pravastatin (Pravachol)	Initially: 10–20 mg/d orally at bedtime. Followed by: 5–40 mg/day orally at bedtime.	8–13 years: 20 mg/day orally. 14–18 years: 40 mg/day orally.
Fluvastatin (Lescol)	Initially: 20–30 mg/day orally at bedtime. Followed by: 20–80 mg/day orally at bedtime; for 80 mg/day, divided twice daily.	10–16 years: 20 mg/day orally initially; maintenance dosage ranges from 20–80 mg/day.
Atorvastatin (Lipitor)	Initially: 10 mg/d orally at bedtime. Followed by: 10–80 mg/day orally at bedtime.	10–17 years: 10 mg/day orally initially; maintenance dosages not to exceed 20 mg/day.
Rosuvastatin (Crestor)	10–20 mg/day orally initially; maintenance dosage range is 5–40 mg/day.	Not established.

CVD risk factors (i.e., overweight, hypertension, insulin resistance, or smoke exposure), or (c) a primary disease associated with a moderately or mildly increased risk of CVD. Statins can also be used if the LDL is greater than 130 mg/dL and the patient has moderate-risk underlying disease, such as heterozygous FH or type II diabetes mellitus, or if the LDL is greater than 100 mg/dL and the patient has high-risk underlying disease, such as homozygous FH or diabetes mellitus type I.

Currently only lovastatin (Altocor, Altoprev, Mevacor), simvastatin (Zocor), pravastatin (Pravachol), and atorvastatin (Lipitor) are approved by the U.S. Food and Drug Administration (FDA) for use in children. Pravastatin, simvastatin, and lovastatin are available in generic forms. Statins should be started at the lowest dose and given at bedtime to take advantage of the fact that most LDL synthesis occurs at night. The patient should be reassessed within a month to monitor the effectiveness of the medication as well as its side effects. Major side effects of statins include rhabdomyolysis (breakdown of muscle tissue resulting in renal impairment) and hepatic dysfunction. Creatine phosphokinase (CPK) levels and liver function should be monitored during initiation of therapy and if symptoms develop.

Although all statins affect the same pathway, there are subtle differences in how individuals respond. Typically a parent or sibling of the young patient is also on a statin, so the clinician starts with the same agent if it is working for the relative. The efficacy of the different statins in summarized in ▶Tab. 10.4. The ability to lower LDL level does not necessarily equate to reduced risk for CAD. However, statins have other beneficial effects, such as improved arterial compliance, reduction in inflammatory response, decreased thrombus formation, and improved plaque stability. Lovastatin and simvastatin are generic and less expensive. Atorvastatin and fluvastatin are not eliminated by the kidneys and can, therefore, be used in patients with renal impairment.

All statins have similar safety profiles. Rhabdomyolysis occurs in less than 1 in 10,000 patients. Higher doses (particularly of simvastatin) and renal impairment can

Tab. 10.4: Percentage lowering of LDL-cholesterol by statins.

Statin	Name of drug	Daily dose of drug				
		5 mg	10 mg	20 mg	40 mg	80 mg
Atorvastatin	Lipitor Torvast	31%	37%	43%	49%	55%
Fluvastatin	Lescol	10%	15%	21%	27%	33%
Lovastatin	Mevacor Altocor	–	21%	29%	37%	45%
Pravastatin	Pravachol Lipostat Selektine	15%	20%	24%	29%	33%
Rosuvastatin	Crestor	38%	43%	48%	53%	58%
Simvastatin	Zocor Lipex	23%	27%	32%	37%	42%

Law MR, Wald NJ, Rudnicka AR. Quantifying effect of statins on low density lipoprotein cholesterol, ischaemic heart disease, and stroke: systemic review and meta-analysis. BMJ 2003; 326:1423–27.

increase the levels of statins and place the individual at greater risk. Fluvastatin and pravastatin are recommended in individuals who are taking other medications because these agents have the fewest drug interactions.

Ezetimibe (Zetia) acts on the brush border of the small intestine, inhibiting the absorption of cholesterol. It is available alone or in combination with simvastatin (as Vytorin). The typical adult dose is 10 mg once a day; no pediatric dose is available. Bile acid sequestrants (▶Tab. 10.5) have the advantage of no systemic absorption, but poor palatability decreases patient compliance. These should be offered but realistically are not used as much as other medications.

Niacin is usually used in cases of hypertriglyceridemia or mixed hyperlipidemia and usually in conjunction with a statin. Side effects of flushing, headaches, and liver toxicity tend to limit its use. Aspirin (325 mg) given 30 minutes before the niacin does help diminish the flushing. Niacin is indicated in type IV and V hyperlipidemias with an adult dose of 100 to 250 mg three times a day, then increased 100 mg/day each week as tolerated based on liver function testing. The dosage for the extended release formulation is 500 mg at bedtime.

10.5.2 Anticoagulants

Advances in pediatric cardiac surgery and interventional cardiology have dramatically increased the use of anticoagulants (12). Warfarin (Coumadin) has been the standard oral anticoagulant, whereas aspirin is commonly used for its antiplatelet effect (see chapter 6). Enoxaparin (Lovenox) achieves more stable levels than warfarin; although patients may be reluctant to give injections, most youths and parents quickly adapt. Newer oral anticoagulants that act via direct thrombin inhibition (ximelagatran [Exanta]) or direct factor Xa inhibition (rivaroxaban [Xarelto]) offer stable pharmokinetics similar to enoxaparin but as oral agents. These are not used as frequently, so experience and safety data are not as extensive as for the other medications.

Warfarin

Warfarin (Coumadin, Jantoven, Marfarin) is the oldest and most commonly used vitamin K antagonist (VKA) (see chapter 6). Warfarin interferes with the cyclic interconversion of

Tab. 10.5: Bile acid sequestrants.

Drug	Adult dose	Pediatric dose
Cholestyramine	Begin with 1 scoop (4 g) or pouch mixed with water or juice; advance slowly to 8–16 g/day (usually divided twice daily immediately before major meals).	240 mg/kg per day divided in 2–3 doses, not to exceed 8 g/day.
Colestipol	2 g once or twice daily, with increases of 2 g once or twice daily over periods of 1–2 months.	1 g once or twice daily, with increases of 1 g once or twice daily over periods of 1–2 months.

vitamin K and its 2, 3 epoxide. Vitamin K is a cofactor for the carboxylation of glutamate residues of coagulation proteins (factors II, VII, IX, and X). Warfarin can inhibit carboxylation of the regulatory anticoagulant proteins C and S; therefore it has the potential to exert a procoagulant effect.

Dosages for warfarin range from 0.3 mg/kg in infants to 0.09 mg/kg in older children. Improved hepatic metabolism as a child develops is responsible for the difference between doses for infants and older children, which may also explain the lower doses needed in patients with Fontan circulation (13). Bleeding is the most serious side effect, with a relative risk of 0.5 percent per patient year. Warfarin is titrated to achieve an international normalized ratio (INR) in the range of 2 to 3 in most instances (▶Tab. 10.6). Patients with mechanical prosthetic mitral valves usually have an INR in the range of 2.5 to 3.5. Warfarin dosages must usually be decreased by 10 to 15 percent when antibiotics are taken. Many electronic medical record systems have the ability to track INR levels and warfarin dosages, making following a patient's anticoagulant therapy easier.

Aspirin

Aspirin is used to decrease platelet adhesion in Kawasaki disease and after hemi-Fontan and Fontan palliation. Aspirin is also frequently used in patients with arteriopulmonary shunts and as an adjunct to other anticoagulants. The dosage ranges from 3 to 10 mg/kg per day rounded up to the most convenient dose. Typical dosages range from 40.5 mg, 81 mg, and 162 mg up to a maximum of 325 mg. Since the effects of aspirin are irreversible for the life of the platelet, therapy can easily be suspended for up to a week with no significantly increased risk of coagulation. This is beneficial, since many physicians will halt aspirin therapy when a patient has influenza so as to decrease the risk of Reye's syndrome.

Tab. 10.6: INR dosing and schedules.

International normalized ratio (INR)	Dose
Loading dose if INR 1–1.3	0.2 mg/kg (maximum 10 mg)
Day 2–4 dependent on INR	
1.1–1.3	Repeat loading dose
1.4–3	Repeat 50% loading dose
3.1–3.5	Repeat 25% loading dose
>3.5	Hold dose until INR <3.5
Maintenance dose after day 5	
1.1–1.4	Increase dose 20%
1.5–1.9	Increase dose 10%
2–3	No change
3.1–3.5	Decrease dose 10%
>3.5	Hold dose until <3.5, then restart dose decreased by 20%

Other anticoagulants

Dipyridamole also decreases platelet adhesion, but through a different mechanism than aspirin. It can be used as adjunctive therapy to other oral anticoagulants and aspirin. Dosage is 3 to 6 mg/kg per day divided in three doses. The newer oral anticoagulant ximelagatran acts by direct thrombin inhibition. It is dosed twice daily and has the advantage of a predictable, stable anticoagulant effect. Ximelagatran has not been studied in pediatric patients. Rivaroxaban is another oral anticoagulant that acts by direct inhibition of activated factor X.

10.6 Syncope

Syncope is defined as a temporary loss of consciousness secondary to a decrease in cerebral blood flow. It is one of the more common complaints of adolescents seen in the office and the incidence ranges from 0.03 to 0.5 percent. According to one survey, 20 percent of males and 50 percent of females have had at least one syncopal episode by the age of 20 (14). In 90 percent of cases, syncope is mediated by the vagal response and, although benign, can cause considerable anxiety in both the adolescent and parents, thereby generating more testing and expense for reassurance. History is the key factor in evaluating syncope, with the physical examination and testing usually being normal. Orthostatic blood pressure measurement and a 12-lead electrocardiogram (ECG) are considered standard in the workup of syncope. Reasons for referral of an adolescent with syncope to a pediatric cardiologist are noted in ▶Tab. 10.7.

10.6.1 Management

Treatment of dizziness and syncope is largely supportive, involving increasing fluid and salt intake as well as recognizing and avoiding precipitating factors. Clinicians should also encourage their patients to avoid skipping meals and eliminate caffeine intake. If patients become dizzy, maneuvers to increase venous return (such as squatting, sitting,

Tab. 10.7: Reasons for cardiology referral in syncope.

R	Recurrent	If there is a history of recurrent syncope.
E	Exercise-related	If dizziness or syncope occurs during exercise. Frequently there may be dizziness or syncope after running if the adolescent does not keep moving.
F	Family history	Many of the cardiac causes of syncope are due to autosomal dominant conditions, so a family history of syncope, sudden death, arrhythmia, cardiomyopathy, etc., is important. Family history is second only to the history of the event in importance when working up syncope.
E	ECG or exam abnormal	If there are abnormalities on the ECG or examination, the risk of cardiac disease as a cause of syncope increases.
R	Rapid onset	Vagally mediated syncope usually has identifiable prodrome of nausea, pallor, dizziness, and visual changes. Any syncope that occurs without a prodrome should be suspected to be cardiac in origin.

or lying down) will help to alleviate the symptoms and avoid syncope. When supportive measures are insufficient, especially when a history of injury is associated with syncope, pharmacologic intervention may be indicated.

Fludrocortisone (Florinef) is the most commonly used medication in treating autonomic syncope. As a mineralocorticoid, it increases sodium reabsorption in the distal loops of the kidney, thereby decreasing water loss and increasing the circulating blood volume. Fludrocortisone at the appropriate dosages does not have a significant glucocorticoid effect but at higher dosages may cause problems. The recommended dosage is 0.1 to 0.2 mg twice daily. Patients should continue to increase their salt and water intake and other supportive measures while on fludrocortisone. Since adolescents with dizziness and syncope tends to improve with age, a 6-month to 1-year trial on medication can be followed by a trial without medication. Drug discontinuation is best accomplished during the summer, when school is not in session.

Midodrine (Amatine, Gutron) can be used either instead of or in addition to fludrocortisone. As an alpha agonist, midodrine increases vasomotor tone and does not stimulate cardiac beta-adrenergic receptors; thus it does not cause tachycardia. Also, midodrine does not cross the blood-brain barrier to exert effects on the central nervous system. Midodrine is very effective in treating orthostatic hypotension, but it can also be useful as therapy for vasovagal syncope. The oral dosage is 0.1 to 0.2 mg four times daily. In addition, the selective serotonin uptake inhibitors (SSRIs), such as paroxetine (Paxil), fluoxetine (Prozac), and sertraline (Zoloft), have been used to treat vasovagal syncope, possibly by reregulating the autonomic nervous system.

Postural orthostatic tachycardia syndrome (POTS) is one of the dysautonomias and can be similar to vasovagal syncope. We view it as an exaggerated response to orthostatic changes. Individuals with POTS have an increased heart rate of over 30 beats per minute when going from supine to standing and frequently have standing heart rates above 120 beats per minute. As in the case of vasovagal syncope, 80 percent of patients with POTS are females 13 to 40 years of age. Individuals can be highly symptomatic, and anxiety can increase the symptoms.

A combination of counseling, lifestyle changes, and medications can effectively treat many of these individuals with POTS. In addition to fludrocortisone and midodrine, beta blockers can be used to treat the tachycardia. Care should be taken since beta blockers may worsen hypotension, especially if the patient is hypovolemic and has significant orthostatic hypotension. For that reason, clinicians usually use beta blockers in conjunction with other medications. Propranolol (Inderal) can be helpful, especially if migraines are part of the constellation. This drug is started at a dose of 10 mg twice daily and titrated upwardon the basis of symptoms. Once the adolescent is stable, longer-acting propranolol (Inderal LA) 60 to 80 mg daily is usually sufficient. Atenolol can also be used, at a dose of 25 to 50 mg daily.

10.7 Cardiac evaluation for ADHD medication

Attention deficit hyperactivity disorder (ADHD) is the most common neurobehavioral disorder of childhood and adolescents, with a prevalence of 4 to 12 percent in community samples of American schoolchildren. (See chapter 11 in Greydanus DE, Patel DR, Omar HA, Feucht C, Merrick J: Adolescent Medicine – Pharmacotherapeutics in

General, Mental and Sexual Health, Berlin: de Gruyter; 2012.) More than 2.5 million children take medications for ADHD yearly. The disorder is more prevalent in children with cardiac disease than in the general pediatric population without heart disease. Mahle et al reported abnormal attention scores in 45 percent of children with heart disease (15), whereas Kishbom reported that 50 percent of children with total anomalous pulmonary venous return displayed evidence of hyperactivity or attention deficit (16). Also, ADHD reportedly affects 35 to 55 percent of children with 22q11 microdeletion (17).

Between 1999 and 2004, according to the FDA voluntary reporting system, 19 children prescribed ADHD medications died suddenly, and 26 children reportedly experienced cardiovascular events, including heart palpitations, strokes, and cardiac arrests. (See chapter 11 in Greydanus DE, Patel DR, Omar HA, Feucht C, Merrick J: Adolescent Medicine – Pharmacotherapeutics in General, Mental and Sexual Health, Berlin: de Gruyter; 2012.) The amount of accurate information about the cause of death, dose of medication, and duration of therapy varied considerably among cases. Some patients had underlying cardiac abnormalities, a family history of ventricular tachycardia, or other medical conditions.

Based upon the data, the estimated rate of sudden death among the 2.5 million children taking stimulant medication in the United States would be 1.9 per 1 million children below 18 years of age, which is substantially lower than the estimated rate in the general pediatric population of 10 to 20 per 1 million children below 18 years of age (18). In a large cohort study, 241,417 patients ages 3 to 17 years using amphetamine, atomoxetine (Strattera), or methylphenidate were matched by gender, database, state, and age to 965,668 nonusers. No statistically significant difference was noted in sudden death, ventricular arrhythmia, stroke, myocardial infarction, and all causes of death, even though the ADHD medication users had a higher incidence of cardiac conditions and/or cardiac risk factors (19).

The AAP and the AHA differ in their opinions regarding screening ECGs for children and adolescents before ADHD medication is prescribed. The AHA published a statement in 2008 saying that screening ECGs may increase the sensitivity for detecting underlying heart disease, and calling for routine ECGs as an indication for starting ADHD medications (class IIA, level of evidence C). The organization subsequently corrected that statement, recommending ECGs but not requiring them before starting ADHD medications (20).

The AAP statement that same year reported the incidence of cardiac events as extremely low and no higher than that seen in the general population. It classified routine ECGs as supported by class IIB, level of evidence D (21). Both groups agree that a careful history and physical examination directed to the cardiac system is needed. The author of this discussion agrees that with the extremely low incidence of sudden death due to stimulant medication, the low positive predictive value of ECGs make them a poor screening tool. The practitioner is encouraged to follow the AAP guidelines, obtaining a careful history and physical exam and using an ECG when there is suspicion of heart disease. (See chapter 11 in Greydanus DE, Patel DR, Omar HA, Feucht C, Merrick J: Adolescent Medicine – Pharmacotherapeutics in General, Mental and Sexual Health. Berlin: de Gruyter, 2012.)

Even in children or adolescents with known palliated congenital heart disease, ADHD medications can frequently be used without undue concern. There are no studies that have demonstrated an increased risk of sudden cardiac death (SCD) in pediatric patients with congenital heart disease on stimulant medication. The AHA felt that stimulant medication was reasonable in patients with known risk factors for SCD (long-QT syndrome, hypertrophic cardiomyopathy) even with a history of arrhythmia requiring cardiopulmonary resuscitation (CPR) after other methods had been considered or attempted (20). Nevertheless, one should try to avoid stimulant medication in patients with long QT intervals, known tachyarrhythmia, or cardiac conditions that place them at a high risk for arrhythmia. Consultation with the cardiologist taking care of the adolescent is warranted before starting or if planned dosages are in the high therapeutic range.

10.8 Conclusions

Many advances have occurred in the field of pediatric cardiology that have remarkable benefit for adolescents with cardiac disease. An important part of this progress is the development of pharmacologic approaches to disorders that have a profound impact on the adolescents themselves and the adults they will become in later life. Although often use off label, these drugs are beneficial. This discussion reviews pharmacologic approaches to dyslipidemias, anticoagulation, and syncope. Also considered is the controversial role of stimulant medication in youth with both cardiac disorders and attention-deficit/hyperactivity disorder.

References

1. Pasquali SK, Hall M, Slonim AD, Jenkins KJ, Marino BS, Cohen MS, et al. Off-label use of cardiovascular medications in children hospitalized with congenital and acquired heart disease. Circ Cardiovasc Qual Outcomes 2008;1:74–83.
2. Alexander DC, Bundy DG, Shore AD, Morlock L, Hicks RW, Miller MR. Cardiovascular medication errors in children. Pediatrics 2009;124:324–32.
3. Newman WP III, Freedman DS, Voors AW, Gard PD, Srinivasan SR, Cresanta JL, et al. Relation of serum lipoprotein levels and systolic blood pressure to early atherosclerosis: the Bogalusa Heart Study. N Engl J Med 1986;314(3):138–44.
4. Berenson GS, Srinivasan SR, Bao W, Newman WP III, Tracy RE, Wattigney WA. Association between multiple cardiovascular risk factors and atherosclerosis in children and young adults. The Bogalusa Heart Study. N Engl J Med 1998;338(23):1650–56.
5. McMahan CA, Gidding SS, Malcom GT, Tracy RE, Strong JP, McGill HC, Jr. Pathobiological determinants of atherosclerosis in youth risk scores are associated with early and advanced atherosclerosis. Pediatrics 2006;118(4):1447–55.
6. Kanani PM, Sperling MA. Hyperlipidemia in adolescents. Adolesc Med 2002;13:37–52.
7. Third Report of the National Cholesterol Education Program (NCEP) Expert Panel on Detection, Evaluation, and Treatment of High Blood Cholesterol in Adults (Adult Treatment Panel III) final report. Circulation 2002;106(25):3143–421.
8. Daniels SR, Greer FR and the Committee on Nutrition. Lipid screening and cardiovascular health in childhood. Pediatrics 2008;122:198–208.
9. American Heart Association. Heart Disease and Stroke Statistics: 2006 Update. Dallas, TX: American Heart Association; 2006.
10. de Jongh S, Lilien MR, op't Roodt J, Stroes ES, Bakker HD, Kastelein JJ. Early statin therapy restores endothelial function in children with familial hypercholesterolemia. J Am Coll Cardiol 2002;40(12):2117–21.

11. Laufs U, LaFata V, Plutzky J, Liao K. Upregulation of endothelial nitric oxide synthase by HMG CoA reductase inhibitors. Circulation 1998;97:1129–35.
12. Jain S, Vaidyanathan B. Oral anticoagulants in pediatric cardiac practice: A systemic review of the literature. Ann Pediatr Cardiol 2010;3:31–34.
13. Streif W, Andrew M, Marzinotto V, Massicotte P, Chan AKC, Julian JA, et al. Analysis of warfarin therapy in pediatric patients: A prospective cohort study of 319 patients. Blood 1999;94(9):3007–14.
14. Ganzeboom KS, Colman N, Reitsman JB. Prevalence and triggers for syncope in medical students. Am J Cardiol 2003;91:1006–8.
15. Mahle WT, Clancy RR, Moss EM, Gerdes M, Jobes DR, Wernovsky G. Neurodevelopmental outcome and lifestyle assessment in school-aged and adolescent children with hypoplastic left heart syndrome. Pediatrics 2000;105:1082–89.
16. Kirshborm PM, Flynn TB, Clancy RR, Ittenbach RF, Hartman DM, Paridon SM, et al. Late neurodevelopmental outcome after repair of total anomalous pulmonary venous connections. J Thorac Cardiovasc Surg 2005;129:1091–97.
17. Gothelf D, Gruber R, Presburger G, Dotan I, Brand-Gothelf A, Burg M, et al. Methylphenidate treatment for attention-deficit/hyperactivity disorder in children and adolescents with the velocardiofacial syndrome: An open-label study. J Clin Pschiatry 2003;64:1163–69.
18. Nissen SE. ADHD drugs and cardiovascular risk. N Engl J Med 2006;354:1445–48.
19. Schelleman H, Bilken WB, Strom BL, Kimmel SE, Newcomb C, Guevara JP, et al. Cardiovascular events and death in children exposed and unexposed to ADHD agents. Pediatrics 2011;127:1102–10.
20. Vetter VL, Elia J, Erickson C. Cardiovascular monitoring of children and adolescents with heart disease receiving medications for attention deficit disorder. Circulation 2008;117(18):2407–23.
21. Perrin JM, Friedman RA, Knilans TK, The Black Box Working Group. The Section on Cardiology and Cardiac Surgery. Cardiovascular monitoring and stimulant drugs for Attention-Deficit/Hyperactivity Disorder. Pediatrics 2008;122:451–53.

11 Pulmonary disorders

John H. Marks

Pulmonary disorders in adolescents represent an important cause of morbidity and mortality; thus appropriate care of these conditions is critical to the overall health of these individuals. The most common pulmonary condition in youth is asthma, a problem that continues to increase in prevalence and severity around the world. Other disorders considered here include community-acquired pneumonia and cystic fibrosis. Management is generally based on national or international guidelines developed by expert panels and published in professional journals.

11.1 Introduction

This chapter reviews the pharmacologic management of major respiratory conditions in the adolescent patient: community-acquired pneumonia, asthma, and cystic fibrosis. A brief discussion of the definition, epidemiology, and differential diagnosis precedes consideration of the pharmacologic management of each disorder.

The Management is generally based on national or international guidelines developed by expert panels of professional groups including the American Thoracic Society, the U.S. Infectious Disease Society and the British Thoracic Society (for community-acquired pneumonia), the U.S. National Asthma Education and Prevention Program (NAEP) of the National Institutes of Health, and the U.S. Cystic Fibrosis Foundation.

11.2 Community-acquired pneumonia

Community-acquired pneumonia (CAP) is pneumonia acquired outside of the hospital setting, as opposed to nosocomial pneumonia, which is acquired in the hospital (1). *Streptococcus pneumoniae Mycoplasma pneumoniae,* and *Chlamydophila* (formerly *Chlamydia*) *pneumoniae* appear to be the most frequently encountered pathogens in CAP. These organisms also cause CAP in adults. Other bacterial pathogens that can cause CAP include *Staphylococcus aureus* and *Haemophilus influenzae Legionella pneumophila* is a less common pathogen.

The term *atypical pneumonia* refers to pneumonia that does not present with the usual clinical picture (including high fever, productive cough, and chills) of "typical" pneumonia due to *S. pneumoniae* infection. The term *atypical pneumonia* is frequently used to describe the illness of adolescents with CAP. The clinical presentation of CAP can be highly variable, depending on the causative agent. However, the clinical picture does not always predict the infecting organism. It is probably inaccurate to use the term *atypical pneumonia* and preferable instead to refer to more atypical pathogens as common causes of CAP.

CAP may also be caused by several viruses, which cause 20 percent of CAP cases. The most common viruses are influenza, parainfluenza, respiratory syncytial virus, metapneumovirus, and adenovirus. Less common viral infections causing significant illness include chickenpox, severe acute respiratory syndrome (SARS), avian flu, and hantavirus infection.

11.2.1 Epidemiology

The incidence of pneumonia caused by specific pathogens is not well known for the adolescent population with CAP. Adolescents are often grouped together with young children or adults in epidemiologic studies, which may obscure the results (2). Wide variability in diagnostic testing methods may also affect the incidence reported in studies (3).

An estimated annual incidence of CAP in older children and adolescents is 6 to 12 cases per 1,000. In patients between 10 and 16 years of age, *S. pneumoniae* cause approximately 30 percent of cases of CAP. *Mycoplasma pneumoniae* is the cause in 15 to 40 percent of cases and *C. pneumoniae* comprises 14 to 35 percent of cases. Non-typable *H. influenzae*, influenza A or B, adenovirus, metapneumovirus, and other respiratory viruses are found less frequently.

11.2.2 Diagnosis

The diagnosis of CAP is based on clinical history, physical examination, radiographic studies, and laboratory evaluation (1,4). For teaching purposes, clinical features have been classified to differentiate between bacterial pneumonia, atypical bacterial pneumonia, and viral pneumonia. However, the clinical features of pneumonias caused by different microorganisms frequently overlap and cannot be used reliably to establish etiology. In addition, as many as 50 percent of infections may be mixed bacterial/viral infections.

Typical bacterial pneumonia, usually resulting from *S. pneumoniae* infection, is abrupt in onset, with fever and an ill-appearing, sometimes toxic patient. Respiratory distress may be moderate or severe; auscultation may reveal crackles and egophony limited to the involved anatomic segment. Pleural involvement with pleuritic pain and a pleural friction rub on auscultation are suggestive of a bacterial etiology, as these findings are rarely present in nonbacterial pneumonia. These symptoms may follow days of symptomatic upper respiratory tract infection.

Atypical bacterial pneumonia, resulting from *M. pneumoniae* or *C. pneumoniae* infection, often presents with an abrupt onset of fever, malaise and myalgia, headache, photophobia, sore throat, and gradually worsening nonproductive cough despite improvements in other symptoms. Although hoarseness may be seen in disease caused by both agents, it is more frequently seen with *C. pneumoniae* infection. Wheezing is a frequent finding in atypical bacterial and viral pneumonias.

Differential diagnosis

The differential diagnosis of CAP includes conditions that may present with fever, cough, dyspnea, chest pain, hypoxemia, crackles on auscultation, and radiographic infiltrates. Possible diagnoses include noninfectious lower respiratory syndromes such as asthma, hypersensitivity pneumonitis, pulmonary involvement in collagen vascular disease (see chapter 13), aspiration, and cardiac causes of tachypnea and crackles.

11.2.3 Pharmacologic management

In considering pharmacologic management of CAP, the first decision is whether the patient can be managed as an outpatient or is ill enough to require hospitalization. This determination is based on clinical presentation, severity of symptoms, and, in some cases, laboratory and radiologic evaluation. Administration of an oral macrolide antibiotic (erythromycin, clarithromycin, or azithromycin) is acceptable for treatment of the outpatient who is not seriously ill. Doxycycline is also acceptable for these patients (see ▶Tab. 11.1). These drugs will treat most of the common causes of CAP in adolescents, including the atypical pathogens (4,5,6,7).

It should be noted that up to 50 percent of *S. pneumoniae* strains are resistant to macrolides. Patients should be monitored for response to therapy and, if they are not improving or are worsening, a change should be made in antibiotic coverage. For outpatients, a beta-lactam (amoxicillin or cephalosporin) antibiotic should be instituted (see ▶Tab. 11.2). Oral fluoroquinolones (levofloxacin or moxifloxacin) are alternatives in stable outpatients, even with penicillin-resistant *S. pneumoniae* (see ▶Tab. 11.3).

Adolescents with CAP who are ill enough to be hospitalized should be treated with an intravenous penicillin or cephalosporin (▶Tab. 11.4). For treatment of

Tab. 11.1: Antibiotic treatment of suspected atypical organisms (*M. pneumoniae C. pneumoniae*) in outpatients not seriously ill (all given for 7–10 days).

Medication	Dosage
Erythromycin	50 mg/kg per day divided every 6 hours; maximum dose 2 g/day as base, 3.2 g/day as ethyl succinate
Clarithromycin	15 mg/kg per day divided every 12 hours; maximum dose 1 g/day
Azithromycin	10 mg/kg administered once on day 1 (maximum dose 500 mg) followed by 5 mg/kg once daily on days 2–5 (maximum dose 250 mg/day)
Doxycycline	4 mg/kg per day in two divided doses; maximum 200 mg/day

Tab. 11.2: Antibiotic treatment of suspected drug-resistant *S. pneumoniae* (all given for 7–10 days).

Medication	Dosage
Amoxicillin	80–100 mg/kg per day by mouth in three divided doses; maximum dose 2–3 g/day; this regimen is preferred because of superior in vitro activity against *S. pneumoniae*.
Cefdinir	14 mg/kg per day by mouth in one or two divided doses; maximum dose 600 mg/day
Cefpodoxime	10 mg/kg per day by mouth in one or two divided doses; maximum dose 800 mg/day

Tab. 11.3: Antibiotic treatment of suspected atypical organisms or possible drug resistant *S. pneumoniae* (all given for 7–10 days).

Medication	Dosage
Levofloxacin	500 mg once per day
Moxifloxacin	400 mg once per day

Tab. 11.4: Antibiotics for treatment of hospitalized adolescents with CAP (all given for 7–10 days).

Medication	Dosage
Cefuroxime	150 mg/kg per day divided every 8 hours
Ceftriaxone	50–75 mg/kg per day in a single dose
Ampicillin	50 mg/kg per day divided every 6 hours
Vancomycin	40–60 mg/kg per day divided every 6 hours
Linezolid	600 mg (IV/PO) divided every 12 hours

penicillin-resistant *S. pneumoniae*, vancomycin or linezolid can be used. These anti-biotics also cover methicillin-resistant *S. aureus* (MRSA). Oral or intravenous azithro-mycin should be added to cover the possibility of an atypical pathogen. Whether the adolescent with CAP is treated as an outpatient or is hospitalized, the importance of monitoring clinical response cannot be stressed too much. The role of immunomodu-latory agents (i.e., macrolides, statins, aspirin, corticosteroids) requires further research to elucidate (8).

11.3 Cystic fibrosis

Cystic fibrosis (CF) is an autosomal recessive disorder in which the gene that codes for a protein, called the cystic fibrosis transmembrane conductance regulator (CFTR), is defective (9). The CFTR facilitates the transport of chloride ions across the apical mem-brane of epithelium-lined cells. The altered chloride transport results in altered sodium and water distribution, causing thickened, dehydrated epithelial secretions and mucus. As a result, CF has pulmonary, gastrointestinal, pancreatic, and hepatic manifestations. Obstructive pulmonary disease is the leading cause of morbidity and mortality in CF patients.

The pulmonary aspect of cystic fibrosis has four major components: airway obstruc-tion, infection, inflammation, and ultimately lung tissue damage. Because of the extremely thick mucous secretions, airway clearance is impaired. The thick, stagnant mucus facilitates the growth of bacteria and other pathogens that colonize the airways. The presence of bacteria such as *S. aureusPseudomonas aeruginosaH. influenzae*, and *Burkholderia cepacia* contributes to the destruction of lung tissue and compounds the inflammatory process. Cellular debris becomes trapped and accumulates in the spu-tum, resulting in more inflammation. As neutrophils die, they release large amounts of DNA, which contributes to the viscosity of the already thick sputum.

Manifestations of CF include bronchiectasis, frequent exacerbations, air trapping with an increase in the anterior-posterior chest diameter (barrel chest), a flattened diaphragm, pulmonary hypertension, and ultimately right-sided heart failure (6). Common signs are decreased hemoglobin oxygen saturation, leukocytosis, tachypnea, and fever. Serious complications include hemoptysis and pneumothorax. Digital clubbing and nasal polyps are common in CF patients.

11.3.1 Epidemiology

The incidence of CF varies according to ethnic group. This disease is the most common lethal autosomal recessive disorder in Caucasians, who make up an estimated 90 percent of the patients diagnosed with CF. Hispanics represent 5 percent of the diagnosed cases, while African Americans account for approximately 4 percent. Cystic fibrosis occurs in 1 of every 2,500 Caucasian infants and 1 of every 17,000 African American infants. The disease has been reported in Asians as well as Native Americans but is rare in these groups. Life expectancy for patients with CF is now longer than 35 years and death is often due to such causes as infection (*Pseudomonas*) and pulmonary hypertension (10).

11.3.2 Differential diagnosis

CF is now diagnosed routinely by newborn screening; however, in older children and adolescents born before implementation of newborn screening, diagnosis was based on clinical suspicion, sweat chloride testing, and/or gene mutation analysis. The differential diagnosis includes conditions causing chronic cough and progressive obstructive lung disease, such as immune deficiency, primary ciliary dyskinesia, and recurrent aspiration. CF-related diabetes mellitus (CFRD) is a common comorbid condition (see chapter 3) (11). Also, chronic (polypoid) sinusitis is a nearly universal aspect of CF owing to chronic bacterial infection but also allergic mechanisms to some extent (12).

11.3.3 Pharmacologic management

Acute pulmonary exacerbations

Acute exacerbations occur because of flare-up of infections within the airways. Frequent signs and symptoms of an acute exacerbation include cough with sputum production, weight loss, a decrease in pulmonary function, and reduced energy levels. Treatment of pulmonary exacerbations consists of airway clearance techniques, nutritional support, and antibiotic therapy. The specific antibiotics used in treatment are determined by the known or suspected organisms in the most recent sputum culture (13,14,15,16,17). *S. aureus* and *P. aeruginosa* are the most common pathogens in adolescents and adults. Often sputum samples reveal different strains of *P. aeruginosa* with varying degrees of susceptibility.

Another highly resistant organism that eventually emerges as CF progresses is *Burkholderiacepacia*. Patients colonized with this pathogen generally have a faster rate of pulmonary decline and a shorter life span. Evolving data suggest that the pathogenicity of this organism depends on the specific genomovar (subspecies of microbe) present.

Preliminary epidemiologic data indicate that *B. cepacia* (genomovar III) carries the greatest risk for increased morbidity and mortality.

Initial treatment generally consists of 2 to 3 weeks of antibiotic therapy (9,18,19). The patient is hospitalized if symptoms are moderate to severe, whereas mild exacerbations are often managed in the home setting. ▶Tab. 11.5 lists frequently prescribed intravenous antibiotics and their dosing regimens. Ampicillin/sulbactam or cefuroxime are reasonable empiric choices when *S. aureus* and *H. influenzae* are suspected pathogens. Treatment of exacerbations involving *S. aureus* typically includes a first-generation cephalosporin (cefazolin, cephalothin) or a penicillinase-resistant penicillin such as nafcillin (20). When MRSA is the causative agent, vancomycin or linezolid may be used.

Treatment of exacerbations involving *P. aeruginosa* requires a combination of an antipseudomonal beta-lactam antibiotic (piperacillin, ceftazidime, cefepime, imipenem, or meropenem) and an aminoglycoside (gentamicin or tobramycin) or fluoroquinolone (ciprofloxacin or levofloxacin). Combination therapy is used to provide

Tab. 11.5: Intravenous antibiotic dosage recommendations for the treatment of pulmonary exacerbations in CF.

Antibiotic	Dosage (mg/kg per day)	Doses per day	Maximum daily dose (g) or desired serum concentration
Amikacin	30	2–3	Peak 25–30 Trough <5
Ampicillin-sulbactam	100–150	4	9 g
Aztreonam	150–200	3–4	8 g
	100	c.i.	8 g
Cefepime	150–200	3–4	8 g
Ceftazidime	150–200	3–4	8 g
	100	c.i.	8 g
Cefuroxime	100–150	3	4.5 g
Ciprofloxacin	20–30	2–3	1.2
Colistin	5–8	3	0.45
Gentamicin	10	2–3	Peak 8–12 Trough <2
Imipenem-cilastatin	50–100	4	4 g
Nafcillin	100–200	4	12 g
Piperacillin ± tazobactam	400*	4	18 g
Ticarcillin ± clavulanate	400*	4	18 g
Tobramycin	10–15	2–3 1	Peak 8–12 Trough <2
Trimethoprim/ sulfamethoxazole	10–15	2	0.64 (TMP)

c.i., continuous infusion regimen; TMP, trimethoprim.
*Refers to dosing of piperacillin and ticarcillin components.

synergistic activity and reduce the potential for development of resistance. Oral cipro-floxacin or levofloxacin are widely used in the management of mild exacerbations involving *P. aeruginosa*; however, owing to increased resistance over the past decade, they may no longer be effective as monotherapy.

The antibiotic dosages for CF patients tend to be higher than those for non-CF patients for a number of reasons. Patients with CF possess an increased clearance and volume of distribution for the aminoglycosides and many beta-lactam compounds. In addition, because of chronic colonization and frequent antibiotic courses, antibiotic resistance is inevitable. Also, the microenvironment within the airways contains mucin, DNA, cations, and other factors that interfere with antibiotic activity. These factors explain the rationale for more aggressive therapy when exacerbations occur.

The larger volume of distribution, expressed as liters per kilogram of body weight, may be a result of the patient's nutritional status. Beta-lactam antibiotics and aminoglycosides are distributed into lean body mass. Patients with CF tend to have an increased lean body mass and relatively low amounts of adipose tissue because of weight loss and malnutrition. The increased clearance of certain drugs exhibited by CF patients may be due to other mechanisms, including increased renal clearance, increased nonrenal clearance, and decreased protein binding.

11.3.4 Management of chronic cystic fibrosis

Anti-inflammatory agents

The presence of bacterial organisms within the airway creates a chronic inflammatory state that leads to the eventual destruction of the airways themselves (21). Early studies showed that low-dose oral corticosteroids given on alternate days slowed the pulmonary decline in CF patients. Because doses of 1 mg/kg every other day were used, adverse events were dramatically decreased but not totally eliminated. In a 4-year multicenter trial, 285 patients were randomly assigned to receive prednisone 1 mg/kg, 2 mg/kg, or placebo every other day (7,17). The study demonstrated evidence of a significant increase in glucose intolerance among patients receiving 2 mg/kg compared with those receiving 1 mg/kg. A significant increase in growth retardation was also observed in both treatment groups Versus

the placebo group. The beneficial effects of alternate-day prednisone, as measured by a decrease in serum IgG and pulmonary function (FEV1 and FVC) and a decline in hospitalization, reached a plateau after 6 months of therapy. The authors recommended that therapy be limited to less than 1 year to decrease the risk of adverse effects (growth retardation and glucose intolerance) (7,17,18,21). Prednisone 2 mg/kg could not be recommended because of adverse effects (17,18,21).

In general, chronic therapy with prednisone is not a common event simply because the risks appear to outweigh the benefits. Studies examining the use of inhaled corticosteroids (ICSs) have shown conflicting results. At this point the role of ICSs for maintenance therapy in CF patients is not clearly defined. As a result, there is general consensus that ICSs should not be used unless the patient is concurrently diagnosed with asthma.

Nonsteroidal anti-inflammatory drugs (NSAIDs) are used in the treatment of CF to inhibit neutrophil activation and migration (21). The effects of high-dose ibuprofen were examined in a 4-year clinical trial of 85 patients with mild lung disease (17). The study resulted in a slower rate of decline in pulmonary function in patients treated with ibuprofen. However, the most benefit was noted in patients ages 5 to 13, who showed a decline in FEV1 of only 2 percent over the 4-year period versus a 15 percent decline during the same period in the placebo group. Patients treated with ibuprofen also maintained their body weight while patients in the placebo group lost weight. Despite the significant efficacy demonstrated in this study, ibuprofen is not routinely prescribed in all centers owing to concerns for serious bleeding or renal insufficiency, especially when this agent is given with an aminoglycoside. In patients who are started on ibuprofen, blood testing is recommended to ensure optimal therapy.

Azithromycin, an antibiotic with both antimicrobial and anti-inflammatory activity, has been shown to be beneficial in treating CF. Although the mechanism of action of azithromycin in CF is not understood, four randomized placebo-controlled trials have been conducted in adults and children with CF, most of whom had chronic infection with *P. aeruginosa* (17,18). These studies demonstrated that azithromycin was associated with reduced pulmonary exacerbations, increased weight gain, and improved lung function. Azithromycin is currently recommended for people with CF 6 years of age or older who have had *P. aeruginosa* in their sputum for at least 1 year. The dosage is 250 mg or 500 mg based on body weight taken 3 days per week.

Aerosolized antibiotics

The purpose of aerosolized antibiotics is to deliver large quantities of medication to the lungs while decreasing the risk of side effects from systemic absorption. Aerosolized antibiotics have been used as adjunctive treatment with intravenous antibiotics for acute pulmonary exacerbations, as chronic suppressive therapy in patients colonized with *P. aeruginosa*, and, more recently as early treatment to eradicate *P. aeruginosa* after initial positive sputum culture.

Tobramycin solution for inhalation (TOBI) was introduced in 1998. The efficacy and safety of chronic maintenance therapy were established based on a large multicenter randomized controlled trial in CF patients persistently colonized with *P. aeruginosa* (17,18,22). Patients were treated with aerosolized tobramycin 300 mg twice a day, in three cycles of 28 days on therapy and 28 days off therapy. This study showed a significant increase in pulmonary function over baseline measurements. The greatest effect was seen in patients aged 13 to 17 years. The secondary endpoints of the study were to evaluate the need for hospitalization and antipseudomonal antibiotics. Patients who received aerosolized tobramycin had fewer hospitalizations and required less use of antipseudomonal antibiotics (17,22). The use of TOBI did not result in significant increases in ototoxicity or nephrotoxicity.

Aztreonam for inhalation solution (Cayston 75 mg) is an inhaled antibiotic for patients with CF who have *P. aeruginosa* infection. Aztreonam has potent in vitro activity against gram-negative aerobic pathogens, including *P. aeruginosa*. Cayston contains aztreonam formulated with lysine, a proprietary formulation developed specifically for inhalation. The medication was approved by the U.S. Food and Drug Administration (FDA) in 2010 after reviewing results of safety and efficacy studies. Cayston had positive effects on the maintenance of pulmonary function and delayed the onset of acute pulmonary exacerbations. It is administered three times a day using a proprietary nebulizer system that delivers the dose in 2 to 3 minutes. Therapy is given daily for a 28-day course, followed by 28 days off. Other antibiotics delivered by inhalation aerosol are being studied for the treatment of pulmonary infection in patients with CF. These include levofloxacin, ciprofloxacin, amikacin, and fosfomycin/tobramycin.

Mucolytic agents

Mucolytic agents loosen sputum by cleaving DNA remnants left behind by degenerating neutrophils (23). Currently dornase alpha (Pulmozyme) is the only FDA-approved mucolytic agent use in the United States (24). A mucolytic is a well-accepted adjunct to standard airway clearance and antibiotic therapy. By using this agent, clinicians hope to prevent or delay the bronchiectasis that results from obstruction of the airways. The typical dose is 2.5 mg nebulized daily over a period of 15 to 20 minutes. Side effects include rash, pharyngitis, laryngitis, chest pain, and conjunctivitis. Dornase alpha received approval from the FDA when its safety and efficacy were established in a phase III clinical trial involving 968 patients with mild to moderate lung disease (17). Compared with the control group, patients receiving 2.5 mg of dornase alpha daily showed a 5.8 percent increase in pulmonary function as measured by mean FEV1 and a 31 percent decrease in the risk of pulmonary exacerbations (17).

Hypertonic saline (7%) inhalation has been found in controlled clinical trials to improve lung function and decrease the number of pulmonary exacerbations compared with normal saline (0.9%) (25). It is thought to increase airway surface liquid by osmosis, thus aiding airway clearance. Side effects are cough and bronchospasm; thus a nebulized bronchodilator should be used prior to saline inhalation. Mannitol, a nonionic osmotic agent, has been shown to be as effective as hypertonic saline when given as a dry-powder inhalation. As of this writing it has not been approved by the FDA.

Potential newer treatments

Several agents that modulate CFTR function or stimulate chloride secretion via non-CFTR pathways are being investigated. These agents are meant to return the airway surface liquid to normal or near normal, thereby limiting the degree of airway obstruction, infection, and inflammation in the lungs of patients with CF (13,14,15,16,17). Although caring for adolescents with CF is challenging, the prospect of newer therapies that will improve the quality of life and survival of these patients is exciting. Dealing with comorbid depression and anxiety is important, as well as ensuring proper transitioning to adult care (26,27,28,29).

11.4 Asthma

Asthma is the most common chronic disease of children and adolescents (30). It is characterized by recurrent episodes of reversible airway obstruction, hyperreactivity, and inflammation (31,32,33). Increased airway responsiveness to a variety of immunologic challenges (e.g., pollen, dust mites) and nonimmunologic stimuli (e.g., exercise, smoke, cold air, viral respiratory infection) is characteristic of asthma. Exposure results in the release of inflammatory mediators, such as leukotrienes, from eosinophils, causing bronchial smooth muscle constriction, airway mucosal edema, and mucus secretion. This leads to symptoms of wheezing, coughing, chest tightness, and dyspnea. Recurrent episodes lead to bronchial smooth muscle hypertrophy, subepithelial fibrosis, and often airway remodeling, with collagen deposition in the basement membrane.

11.4.1 Epidemiology

Nine million children under the age of 18 years in the United States have been diagnosed with asthma (30). In 2005, some 8.9 percent of children in the United States currently had asthma. Children and adolescents with asthma miss about 10 school days per year and account for 3 million sick visits to health care providers and 200,000 hospitalizations annually. Asthma prevalence and morbidity are higher among poor, disadvantaged minority children and adolescents living in urban areas. Research is identifying a link between asthma and obesity, two conditions that are both increasing in prevalence (34).

11.4.2 Differential diagnosis

The differential diagnosis of asthma in adolescents includes conditions that cause acute or chronic respiratory symptoms, such as wheezing, coughing, dyspnea, and chest pain. These include CF, pneumonia, aspiration, pulmonary edema, airway compression from tumors or lymph nodes, vocal cord dysfunction, and anxiety/hyperventilation.

11.4.3 Pharmacological management

Treatment of asthma is based on a classification of severity based on symptom frequency and pulmonary function (31–33,). Asthma management guidelines were initially published by the National Institutes of Health, National Heart, Lung, and Blood Institute Expert Panel Report 1 in 1991 as the National Asthma Education and Prevention Program (NAEPP). The latest revision of the report was published in 2007 (33).

Asthma severity is classified as intermittent, mild persistent, moderate persistent, or severe persistent, as illustrated in ▶Tab. 11.6. Severity is usually classified initially, before long-term controller medications are started. After asthma classification, the NAEPP recommends a stepwise approach to therapy (▶Fig. 11.1), with aggressive attempts to control symptoms quickly and subsequent adjustment of therapy in a stepwise fashion as symptoms require. The principal goals of the treatment of asthma are to minimize symptoms, normalize pulmonary function, prevent exacerbations, and improve health-related quality of life. A theoretical goal is to prevent long-term consequences of airway inflammation, particularly airway remodeling and chronic persistent airway obstruction. Dealing with asthma's comorbidities (i.e., depression, anxiety, posttraumatic stress disorder) is important to improve compliance with recommended treatment guidelines (35,36).

Intermittent asthma does not require daily controller medications and is usually managed with as-needed use of a short-acting beta agonist (SABA), such as albuterol, given by metered-dose inhaler (37). Available SABAs are shown in ▶Tab. 11.7. A patient with intermittent asthma may have exacerbations requiring anti-inflammatory medications such as oral corticosteroids.

Tab. 11.6: Classification of asthma severity and initiating treatment in youths greater than or equal to 12 years of age and adults.

Components of severity		Classification of asthma severity (≥12 years of age)			
		Intermittent	Persistent		
			Mild	Moderate	Severe
Impairment Normal FEV1/FVC:	Symptoms	≤2 days per week	>2 days per week but not daily	Daily	Throughout the day
8–19 years, 85%	Nighttime awakenings	≤2 times per month	3–4 times per month	>1 time per week but not nightly	Often 7 times per week
20–39 years, 80%	Short-acting beta2-agonist use for symptom control (not prevention of EIB)	≤2 days per week	>2 days per week but not daily, and not more than once on any day	Daily	Several times per day
	Interference with normal activity	None	Minor limitation	Some limitation	Extremely limited
40–59 years, 75%	Lung function	Normal FEV1 between exacerbations FEV1 >80% predicted FEV1/FVC normal	FEV1 ≥80% predicted FEV1/FVC normal	FEV1 >60 but <80% predicted FEV1/FVC reduced 5%	FEV1 <60% predicted FEV1/FVC reduced >5%
60–80 years, 70%					
Risk	Exacerbations requiring oral systemic corticosteroids	0–1 per year (see section 11.4.3)	≥2 per year		
		Consider severity and interval since last exacerbation. Frequency and severity may fluctuate over time for patients in any severity category. Relative annual risk of exacerbations may be related to FEV1.			
Recommended step for initiating treatment		Step 1	Step 2	Step 3 And consider a short course of oral systemic corticosteroids.	Step 4 or 5
		In 2–6 weeks, evaluate level of asthma control that is achieved and adjust therapy accordingly.			

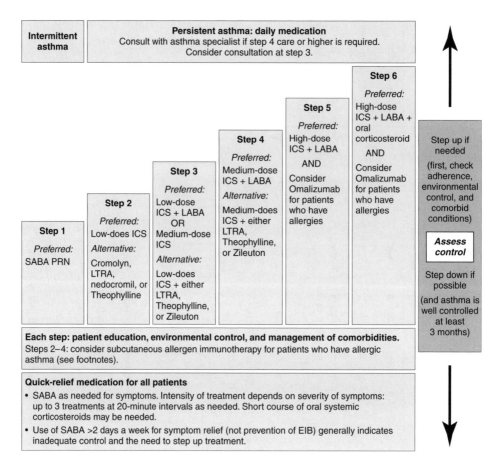

| Intermittent asthma | Persistent asthma: daily medication Consult with asthma specialist if step 4 care or higher is required. Consider consultation at step 3. | | | | |

Step 1
Preferred:
SABA PRN

Step 2
Preferred:
Low-does ICS
Alternative:
Cromolyn, LTRA, nedocromil, or Theophylline

Step 3
Preferred:
Low-dose ICS + LABA
OR
Medium-dose ICS
Alternative:
Low-does ICS + either LTRA, Theophylline, or Zileuton

Step 4
Preferred:
Medium-dose ICS + LABA
Alternative:
Medium-does ICS + either LTRA, Theophylline, or Zileuton

Step 5
Preferred:
High-dose ICS + LABA
AND
Consider Omalizumab for patients who have allergies

Step 6
Preferred:
High-dose ICS + LABA + oral corticosteroid
AND
Consider Omalizumab for patients who have allergies

Step up if needed
(first, check adherence, environmental control, and comorbid conditions)

Assess control

Step down if possible
(and asthma is well controlled at least 3 months)

Each step: patient education, environmental control, and management of comorbidities.
Steps 2–4: consider subcutaneous allergen immunotherapy for patients who have allergic asthma (see footnotes).

Quick-relief medication for all patients
- SABA as needed for symptoms. Intensity of treatment depends on severity of symptoms: up to 3 treatments at 20-minute intervals as needed. Short course of oral systemic corticosteroids may be needed.
- Use of SABA >2 days a week for symptom relief (not prevention of EIB) generally indicates inadequate control and the need to step up treatment.

Fig. 11.1: Stepwise approach for managing asthma in youths greater than or equal to 12 years of age and adults..

When the adolescent with asthma presents with decreased lung function and poorly controlled symptoms, a short course or "burst" of an oral corticosteroid such as prednisone or prednisolone is started at a dose of 1 to 2 mg per kg given for 5 to 7 days. This is done while starting an aggressive program of anti-inflammatory controller medications in addition to SABA rescue medication. Inhaled corticosteroids are the daily controller medications of choice.

Several randomized prospective studies demonstrate that inhaled ICSs improve lung function, diminish symptoms, decrease need for SABAs, and improve airway responsiveness to methacholine in patients with all levels of persistent asthma (17). In patients with stable but not well-controlled asthma, a medium-dose ICS is prescribed initially. Several ICSs are available in metered-dose inhalers or dry-powder inhalers (▶Tab. 11.8). If a daily ICS is not achieving adequate control of symptoms, an additional controller should be added, such as a long-acting beta-agonist (LABA; formoterol or salmeterol) or a leukotriene modifier (montelukast or zafirlukast) (17). Short-acting beta-agonist "rescue" inhalers are prescribed to all patients with persistent asthma.

Tab. 11.7: Short-acting inhaled beta agonists.

Drug	Approved age range	Formulation	Adult dosage
Short-acting inhaled beta-2 agonists			
Albuterol			
Proventil, Ventolin, or generic solution	≥2 years old	Nebulizer solutions: 0.021% (0.63 mg/3 mL), 0.042% (1.25 mg/3 mL), 0.083% (2.5 mg/3 mL), 0.5% (0.5 mg/20 mL)	2.5 mg every 4–6 hours as needed
Proventil-HFA, Ventolin-HFA, or ProAir	≥4 years old	MDI: 90 mcg per puff	2 puffs every 4–6 hours as needed
Levalbuterol			
Xopenex solution	≥6 years old	Nebulizer solution: 0.31, 0.63, or 1.25 mg/3 mL	0.63 to 1.25 mg, two to four times daily as needed
Xopenex-HFA-	≥6 years old	45 mcg per puff	2 puffs every 4–6 hours as needed
Pirbuterol			
Maxair Autohaler	≥12 years old	Breath-actuated MDI: 200 mcg per puff	2 puffs every 4–6 hours as needed
Long-acting, beta-2 agonists			
Salmeterol			
Serevent Diskus	>4 years old	DPI: 50 mcg per inhalation	1 inhalation every 12 hours
Formoterol			
Foradil aerolizer	≥5 years old	DPI: 12 mcg per inhalation	1 inhalation every 12 hours

MDI, metered-dose inhaler; DPI, dry-powder inhaler; HFA, hydrofluoroalkane; h, hour.

Inhaled LABAs help maintain bronchodilation for 8 to 12 hours and are taken twice daily (▶Tab. 11.9) (38,39). Salmeterol has a slow onset of action, while formoterol has a rapid onset of action, 5 to 15 minutes, similar to albuterol. The LABAs should not be prescribed as rescue medications, and should not be used without concurrently using an ICS. These medications have an FDA "black box" warning due to results of a placebo-controlled study of salmeterol that showed a significantly increased risk of asthma-related deaths in the salmeterol group (17). This risk was greater in African-Americans; however, only 38 percent of African Americans in the study were using an inhaled ICS (17). Combination inhalers containing both an ICS and a LABA can be prescribed for patients not controlled on medium- or high-dose ICSs alone. The combination of a LABA plus an inhaled ICS is more effective than higher doses of inhaled ICSs in most patients.

Tab. 11.8: Estimated comparative daily doses for inhaled glucocorticoids in adolescents and adults.

Drug	Low dose	Medium dose	High dose
Beclomethasone HFA	80–240 mcg	240–480 mcg	>480 mcg
• 40 mcg/dose	(2–6 puffs)	–	–
• 80 mcg per dose	(1–3 puffs)	(3–6 puffs)	(>6 puffs)
Budesonide DPI (Flexhaler®)	180–600 mcg	600–1200 mcg	>1200 mcg
• 90 mcg per dose	(2–6 inhalations)	–	–
• 180 mcg per dose	(1–3 inhalations)	–	–
	200–600 mcg	600–1200 mcg	>1200 mcg
• 100 mcg per dose	(2–6 inhalations)	–	–
• 200 mcg per dose	(1–3 inhalations)	(3–6 inhalations)	(>6 inhalations)
• 400 mcg per dose	(1 inhalation)	(2–3 inhalations)	(>3 inhalations)
Ciclesonide HFA	80–320 mcg	320–640 mcg	>640 mcg
• 80 mcg per puff	(1–4 puffs)	(4–8 puffs)	(>8 puffs)
• 160 mcg per puff	(1–2 puffs)	(2–4 puffs)	(>4 puffs)
Flunisolide HFA*	320 mcg	320–640 mcg	>640 mcg
• 80 mcg per puff	(4 puffs)	(4–8 puffs)	(>8 puffs)
Flunisolide CFC*	500–1000 mcg	1000–2000 mcg	>2000 mcg
• 250 mcg per puff	(2–4 puffs)	(4–8 puffs)	(>8 puffs)
Fluticasone HFA	88–264 mcg	264–440 mcg	>440 mcg
• 44 mcg per puff	(2–6 puffs)	–	–
• 110 mcg per puff	(2 puffs)	(3–4 puffs)	(>4 puffs)
• 220 mcg per puff	–	–	(>2 puffs)
Fluticasone DPI	100–300 mcg	300–500 mcg	>500 mcg
• 50 mcg per dose	(2–6 inhalations)	–	–
• 100 mcg per dose	–	(3–5 inhalations)	(>5 inhalations)
• 250 mcg per dose	–	–	(>2 inhalations)
Mometasone DPI	220 mcg	440 mcg	>440 mcg
• 110 mcg per dose	(2 inhalations)	–	–
• 220 mcg per dose	(1 inhalation)	(2 inhalations)	(>2 inhalations)

The combinations include fluticasone and salmeterol, budesonide and formoterol, and mometasone and formoterol as shown in ▶Tab. 11.10. Combination inhalers are preferred over separate ICS and LABA inhalers because they ensure that patients will not omit the ICS, leaving them on LABA monotherapy.

Leukotriene modifiers may be added to obtain better asthma control with lower doses of ICSs. Montelukast and zafirlukast are leukotriene D4 receptor antagonists, and zileutin is a 5-lipoxygenase inhibitor (▶Tab. 11.11). Leukotriene modifiers may be slightly less effective than a LABA when added to an ICS.

Theophylline in an oral sustained-release form may be added as a long-term controller in some patients. Once a commonly used first-line treatment, theophylline is now used only in selected patients, such as those who cannot tolerate a LABA. Blood levels of the drug must be monitored to avoid side effects.

Tab. 11.9: Long-acting inhaled beta agonists.

Long-acting beta-2 agonists			
Salmeterol			
Serevent Diskus	>4 years old	DPI: 50 mcg per inhalation	1 inhalation every 12 hours
Formoterol			
Foradil aerolizer	≥5 years old	DPI: 12 mcg per inhalation	1 inhalation every 12 hours

DPI, dry-powder inhaler.

Tab. 11.10: Usual doses of combination inhaled glucocorticoids and long-acting beta agonists for the treatment of asthma in adolescents age 12 and older and adults.

Medication	Low dose	Medium dose	High dose
Budesonide/formoterol HFA			
80/4.5 mcg	2 puffs twice a day	–	–
160/4.5 mcg	–	2 puffs twice a day	–
Fluticasone/salmeterol DPI			
100/50 mcg	1 inhalation twice a day	–	–
250/50 mcg	–	1 inhalation twice a day	–
500/50 mcg	–	–	1 inhalation twice a day
Fluticasone/salmeterol HFA			
45/21 mcg	2 puffs twice a day	–	–
115/21 mcg	–	2 puffs twice a day	–
230/21 mcg	–	–	2 puffs twice a day
Mometasone/formoterol HFA			
100/5 mcg	–	2 puffs twice a day	–
200/5 mcg	–	–	2 puffs twice a day

By convention, doses from MDIs are expressed as puffs and doses from DPIs are expressed as inhalations.
HFA, metered dose inhaler with hydrofluoroalkane propellant; DPI, dry powder inhaler.

Tab. 11.11: Usual doses of agents affecting 5-lipoxygenase pathway.

Medication	Dose form	Age 12 through adult
Montelukast (Singulair)	Granules: 4 mg/packet Tablet: 10 mg Chewable tablets: 4 mg, 5 mg	10 mg tablet once daily in evening
Zafirlukast (Accolate)	Tablets: 10 mg, 20 mg	20 mg twice daily
Zileuton (Zyflo CR)	Extended-release tablet: 600 mg	1200 mg twice daily

Tab. 11.12: Assessing asthma control and adjusting therapy in youths greater than or equal to 12 years of age and adults.

Components of control		Classification of asthma control (≥12 years of age)		
		Well controlled	Not well controlled	Very poorly controlled
Impairment	Symptoms	≤2 days per week	>2 days per week	Throughout the day
	Nighttime awakenings	≤2 times per month	1–3 times per week	≥4 times per week
	Interference with normal activity	None	Some limitation	Extremely limited
	Short-acting beta-2 agonist use for symptom control (not prevention of exercise-induced bronchospasm [EIB])	≤2 days per week	>2 days per week	Several times per day
	FEV1 or peak flow	>80 % predicted/personal best	60–80% predicted/personal best	<60% predicted/personal best
Risk	Exacerbations requiring oral systemic corticosteroids	0–1 per year		≥2 per year (see section 11.4.3)
	Consider severity and interval since last exacerbation			
	Progressive loss of lung function	Evaluation requires long-term follow-up care.		
Treatment-related adverse effects		Medication side effects can vary in intensity from none to very troublesome and worrisome. The level of intensity does not correlate with specific levels of control but should be considered in the overall assessment of risk.		
Recommended action for treatment		• Maintain current step. • Regular follow-ups every 1–6 months to maintain control. • Consider step down if well controlled for at least 3 months.	• Step up 1 step. • Reevaluate in 2–6 weeks. • For side effects, consider alternative treatment options.	• Consider short course of oral systemic corticosteroids. • Step up 1–2 steps. • Reevaluate in 2 weeks. • For side effects, consider alternative treatment options.

Assessing control

Assessment of "control," rather than severity, is used to adjust therapy. Control is based on impairment over the past 2 to 4 weeks (based on history or a validated questionnaire), current FEV1 or peak flow, and estimates of risk, as shown in ▶Tab. 11.12. If asthma is not well controlled, therapy should be stepped up. If the asthma is well controlled, therapy can be continued or possibly stepped down to minimize medication side effects. Most patients who are compliant with therapy achieve control of their asthma within a few weeks or months. Achieving control is emphasized, because patients with poor control of asthma symptoms are more likely to require urgent care for asthma than those whose asthma is well controlled. Complementary and alternative medical strategies, although commonly used by patients with asthma, require further research to identify their potential efficacy (40).

11.5 Conclusions

Pulmonary disorders are important yet challenging conditions to treat in adolescents. Three key pulmonary disorders are considered: community-acquired pneumonia, cystic fibrosis, and asthma (17). Improvement in morbidity and mortality includes attention to behavioral issues as well as ever-changing pharmacologic management. Antibiotic resistance presents an ongoing dilemma in managing pulmonary infections. Attention to comorbid conditions is also important.

Improving compliance with recommended treatments remains a challenge for clinicians caring for youth with acute and chronic pulmonary disorders. Successful transitioning to accepting adult care providers is also a critical component in caring for youths with chronic disorders.

References

1. American Thoracic Society. Guidelines for the initial management of adults with community-acquired pneumonia: diagnosis, assessment of severity, and initial antimicrobial therapy. Am J Resp Crit Care Med 2001;163:1730–54.
2. Kronman MP, Hersh Al, Feng R, Huang YS. Lee GE, Shah SS. Ambulatory visit rates and antibiotic prescribing for children with pneumonia, 1994–2007. Pediatrics 2011; 127:411–18.
3. Bartlett JG. Diagnostic tests for agents of community-acquired pneumonia. Clin Infect Dis 2011;52(Suppl 4):S296–304.
4. British Thoracic Society Standards of Care Committee. British Thoracic Society guidelines for the management of community acquired pneumonia in childhood. Thorax 2002;57(suppl 1):i1.
5. Community acquired pneumonia guideline team, Cincinnati Children's Hospital Medical Center. Evidence-based care guidelines for medical management of community acquired pneumonia in children 60 days to 17 years of age. Accessed 2011 Jun 08. URL: www.cincinnatichildrens.org/svc/alpha/h/health-policy/ev-based/pneumonia.htm
6. File TM, Niederman MS. Antimicrobial therapy of community-acquired pneumonia. Infect Dis Clin North Am 2004;18:993–1016.
7. Mandell LA, Wunderink RG, Anzueto A, Bartlett JG, Campbell GD, Dean NC, et al. Infectious Diseases Society of America/American Thoracic Society consensus guidelines

on the management of community-acquired pneumonia in adults. Clin Infect Dis 2007;44(suppl 2):S27–S72.

8. Corrales-Medina VF, Musher DM. Immunomodulatory agents in the treatment of community-acquired pneumonia: A systemic review. J Infect 2011 Jul 5. [Epub ahead of print]

9. Nasr SZ. Cystic fibrosis in adolescents and young adults. Adolesc Med 2000;11:589–603.

10. Baghale N, Kalilzedeh S, Hasssanzad M, Parsanejad N, Velayati A. Determination of mortality from cystic fibrosis. Pneumologia 2010;59(3):170–73.

11. Laguna TA, Nathan BM, Moran A. Managing diabetes in cystic fibrosis. Diabetes Obes Metabol 2010;12:858–64.

12. Schraven SP, Wehrmannn M, Wagner W, Blumenstock G, Koitschev A. Prevalence and histopathology of chronic polypoid sinusitis in pediatric patients with cystic fibrosis. J Cyst Fibros 2011; 10:181–86.

13. Davis SD, Ferkol TW. Hitting the target: new treatments for cystic fibrosis. Am J Respir Crit Care Med 2010;182:1460–61.

14. Bais R, Hubert D, Tümmler B. Antibiotic treatment of CF lung disease: from bench to bedside. J Cyst Fibros 2011;10(Suppl 2):S146–51.

15. Van Westreenen M, Tiddens HA. New antimicrobial strategies in cystic fibrosis. Paediatr Drugs 2010;12:343–52.

16. Rogers GB, Hoffman LR, Döring G. Novel concepts in evaluating antimicrobial therapy for bacterial lung infections in patients with cystic fibrosis. J Cyst Fibros 2011 Jul 11. [Epub ahead of print]

17. Light MJ, Blaisdell Cj, Homnick DN, Schechter MS, Wienberger MM, eds. Pediatric pulmonology. Elk Grove Village, IL: American Academy of Pediatrics, 2011.

18. Flume PA, O'Sullivan BP, Robinson KA, Goss CH, Mogayzel PJ, Willey-Courand DB, et al. Cystic Fibrosis Foundation, Pulmonary Therapies Committee. Cystic fibrosis pulmonary guidelines: chronic medications for maintenance of lung health. Am J Respir Crit Care Med 2007;176(10):957–69.

19. Breen L, Aswani N. Elective versus symptomatic intravenous antibiotic therapy for cystic fibrosis. Cochrane Database Syst Rev 2001;1:CD001747.

20. Goss CH, Muhlebach MS. Review: Staphylococcus aureus and MRSA in cystic fibrosis. J Cyst Fibros 2011 Jun 28. [Epub ahead of print]

21. Chmiel JF, Konstan MW. Inflammation and anti-inflammatory therapies for cystic fibrosis. Clin Chest Med 2007;28(2):331–46.

22. Konstan MW, Flume PA, Kappler M, Chiron R, Higgins M, Brockhaus F, et al. Safety, efficacy and convenience of tobramycin inhalation powder in cystic fibrosis patients: The EAGER trial. J Cyst Fibros 2011;10:54–61.

23. Jones AP, Wallis CE. Recombinant human deoxyribonuclease for cystic fibrosis. Cochrane Database Syst Rev 2003;3:CD001127.

24. Dentice R, Elkins M. Timing of dornase alfa inhalation for cystic fibrosis. Cochrane Database Syst Rev 2011;5:CD007923.

25. Donaldson SH, Bennett WD, Zeman KL, Knowles MR, Tarran R, Boucher RC. Mucus clearance and lung function in cystic fibrosis with hypertonic saline. N Engl J Med 2006;354(3):241–50.

26. Modi AC, Driscoll KA, Montaq-Leifling K, Acton JD. Screening for symptoms of depression and anxiety in adolescents and young adults with cystic fibrosis. Pediatr Pulmonol 2011;46:153–59.

27. Casier A, Goubert L, Theunis M, Huse D, De Baets F, Matthys D, et al. Acceptance and well-being in adolescents and young adults with cystic fibrosis: a prospective study. J Pediatr Psychol 2011;36:476–87.

28. Barker DH, Driscoll KA, Modi AC, Light MJ, Quittner AL. Supporting cystic fibrosis disease management during adolescence: the role of family and friends. Child Care Health Dev 2011 Jul 19. [Epub ahead of print]

29. Towns SJ, Bell SC. Transition of adolescents with cystic fibrosis from paediatric to adult care. Clin Respir J 2011;5:64–75.

30. Centers for Disease Control and Prevention. Vital signs: asthma prevalence, disease characteristics, and self-management education: United States, 2001–2009. MMWR 2011;60:547–52.

31. Bateman ED, Boushey HA, Bousquet J, Busse WW, Clark TJ, Pauwels RA, Pedersen SE. Can guideline-defined asthma control be achieved? The Gaining Optimal Asthma Control study. GOAL Investigators Group Am J Respir Crit Care Med 2004;170(8):836–44.

32. Global Initiative for Asthma (GINA). Global strategy for asthma management and prevention: NHLBI/WHO Workshop Report: Bethesda, MD: National Heart Lung Blood Institute, 02-3659, 2002.

33. National Asthma Education and Prevention Program: Expert panel report III: Guidelines for the diagnosis and management of asthma. Bethesda, MD: 08-4051, 2007.

34. Jensen ME, Collins CE, Gibson PG, Wood LG. The obesity phenotype in children with asthma. Paediatr Respir Rev 2011;12:152–59.

35. Sadof M, Kaslovsky R. Adolescent asthma: A developmental approach. Curr Opin Pediatr 2011;23:373–78.

36. Arellano FM, Arana A, Wentworth CE, Vidaurre CF, Chipps BE. Prescription patterns for asthma medications in children and adolescents with health care insurance in the United States. Pediatr Allergy Immunol 2011;22:469–76.

37. Panontin E, Longo G. Treatment of mild persistent asthma in children. Lancet 2011;377:1743–44.

38. Ducharme FM, Lasserson TJ, Cates CJ. Addition to inhaled corticosteroids of long-acting beta2-agonists versus anti-leukotrienes for chronic asthma. Cochrane Database Syst Rev 2011;5:CD003137.

39. Robinson PD, Van Asperen P. Update in paediatric asthma management: Where is evidence challenging current practice? J Paediatr Child Health 2011 Apr 6. [Epub ahead of print]

40. Cotton S, Luberto CM, Yi MS, Tsevat J. Complementary and alternative medicine behaviors and beliefs in urban adolescents with asthma. J Asthma 2011;48:531–38.

12 Musculoskeletal disorders and sports injuries

Cynthia L. Feucht and Dilip R. Patel

12.1 Introduction

Musculoskeletal injuries account for most sports-related injuries (1). Overuse musculoskeletal injuries account for more than half of all sport-related injuries in adolescents and young adults. Overuse injuries can result in chronic or intermittent symptoms depending on the athlete's level of activity. Acute muscle injuries (i.e., strains, contusions, and lacerations) can lead to significant structural or functional damage to the muscle (1,2,3,4,5,6,7,8,9,10,11). Delayed-onset muscle soreness (DOMS), or exercise-induced muscle damage (EIMD), is typically associated with new or unaccustomed exercise and often results from intense eccentric muscle activity; it manifests with pain, discomfort, and decreased performance 24 to 48 hours after exercise (1,4).

Nonpharmacologic approaches are often considered as first-line treatment for musculoskeletal injuries and may include relative rest, ice, compression, and elevation (3). Moderate to severe injuries to the athlete may result in several weeks of an inability to train or compete. Even after resuming the physical activity or sport, the athlete may continue to experience difficulties with muscle weakness and decreased flexibility (1). As a result, treatment is often sought to alleviate pain, restore function, and allow the athlete to resume activities more quickly. Treatment options include analgesics such as nonsteroidal anti-inflammatory drugs (NSAIDs), acetaminophen, and topical over-the-counter (OTC) preparations. These classes of drugs are reviewed in this chapter, including their mechanisms of action, side effects, and efficacy in treating pain and inflammation associated with acute and overuse musculoskeletal injuries.

Mechanism of action

Arachidonic acid is released from cellular membranes as a result of tissue injury. Arachidonic acid is broken down by cyclooxygenase (COX) enzymes to produce prostaglandins and thromboxane A2 and by lipoxygenase (LOX) enzymes to produce leukotrienes. (See chapter 17 in Greydanus DE, Patel DR, Omar HA, Feucht C, Merrick J: Adolescent Medicine – Pharmacotherapeutics in General, Mental and Sexual Health. Berlin: de Gruyter; 2012.) Prostaglandins are localized hormones that, once released within the intracellular space, can produce fever, inflammation, and pain (12). Thromboxanes are released in response to tissue injury and are responsible for producing platelet aggregation as well as clot formation and for the regulation of vascular tone (12). Pain relief and decreased inflammation occur from the blockade of COX enzymes, thereby inhibiting prostaglandin E2 and prostacyclin (PGI2) formation (12,13).

Two forms of COX enzymes are cyclooxygenase-1 (COX-1) and cyclooxygenase-2 (COX-2). COX-1 is expressed in most normal tissues and cells and is the predominant form within gastric epithelial cells (12,14). Prostaglandin production within the gastrointestinal tract protects the gastrointestinal mucosa from gastric acidity. COX-2 is expressed when tissue damage occurs; its release is induced by cytokines and inflammatory mediators during inflammation (12,14). NSAIDs are a heterogeneous class of medications that are chemically unrelated but known to have similar therapeutic effects, including antipyretic, analgesic, and anti-inflammatory activity (see chapter 13).

Prostaglandin synthesis is inhibited due to inhibition of COX-2. In addition, the primary therapeutic effect of NSAIDs is due to the inhibition of prostaglandin synthesis as well as COX-2 activity; there is also a correlation between COX-2 inhibition and anti-inflammatory activity (15). Bradykinin and cytokines (i.e., tumor necrosis factor-alpha [TNF-a] and interleukin-1 [IL-1]) are thought to be responsible for inducing pain with inflammation and releasing prostaglandins, which enhance pain sensitivity (16). Other mediators, such as neuropeptides (i.e., substance P), are also involved in inducing pain. The gastrointestinal adverse effects of NSAIDs are predominantly but not exclusively due to the inhibition of COX-1. NSAIDs are considered competitive reversible inhibitors of COX enzymes (unlike aspirin, which is considered an irreversible inhibitor of COX enzymes) and do not affect the LOX pathway (17).

12.2 Salicylated NSAIDs

Derivatives of salicylic acid include aspirin (acetylsalicylic acid), diflunisal (difluorophenyl derivative), salsalate, magnesium salicylate, and choline magnesium salicylate (▶Tabl. 12.1 and 12.2). Aspirin continues to be the most widely used drug and is the standard to which other NSAIDs are compared (18). Owing to its widespread availability, aspirin's potential for toxicity often goes underrecognized, and it continues to be a cause of fatal poisonings in children (14).

Salicylates are rapidly absorbed from the gastrointestinal tract, are widely distributed throughout the body, and are highly protein-bound (especially albumin) (16). Because of their high protein binding, salicylates may compete for binding with other compounds, including thyroxine, penicillin, phenytoin, bilirubin, uric acid, and other NSAIDs such as naproxen (14). Salicylates are metabolized in the liver and excreted by the kidneys, with free salicylate excretion dependent on urinary pH and salicylate dose (16).

Gastrointestinal adverse effects are common with salicylates and may include dyspepsia, nausea, vomiting and, more seriously, gastric ulceration, gastrointestinal hemorrhage, and erosive gastritis (14,16). Aspirin irreversibly inhibits platelet aggregation and leads to a prolongation in the bleeding time. Gastrointestinal and platelet effects are less likely to occur with nonacetylated salicylates (i.e., salsalate, magnesium salicylate, and so forth) because they cannot acetylate COX (16). Owing to aspirin's effect on platelet aggregation, it should be avoided in patients with hepatic impairment, hypoprothrombinemia, vitamin K deficiency, hemophilia, and within 1 week of a surgical procedure (14).

Salicylates have been shown to have a dose-dependent effect on uric acid excretion and in elevated doses can result in pulmonary edema, hepatotoxicity, and hyperglycemia (14). Hypersensitivity to salicylates can result in hives, flushing, bronchoconstriction, angioedema, low blood pressure, and shock (14). Hypersensitivity is thought to be due to COX inhibition, and cross-sensitivity occurs with other agents in the class as well as with nonsalicylated NSAIDs (14). Patients with asthma, nasal polyps, and sensitivity to tartrazine dyes are at an increased risk for salicylate sensitivity (20). In

Tab. 12.1: Salicylated NSAIDs (13,14,19).

Drug	Onset of action and duration of effect (hours)	Comments
Diflunisal	Onset: about 1 Duration: Analgesic: 8–12 Anti-inflammatory: ≤12	Some four to five times more potent analgesic and anti-inflammatory effects than aspirin; fewer platelet/GI side effects compared with aspirin; not metabolized to salicylic acid
Salsalate	Onset: N/A Duration: N/A	Fewer platelet and GI side effects than aspirin
Choline magnesium trisalicylate	Onset: about 2 Duration: N/A	Less effect on platelet aggregation and fewer GI side effects than aspirin; avoid or use with caution in renal insufficiency due to magnesium content
Magnesium salicylate	Onset: N/A Duration: 4–6	Available OTC; less effect on platelet aggregation and fewer GI side effects than aspirin; to be avoided or used with caution in renal insufficiency, because of magnesium content

Abbreviations: GI, gastrointestinal; N/A, no data available; OTC, over-the-counter.

Tab. 12.2: Common doses of salicylated NSAIDs (19,20).

Generic name	Trade name	Adult dose	Comments
Diflunisal		1000 mg, then 500 mg every 12 hours Age ≥12 years: same as adult	Tablet must not be crushed or chewed; maximum, 1.5 g daily
Salsalate	Amigesic	1 g three times daily	Tablet must not be crushed or chewed; urinary acidification can decrease clearance and increase risk for toxicity
Choline magnesium trisalicylate	Trilisate	500 mg–1.5 g two to three times daily	Maintenance dose: 1–4.5 g daily; available as liquid formulation; urinary acidification can decrease clearance and increase risk for toxicity
Magnesium salicylate	Doan's Extra Strength, Keygesic	Doan's (467 mg): 2 caplets every 6 hours as needed Keygesic (650 mg): 1 tablet every 4 hours as needed Age ≥12 years: same as adult	Available OTC; Doan's maximum, 8 caplets in 24 h Keygesic maximum, 4 tablets in 24 hours

general, salicylates are avoided during pregnancy, especially the third trimester, because of an increased risk for perinatal death, anemia, antepartum and postpartum hemorrhage, prolonged gestation, and premature closure of the ductus arteriosus (14).

Drug interactions can occur when salicylates displace other agents from plasma-binding proteins. Dosages of NSAIDs, sulfonylureas, and methotrexate may have to be adjusted to prevent toxicity due to displacement. NSAIDs given concurrently with corticosteroids and warfarin may increase the risk for bleeding. NSAIDs should not be given concomitantly with the following herbals owing to their anticoagulant or anti-platelet activity and increased risk for bleeding: danshen, dong quai, evening primrose, feverfew, garlic, ginger, ginkgo, red clover, horse chestnut, green tea, policosanol, and willow bark (20,21). In addition, NSAIDs decrease the effectiveness of angiotensin converting enzyme (ACE) inhibitors because of the blockade of renal prostaglandin production.

Salicylates have fallen out of favor for use in adolescents and young adults because of their association with Reye's syndrome, which is characterized by toxic hepatitis and has been associated with encephalopathy, prolonged prothrombin time, fatty infiltration of the liver, and intracranial hypertension in advanced stages (22). Aspirin and other salicylates are contraindicated in children and young adults younger than 20 years who have a fever associated with a viral illness (14).

12.3 Nonsalicylated NSAIDs

Various classes of nonsalicylated NSAIDs (▶Tabs. 12.3 and 12.4) are among the most widely used drugs, with yearly sales in the United States for OTC drugs estimated at $30 billion (13,23). Nonsalicylated NSAIDs are considered effective for mild to moderate pain and have been used for a variety of musculoskeletal disorders including osteoarthritis, rheumatoid arthritis (see chapter 13), and sports-related injuries. The choice of a particular nonsalicylated NSAID depends on its onset of action, tolerability, cost, and insurance coverage. An agent with a short onset of action, minimal adverse effects, low cost, and wide acceptability would make for an ideal nonsalicylated NSAID.

As a class, nonsalicylated NSAIDs are usually well absorbed and highly bound to plasma proteins; they are excreted via either glomerular filtration or tubular secretion (14). These agents accumulate at sites of inflammation and most exhibit nonselectivity for COX-1 and COX-2 enzymes. The last decade has seen the emergence of COX-2 selective inhibitors designed to minimize gastrointestinal effects that occur due to COX-1 inhibition. Other older nonsalicylated NSAIDs have also been found to have COX-2 selectivity similar to the currently available celecoxib, based on whole blood assays (14). Most studies on nonsalicylated NSAIDs are done in adults; however, some findings are of relevance to the adolescent age group.

12.3.1 Side effects of nonsalicylated NSAIDs

Gastrointestinal

Gastrointestinal adverse effects are common with nonsalicylated NSAIDs and are often the leading reason for their discontinuation. The gastrointestinal toxicity is often dose

Tab. 12.3: Nonsalicylated NSAIDs (13,14,19).

Drug	Onset of action and duration of effect	Comments
Propionic acids		
Fenoprofen	Onset: about 72 hours Duration: 4–6 hours	Some 15% of patients will have side effects but few stop therapy.
Flurbiprofen	Onset: about 1–2 hours Duration: variable	Strong inhibitor of CYP 450 2C9 isoenzyme; substrate CYP 2C9 (minor).
Ibuprofen	Onset: Analgesic: 0.5–1 hours Anti-inflammatory: ≤7 days Duration: 4–6 hours	Strong inhibitor of CYP 450 2C9 isoenzyme; substrate CYP 2C9 and 2C19 (minor); equal efficacy to aspirin; some 10%–15% of patients stop therapy because of to side effects.
Ketoprofen	Onset: 0.5 hours Duration: 6 hours	Some 30% of patients develop side effects, with GI as the most common.
Naproxen	Onset: Analgesic: 1 hour Anti-inflammatory: 2 weeks Duration: Analgesic: ≤7 hours Anti-inflammatory: ≤12 hours	Available as OTC product; more potent than aspirin in vitro, likely better tolerated than aspirin; may provide cardioprotection for some individuals with heart disease.
Oxaprozin	Onset: ~0.5–4 hours Duration: variable	Slower onset of effects compared with others; longer half-life allows for once-a-day dosing.
Acetic acids		
Diclofenac	Onset: 1–4.5 hours Duration: 12–24 hours	More potent than aspirin; side effects experienced by some 20% and 2% stop therapy; about 15% of patients will experience an increase in liver function tests; available as topical patch and gel as well as in combination with misoprostol.
Etodolac	Onset: Analgesic: 2–4 hours Anti-inflammatory: several days Duration: N/A	In vitro COX-2 selectivity; 100 mg of etodolac provides similar efficacy to aspirin 650 mg but may have fewer side effects.
Sulindac	Onset: N/A Duration: N/A	Similar efficacy to aspirin; active metabolite; side effects experienced by about 20% (GI) and 10% (CNS).
Tolmetin	Onset: Analgesic: 1–2 hours Anti-inflammatory: days to weeks Duration: variable	Similar efficacy to aspirin; side effects experienced by about 25%–40% and 5%–10% stop therapy.

(Continued)

Tab. 12.3: Nonsalicylated NSAIDs (13,14,19). (*Continued*)

Drug	Onset of action and duration of effect	Comments
Indomethacin	Onset: ~0.5 hours Duration: 4–6 hours	Compared with aspirin 10–40 times more potent; incidence of side effects 3%–50%; some 20% of patients stop therapy owing to side effects.
Ketorolac	Onset: Analgesic: about 10 min (IM) Duration: Analgesic: 6–8 hours	Maximum duration of 5 days (oral and parenteral); strong analgesic activity but weak anti-inflammatory activity; may be given parenterally for acute pain.
Oxicams		
Meloxicam	Onset: N/A Duration: N/A	CYP 450 inhibitor of isoenzyme 2C9 (weak); substrate CYP 2CP and 3A4 (minor); some COX-2 selective action at lower end of dosing range.
Piroxicam	Onset: about 1 hour Duration: variable	Equal efficacy to aspirin; may be better tolerated than aspirin; some 20% of patients will experience side effects and 5% will stop therapy.
Naphthylalkanone		
Nabumetone	Onset: about 72 hours Duration: variable	Prodrug; some COX-2 selectivity; has less GI toxicity than most NSAIDs.
Fenemate		
Meclofenamate	Onset: <1 hour Duration: ≤6 hours	Equal efficacy to aspirin; ~25% of patients will experience gastrointestinal adverse events.
Mefenamic acid	Onset: N/A Duration: ≤6 hours	CYP 450 inhibitor of isoenzyme 2C9 (strong); substrate CYP 2C9 (minor).
COX-2 inhibitor		
Celecoxib	Onset: Analgesic: about 0.75 hours to several months Duration: about 4–8 hours	CYP 450 inhibitor of isoenzymes 2C8 (moderate) and 2D6 (weak); substate CYP 2C9 (major) and 3A4 (minor); does not inhibit platelet aggregation.

dependent and associated with chronic use (14). Dyspeptic symptoms are frequently experienced by patients and may include anorexia, epigastric pain, nausea, bloating, and heartburn. These symptoms have been associated with both selective and nonselective nonsalicylated NSAIDs (13,24). Gastrointestinal toxicity may be related to prostaglandin inhibition, which is important for enhancing mucosal blood flow, mucus and bicarbonate production, and inhibition of acid production. Nonsalicylated NSAIDs also may contribute to gastrointestinal toxicity from local irritation to the gastric mucosa.

More serious complications include gastric and duodenal ulcers, which may occur in up to 15 to 30 percent of regular nonsalicylated NSAID users (25,26). Complications

Tab. 12.4: Common doses of nonsalicylated NSAIDs (19,20).

Generic name	Trade name	Adult dose	Comments
Propionic acids			
Fenoprofen	Naflon	200 mg every 4–6 hours as needed	Maximum, 3.2 g/day; tablets must not be crushed.
Flurbiprofen	Ocufen	50–100 mg 2–3 times daily	Maximum, 300 mg/day; maximum single dose 100 mg; tablets must not be crushed.
Ibuprofen	Motrin Advil	200–400 mg every 4–6 hours Maximum: 3.2 g/day	Available OTC as tablets (regular and chewable), capsules, suspension, and infant drops; chewable tablets may contain phenylalanine.
Ketoprofen	Oruvail	25–50 mg every 6–8 hours as needed	Extended-release formulation is not recommended for acute pain; maximum (immediate release), 300 mg/day; maximum (extended release), 200 mg/day.
Naproxen sodium	Aleve Anaprox Anaprox DS	500 mg initially, then 250 mg every 6–8 hours as needed OTC label: 200 mg every 8–12 hours as needed	Available OTC; dosage recommendations expressed as naproxen base; maximum (adult), 1250 mg/day (naproxen base); OTC formulation not indicated for age <12 years.
Naproxen	Naprosyn Naprelan	500 mg initially, then 250 mg every 6–8 hours as needed	Available as immediate-release, extended-release, and suspension; extended release not recommended for acute pain; extended-release formulation must not be broken, crushed, or chewed; maximum (adult): 1,250 mg/day.
Oxaprozin	Daypro	600–1,200 mg daily	Patients with low body weight should start with 600 mg daily; tablets must not be crushed.
Acetic acids			
Diclofenac	Voltaren	50 mg three times daily	Available as immediate, extended-release formulation and powder for solution; tablets must not be crushed.; powder is mixed in 30–60 mL of water and taken immediately; maximum, 200 mg daily.
Diclofenac patch	Flector patch	Apply one patch twice daily	Patch is applied to most painful area of intact skin; hands washed after applying and after removal; edges of patch may be taped if peeling occurs; not to be worn while sunbathing;

(*Continued*)

Tab. 12.4: Common doses of nonsalicylated NSAIDs (19,20). (*Continued*)

Generic name	Trade name	Adult dose	Comments
			used patches should be folded before disposal.
Etodolac	Lodine	200–400 mg every 6–8 hours	Maximum: 1,000 mg daily (immediate-release) and 1,200 mg daily (extended-release formulation; tablets must not be crushed or capsules broken.
Sulindac	Clinoril	150–200 mg twice daily	Maximum, 400 mg daily
Tolmetin	Tolectin	400 mg three times daily	Maximum: 1,800 mg daily; taking with food decreases bioavailability; do not crush tablets or break capsules
Indomethacin	Indocin	25–50 mg 2–three times daily Age ≥15 years; same as adult	Available as immediate- and extended-release capsules and suspension; maximum (adult): 200 mg/d (immediate-release) and 150 mg/day (extended-release); capsules must not be crushed, broken, or chewed.
Ketorolac	Toradol	20 mg, then 10 mg every 4–6 hours as needed <50 kg: 10 mg, then 10 mg every 4–6 hours as needed	Not to exceed 5 days in duration (injection and oral combined); maximum, 40 mg daily; oral dosing intended to be a continuation of IM/IV therapy; not indicated for minor or chronic pain conditions.
Oxicams			
Meloxicam	Mobic	7.5–15 mg once daily	Available as oral suspension.
Piroxicam	Feldene	10–20 mg once daily	Maximum: 20 mg/day; capsules must not be broken
Naphthylalkanone			
Nabumetone	Relafen	1,000 mg/day daily in one or two divided doses	Maximum, 2 g/day; tablets must not be crushed.
Fenamate			
Meclofenamate		50–100 mg every 4–6 hours as needed Age >14 years: same as adult	Maximum: 400 mg/day.
Mefenamic acid	Ponstel	500 mg, then 250 mg every 4 hours as needed	Maximum duration, usually 1 week.

(*Continued*)

Tab. 12.4: Common doses of nonsalicylated NSAIDs (19,20). (*Continued*)

Generic name	Trade name	Adult dose	Comments
		Age >14 years: same as adult	
COX-2 inhibitor			
Celecoxib	Celebrex	200 mg twice daily as needed	Contents of capsule may be sprinkled onto applesauce for administration; poor metabolizers of CYP 2C9 start at half the recommended dose.

from ulcers include bleeding, perforation, and obstruction. Patients may present with a serious gastrointestinal event but have had no symptoms before presentation (13). Factors that may increase the risk for gastrointestinal complications include the presence of *Helicobacter pylori* (see chapter 8 in Greydanus DE, Patel DR, Omar HA, Feucht C, Merrick J: Adolescent Medicine – Pharmacotherapeutics in General, Mental and Sexual Health. Berlin: de Gruyter; 2012), advanced age, concomitant use of aspirin, anticoagulants (see chapters 6 and 10), or corticosteroids (see chapter 13), and duration of NSAID use (greatest within the first month) (13,27). Lifestyle factors such as smoking and alcohol use also contribute to an increased risk for side effects, but are not independent risk factors (13,27). For those patients at risk, a proton pump inhibitor (PPI) has been shown to be effective at reducing the frequency and severity of upper gastrointestinal symptoms (13,28).

COX-2 inhibitors were developed with the aim of reducing gastrointestinal complications associated with nonselective nonsalicylated NSAIDs. COX-2 inhibitors do not inhibit the COX-1 enzyme, which is responsible for prostaglandin production in the gastrointestinal mucosa; therefore they should pose less risk for gastrointestinal toxicity. The benefit of COX-2 inhibitors with regard to less gastrointestinal toxicity remains controversial. In patients with gastrointestinal disease or risk factors for gastrointestinal complications, risk versus benefit should be assessed. If nonsalicylated NSAIDs are used, the lowest dose for the shortest time period should be considered (25,26, 27,28,29).

Hepatotoxicity

Hepatotoxicity from NSAID use appears to be rare, with estimates between 3 and 23 cases per 10,000 patient-years (30,31). Two older agents (benoxaprofen and bromfenac) have been withdrawn in the United States owing to reports of serious hepatotoxicity (13). Rostom and colleagues (32), in a systematic review, found the rate of hospitalization due to nonsalicylated NSAID-related hepatotoxicity to be 2.7 per 100,000 patients and the rate of death to be 1.9 per 100,000 patients.

A recent case report by Bennett and colleagues details a 16-year-old who was previously healthy and found to be taking ibuprofen for 6 weeks before presentation (30). The first 2 weeks of ibuprofen use involved scheduled dosing and there was sporadic use over the subsequent 4 weeks. The adolescent presented with dark-colored urine, jaundice, and pruritus. Laboratory results were significant for an elevated bilirubin and minimal elevation in liver enzymes (30). The results of a liver biopsy revealed intrahepatic and canalicular cholestasis and histology was suggestive of drug-induced hepatotoxicity (30). Over the following 4 months, the patient's symptoms resolved and laboratory values returned to normal.

Liver dysfunction related to nonsalicylated NSAIDs is rare in otherwise healthy adolescents but should be considered in a patient with recent nonsalicylated NSAID use who presents with cholestasis (30). Thorough medication histories are important in determining the cause and effect in such situations. Despite the potential for hepatotoxicity, current data do not support routine monitoring of liver enzymes in individuals receiving nonsalicylated NSAIDs.

Renal toxicity

Renal insufficiency is well known with nonsalicylated NSAID use and is likely the result of inhibition of renal prostaglandins. Renal insufficiency is estimated to occur in approximately 1 to 5 percent of patients and is usually reversible on discontinuation of the NSAID (13,33). Renal prostaglandins serve an important role in maintaining renal circulation, including vasodilation, renin secretion, and sodium as well as water excretion (13). The disruption in balance between vasoconstriction and vasodilation within the kidneys may predispose a patient to renal failure. Those at the greatest risk for renal toxicity associated with nonsalicylated NSAIDs include patients with heart failure, cirrhosis, chronic kidney disease, and hypovolemic states (13,14) (see chapter 15). Renal toxicity is characterized by elevated serum creatinine, sodium and water retention, hyperkalemia, proteinuria, interstitial nephritis, papillary necrosis, acute renal failure, acute glomerulitis, vasculitis, acute tubular necrosis, and papillary necrosis (13,34,35). In patients at risk for renal toxicity, the risk versus benefit in using a nonsalicylated NSAID should be carefully considered and, if at all possible, NSAIDs, including COX-2 inhibitors, avoided.

There have been several case reports of renal toxicity in adolescents with nonsalicylated NSAID use. Nakahura and colleagues (36) discuss five adolescents (13–19 years old) who developed renal toxicity with the use of nonsalicylated NSAIDs. The first case was a 16-year-old girl who took ibuprofen intermittently over 9 months. Kidney biopsy results were consistent with interstitial nephritis and the patient was treated with corticosteroids. At 1 year she was asymptomatic with a decrease in serum creatinine; however, 2 years later her serum creatinine had risen and results of a repeat kidney biopsy revealed chronic interstitial fibrosis (36). Case 3 in this report describes a 15-year-old girl who used ibuprofen every other day for 6 months. The patient was found to have proteinuria, and results of renal ultrasonography were reported normal. The patient discontinued the nonsalicylated NSAID and was asymptomatic after 1 month (36). The other three cases describe adolescents who used naprosyn (1 week before hospitalization), ibuprofen (daily use for several weeks), and ketorolac (intermittently for 4 months), who all developed an increase in serum creatinine and were found to have urine eosinophilia indicative of nonsalicylated NSAID-associated nephrotoxicity (36). In two of the cases the nephrotoxicity resolved, and the other case showed resolution of symptoms at 1 month but continued elevation in serum creatinine.

These case reports illustrate that nonsalicylated NSAID nephrotoxicity can occur in healthy adolescents. Given the fact that several nonsalicylated NSAIDs are available as

OTC preparations, adolescents should be aware of their potential adverse effects. It is important to use the lowest dose of the nonsalicylated NSAID for the shortest time period necessary and to maintain adequate hydration while on nonsalicylated NSAIDs.

Cardiovascular toxicity

Cardiovascular toxicity related to nonsalicylated NSAID use is generally not of concern in otherwise healthy adolescents. Cardiovascular toxicity came to light with the emergence of the selective COX-2 inhibitors. It has been theorized that the disruption in the balance between prostacyclin and thromboxane formation by selective COX-2 inhibitors may increase this risk. The selective COX-2 inhibitors, via their inhibition of prostacyclin formation, favor increased thromboxane formation and subsequent platelet aggregation.

Current data suggest that selective nonsalicylated NSAIDs may increase cardiovascular risk, but data are conflicting (25,37,38,39). Heterogeneity of the studies – including patient selection, duration of study, agents used, study design, and cardiovascular risk at baseline – makes it challenging to summarize the cardiovascular risks associated with nonsalicylated NSAIDs. Rofecoxib was voluntarily withdrawn from the U.S. market in September 2004, and the U.S. Food and Drug Administration (FDA) requested Pfizer to voluntarily remove valdecoxib from the market in April 2005 because of cardiovascular risks (40). In addition, in 2005 the FDA requested the makers of prescription and OTC nonsalicylated NSAIDs to include a boxed warning highlighting the increased risk for cardiovascular events as well as gastrointestinal toxicity, including the risk for life-threatening gastrointestinal bleeding (40).

12.3.2 Drug interactions

Drug interactions are similar to those already described for salicylated NSAIDs as well as the following additional drug interactions. Nonselective nonsalicylated NSAIDs may decrease the effectiveness of aspirin if given concomitantly owing to blockade of the platelet COX-1 site (14). It is recommended that the nonsalicylated NSAIDs be given at least 2 hours after the dose of aspirin to achieve irreversible platelet inhibition by aspirin (13). Nonsalicylated NSAIDs may also decrease the effectiveness of thiazide and loop diuretics through blockade of renal prostaglandins (19).

In addition, nonsalicylated NSAIDs can reduce renal clearance of lithium, resulting in elevated lithium plasma levels, and the efficacy of nonsalicylated NSAIDs can be reduced with cholestyramine and colestipol owing to blockade of absorption (19). Drug interactions can occur with mefenamic acid, celecoxib, meloxicam, ibuprofen, and flurbiprofen because of their metabolism via cytochrome P450 isoenzymes. With a wide variety of drug interactions, each patient's medication profile should be reviewed – including prescription, OTC, and herbal products – to evaluate for drug-drug interactions before initiating an nonsalicylated NSAID.

12.3.3 Efficacy of NSAIDs in musculoskeletal injuries

NSAIDs have been purported to help in decreasing pain and inflammation, restore musculoskeletal function, decrease time to healing, and allow faster return to previous activity level. The benefit of using NSAIDs in the prevention of myositis ossificans traumatica following deep muscle contusions remains controversial. Concern has been raised that by inhibiting the inflammatory response, NSAIDs may slow phagocytic function and time for muscle regeneration and healing. Animal studies have been conflicting as to the effects of NSAIDs in the musculoskeletal model. Human studies have not always shown a consistent benefit of NSAIDs in treating musculoskeletal injuries. Studies have been limited at times by small sample sizes, the lack of placebo groups, subjective assessment, differing patient populations, and lack of control for confounding factors.

A recent review by Mehallo and colleagues summarized data regarding use of NSAIDs for acute ligament and muscle injuries (3). Rat models for ligament sprains have shown that piroxicam strengthens the medial collateral ligament of the knee at 14 days versus celecoxib, which was found to weaken the medial collateral ligament at 14 days compared with placebo. Other animal studies have not found any benefit with selective and nonselective NSAIDs versus placebo (3). Human studies have provided evidence for a more consistent benefit of NSAIDs in ligament sprains. A variety of NSAIDs have been shown to decrease pain and inflammation associated with acute ankle sprains (3). Several studies have documented the efficacy of NSAIDs in decreasing pain, increasing functional ability, and allowing for a more rapid return to training (3).

Although NSAIDs have been shown to be effective for treating the pain associated with injured ligaments, their efficacy in improving joint stability remains unknown (3). In two animal model studies, piroxicam was shown to improve contractile force and greater maximal failure force early postinjury, but it also slowed deposition of collagen and regeneration of muscle tissue (3). Studies examining NSAIDs in human muscle strains are limited. One trial evaluated meclofenamate and diclofenac versus placebo along with physiotherapy in treating acute hamstring injuries and found no differences among the groups with respect to pain, swelling, and isokinetic muscle performance (3).

Howatson and van Someren reviewed the use of NSAIDs in the treatment and prevention of DOMS (5). In one study, ketoprofen used prophylactically was found to decrease muscle soreness and enhance muscle function, whereas another study evaluated ibuprofen before and after exercise and demonstrated a decrease in muscle damage. In contrast, a study evaluated ibuprofen 45 minutes before downhill running and scheduled dosing for 3 days after the activity and found no effect on muscle soreness or strength (5). Additional studies with oxaprozin and ibuprofen with acetaminophen postexercise failed to provide benefit (5). NSAIDs were found to attenuate loss of muscle strength and muscle soreness postexercise in two studies, whereas another study failed to provide evidence of benefit compared with placebo after elbow flexor eccentric muscle injury (3). Conflicting evidence to support the use of NSAIDs in DOMS may be the result of differences in study methodology, patient selection, and study limitations. NSAIDs may provide benefit in decreasing muscle soreness and improving short-term muscle recovery (3,41). Given the potential ability of NSAIDs to impair muscle healing, risk versus benefit should be considered and, if NSAIDs are used, a short course of 3 to 7 days should be considered (3).

Topical NSAIDs

In addition to oral NSAIDs, topical formulations of NSAIDs have been used for treating musculoskeletal injuries. A systematic review conducted by Moore and colleagues (42) evaluated 37 placebo-controlled trials of topical NSAIDs in the treatment of acute soft tissue injury, sprains, strains, or trauma. Twenty-seven of the trials demonstrated a significant benefit of the topical NSAID over placebo (42). The pooled relative benefit for all trials was 1.7 (95% confidence interval [CI]: 1.5–1.9) (42). For topical NSAIDs evaluated in three or more studies, pooling of data for the individual agents showed ketoprofen, felbinac, ibuprofen, and piroxicam to be superior to placebo (42). Local skin reactions were reported in 3 percent or fewer, systemic adverse effects in less than 1 percent, and discontinuation due to adverse effects in 0.6 percent or less, with no significant difference noted between active treatment and placebo groups (42). The authors note that owing to the small sample size of most of the trials, publication bias may have influenced the results of the systematic review.

Diclofenac gel and topical patch were the first topical NSAIDs approved in 2007 in the United States by the FDA. Diclofenac gel (Voltaren gel) is currently approved for treatment of osteoarthritis and diclofenac topical patch (Flector patch) for the treatment of acute minor sprains, strains, and contusions (20). When applied to the skin, diclofenac accumulates under the application site, leading to a tissue reservoir for localized effects (43). With its topical application, systemic plasma concentrations are in the range of 1 to 3 ng/mL and relative systemic bioavailability compared with oral administration is approximately 1 percent (13). The diclofenac patch is relatively safe, with skin reactions as the most common adverse event (43). Thus the risk for systemic adverse effects is minimal owing to low plasma concentrations.

A randomized double-blind placebo-controlled trial using topical diclofenac in ankle sprains found it to provide a greater reduction in pain on rest and movement from day 2 and faster joint swelling reduction from day 3 (44). Five percent of the patients in the placebo group discontinued treatment owing to lack of efficacy, compared with none in the topical diclofenac group (44). Another randomized double-blind placebo-controlled study compared topical diclofenac to placebo in patients with traumatic blunt soft tissue injury (44). Tenderness at the center of the injured area was produced by pressure applied from calibrated calipers. The primary endpoint was the area under the curve (AUC) for tenderness over the first 3 days of treatment (44). The patch was found to be significantly more effective than placebo for the primary endpoint ($P < 0.0001$) (44). Topical diclofenac also produced a greater pain intensity reduction at rest and with activity (44). There were no significant differences between the groups with respect to adverse events, and topical diclofenac was well tolerated (44). Additional single-blinded or nonrandomized trials have assessed the topical diclofenac patch in acute injuries and have found it to be superior to placebo in relieving pain (44).

Studies support the use of topical diclofenac in alleviating pain related to acute injuries, but its ability to improve muscle recovery and allow participants to return to activity more quickly remains to be appropriately evaluated. Topical diclofenac, because of its low systemic bioavailability, may be beneficial in those patients who are at risk for gastrointestinal or cardiovascular toxicity from oral NSAIDs.

Acetaminophen

Acetaminophen (Tylenol) was initially used in 1893 but did not gain wide acceptance until 1949 (14). Acetaminophen is the active metabolite of phenacetin, which was widely used until the 1980s, when it was withdrawn from the market owing to its association with analgesic-abuse nephropathy and hemolytic anemia (14). Acetaminophen, along with NSAIDs, has largely replaced aspirin as the analgesic of choice in children, adolescents, and young adults because of aspirin's association with Reye's syndrome. Acetaminophen is known to have analgesic and antipyretic activity similar to aspirin; however, acetaminophen has poor anti-inflammatory effects. At typical doses of 1,000 mg, acetaminophen has been shown in whole blood assays of healthy volunteers to inhibit only approximately 50 percent of COX-1 and COX-2 enzymes (14).

Acetaminophen has good bioavailability and is evenly distributed throughout most body fluids (14). Protein binding of acetaminophen is variable, and it undergoes extensive hepatic metabolism with glucuronidation and sulfation to form inactive metabolites that are excreted by the kidneys (14). A small percentage (about 5%–15%) of acetaminophen is metabolized to N-acetyl-p-benzoquinoneimine (NAPQI), which normally reacts with glutathione sulfhydryl groups, is further metabolized, and is then excreted (45). When excessive amounts of acetaminophen are consumed, conjugation pathways become saturated and larger amounts of acetaminophen are converted to NAPQI (14,45). With the shift to NAPQI, glutathione stores become depleted and the excessive NAPQI can lead to hepatotoxicity (14,45).

Acetaminophen has mild to moderate analgesic properties as well as antipyretic activity. It has been used for a wide variety of indications, including fever and pain associated with many different conditions (45). Contributing to acetaminophen's widespread use is its easy tolerability. Unlike NSAIDs, acetaminophen does not affect platelet function or uric acid levels, nor is it associated with significant gastrointestinal toxicity (45). Acetaminophen is felt to be safe in patients with peptic ulcer disease and aspirin hypersensitivity, but it is not a reasonable alternative to NSAIDs in patients with inflammatory conditions such as rheumatoid arthritis (14). Side effects that have been reported, albeit infrequently, include rash, hypersensitivity reactions, blood dyscrasias, and renal toxicity (45).

The most serious adverse event that may occur with acetaminophen is the risk for hepatotoxicity occurring with overdose. The maximum adult dose of acetaminophen is 4,000 mg/day and, for those with chronic alcohol use, 2,000 mg/day (▶Tab. 12.5) (14). Because of the vast number of preparations that contain acetaminophen, including prescription and OTC agents, accidental overdose can occur owing to the consumption of multiple products (i.e., prescription analgesic agents as well as OTC cough and cold preparations). Whether accidental or intentional, acetaminophen overdose is a medical emergency (14). Overdose can occur with single doses of 10 to 15 g, and doses of 20 to 25 g can be lethal (14). Acetaminophen toxicity is divided into four stages.

The first stage can occur within several hours of acute ingestion; is typically associated with nausea, vomiting, and stomach pain; and may resolve within 24 hours (14,45). The second stage can start approximately 12 to 36 hours after acute ingestion and is significant for right-upper-quadrant pain and elevated liver enzymes (45). Stage 3 occurs 72 to 96 hours after ingestion of toxic doses; hepatomegaly, jaundice, and

Tab. 12.5: Acetaminophen formulations and dosing (20).

Formulation	Regular: 80 mg, 160 mg, 325 mg
	Extra strength: 500 mg
	Extended release: 650 mg
	Liquid: 80 mg/0.8 mg, 160 mg/5 mL, 500 mg/15 mL
	Rectal suppository: 80 mg, 120 mg, 325 mg, 650 mg
Dosage (adult and adolescent)	325–650 mg every 4–6 hours as needed
	1000 mg three or four times daily
	Not to exceed 4 g/day
Comments	80 mg and 160 mg available in chewable, oral and disintegrating form as well as "meltaways"
	Shake suspension well before dispensing
	Avoid chronic use in hepatic impairment
	Chewable tablets may contain phenylalanine
	Avoid or limit alcohol to three drinks per day
	Avoid other products with acetaminophen

coagulopathy may be present (14,45). Liver enzyme levels peak during this time period and renal failure can be present. The onset of encephalopathy or worsening coagulopathy after this time period indicates a poor prognosis (14). Stage 4 is the recovery period for those who make it past stage 3 (45). Acetaminophen overdose is best managed when early diagnosis and treatment can occur. It has been estimated that about 10 percent of those who do not receive proper treatment will develop severe hepatic impairment, and 10 to 20 percent of those may eventually die from liver failure (14,45).

Several studies have evaluated acetaminophen and compared it with an NSAID for treating pain. A study by Dalton and Schweinle (46) compared acetaminophen extended release to ibuprofen in 260 patients who presented with grade I or II lateral ankle sprains. At the end of the study, acetaminophen was found to be not inferior to ibuprofen; 78 to 80 percent of patients had resumed normal activities, and mean time to resumption was approximately 4 days in both groups (46).

A study by Woo and colleagues (47) recruited 300 patients who presented to an emergency room with an isolated painful limb injury. Patients were randomized to a 3-day course of acetaminophen, indomethacin, diclofenac, or acetaminophen and diclofenac. Pain reduction was seen in all treatment arms, with score reductions not found to be clinically or statistically significant among the four groups over the course of the 3 days (47). The combination therapy group had the greatest reduction in pain scores at each time point but also produced more side effects, including abdominal pain (47). Although the literature is not as extensive as for NSAIDs regarding the use of acetaminophen for treating musculoskeletal injuries, there is evidence to support its use.

Topical nonprescription analgesics

Nonprescription, or OTC, analgesic agents and external counterirritants are widely used in the United States, with more than $2 billion spent on them each year (48). Because of the easy access without a prescription, OTC topical analgesics are often first used in treating acute injuries before scheduling a visit to the physician. Topical analgesics can have one of several different properties; those with counterirritant effects are indicated for the acute treatment of minor aches and pains. Counterirritants exert their effect by producing a less intense pain than the pain the individual is experiencing (48).

The perception of another sensation distracts the person from the original pain produced by the injury. Counterirritants can fall into one of four categories based on their mechanism: (a) acting as rubefacients, (b) producing a cooling sensation, (c) producing vasodilation, and (d) causing irritation without rubefaction (48). A classification of topical analgesics with counterirritant properties is outlined in ▶Tab. 12.6. The FDA has approved these agents for use in treating minor aches and pain for both adults and children 2 years or older (48). Counterirritants from different categories are often combined in various preparations to enhance the efficacy of the product.

Methyl salicylate

Methyl salicylate is a commonly used rubefacient that is available naturally in wintergreen oil, or it can be produced by esterification of salicylic acid with methyl alcohol (48). Methyl salicylate is thought to exert its effect by producing a local vasodilation, and the counterirritant effect results from the local increase in skin temperature (48). Most of the effects of methyl salicylate are locally mediated; however, systemic absorption can increase with the use of multiple applications, and use with local application of heat and occlusive dressings (48). The most common adverse effects are skin irritation and rash, but more severe skin reactions along with systemic toxicity can occur (48).

The use of heating pads should be avoided while using topical methyl salicylate because tissue and muscle necrosis along with interstitial nephritis have been reported when topical methyl salicylate and menthol were used (49). Methyl salicylate should be avoided in children and in individuals with aspirin sensitivity and asthma, due to the risk for systemic absorption (48). Drug interactions with warfarin have been reported with typical and high-dose topical methyl salicylate, resulting in an elevation of the prothrombin time/international normalized ratio (50,51).

Tab. 12.6: Classification of topical analgesics with counterirritant properties (48).

Group classification	Mechanism	Counterirritant
I	Rubefacients	Methyl salicylate Turpentine oil Ammonia water
II	Cooling sensation	Camphor Menthol
III	Vasodilation	Histamine dihydrochloride Methyl nicotinate
IV	Irritation without rubefaction	Capsaicin Capsicum oleoresina*

*Capsaicin is the major ingredient in capsicum oleoresin.

Camphor

Most camphor is synthetically produced and exerts a counterirritant effect via a cooling sensation. Camphor stimulates skin nerve endings producing mild pain, which allows for a masking of the deeper-seated pain (48). The major toxicity associated with camphor is tonic-clonic seizures. The risk for toxicity correlates with the amount and extent of the camphor ingested (48). In addition to seizures, high doses have also been associated with nausea, vomiting, dizziness, delirium, coma, and death (48). Concentrations of camphor oil at 20 percent and as little as 5 mL can be lethal when ingested by children (48). As a result, in 1982 the FDA ruled that camphorated oil products could no longer be produced and products containing camphor must have concentrations less than 11 percent to be considered safe for nonprescription use (52). Unfortunately pediatric cases of toxicity from acute ingestions have continued to be reported with OTC preparations containing camphor (48,52,53).

Menthol

Menthol, prepared synthetically or derived from peppermint oil, is another counterirritant when used at concentrations greater than 1.25 percent (48). Menthol exerts its cooling effect by activating the transient receptor potential, TRPM8, in sensory neurons (54). Menthol has also been associated with an increase in local blood flow at the application site, resulting in a warm sensation (54). Menthol has been associated with a low incidence of hypersensitivity reactions including itching, erythema, and skin lesions; postmarketing data indicate minimal toxicity (54).

Capsaicin

Capsaicin, which is derived from hot chili peppers, produces an analgesic effect due to its direct irritant properties. Topical application of capsaicin produces a warm sensation locally due to activation of the TRP vanilloid (TRPV1); this effect decreases with repeated administration due to tachyphylaxis (55,56). Capsaicin depletes substance P (neurotransmitter for pain communication) from unmyelinated type C sensory neurons, which can produce an initial burning or itching sensation (57). Blockade of further synthesis of substance P with repeated application leads to persistent desensitization (57). The burning sensation diminishes with repeated use but can lead to an increase in nonadherence and discontinuation of its use.

Topical capsaicin has been recommended for use in osteoarthritis, and pain relief is usually seen within several weeks. Capsaicin is applied routinely three or four times daily to sustain its effect. Gloves should be used to minimize contact with mucous membranes (48). As with other topical analgesics, capsaicin should not be applied to open wounds and should be discontinued if skin breakdown occurs (48). Capsaicin has not been studied in acute sports-related injuries, and the fact that its analgesic effects may not be seen for several weeks may make it less ideal for treatment.

Others

Other counterirritants not widely used include turpentine oil, histamine dihydrochloride, and ammonia water (48). The efficacy of these agents is difficult to evaluate, because they are often used in combination with other counterirritant agents. Few data exist to support the use of eucalyptus oil and trolamine salicylate; however, trolamine salicylate continues to be available in a variety of topical analgesics. Trolamine salicylate is not a counterirritant and has been shown to be systemically absorbed (48). In general trolamine salicylate 10 to 15 percent, is applied to the skin three or four times daily (48). Contraindications, precautions, and drug interactions are similar to those of salicylates. Trolamine may be beneficial for those who are unable to tolerate other counterirritants or find them unacceptable.

Counterirritants are available in a wide variety of single and combination products as nonprescription analgesic agents (▶Tab. 12.7). Counterirritants are indicated for the treatment of mild aches and pains related to acute injury and provide a useful option for self-treatment. General guidelines for the use of topical counterirritant agents are outlined in the following box.

General guidelines for the use of topical analgesics:

- Apply to affected areas of intact skin 3 to 4 times daily.
- Massage or rub gently into the affected area.
- Wash thoroughly with soap and water after application.

For patch application, clean and dry the affected areas and remove film before application.

- Consider using gloves, especially for capsaicin application.
- Capsaicin is contraindicated for those younger than 18 years.
- Follow directions for each product carefully.

12.4 Use and abuse of analgesics

OTC (over-the-counter) medications are widely available and used in the United States. It is not uncommon for individuals to self-treat for a wide variety of ailments, including acute musculoskeletal injuries. It has been estimated that 30 percent of adults have used one or more OTC medications within the past 2 days (59). Children and adolescents are also consumers of OTC medications for cough and cold, headache, fever, menstrual, and joint and muscle pain. Chambers and colleagues (59), administered a questionnaire to 651 junior high school students in Nova Scotia to evaluate the use of OTC medications, indications, and self-administration. Of those who used an OTC medication, 88 percent reported using it for muscle, joint, and back pain; acetaminophen was the most common medication used for each type of pain assessed (59). Self-administration was common, with 58 to 76 percent reporting taking medication within the past 3 months without consulting any knowledgeable professional (59).

With increasing self-administration and easy accessibility, factors that influence consumption of OTC medications have been evaluated. Van den Bulck and colleagues (60) evaluated the association between watching television and analgesic use in 2,545 Belgian students (aged 13–16 years). Using a questionnaire, the investigators found that the use of analgesics differed among school years and between gender. A significant

Tab. 12.7: Topical analgesic agents (58).

Preparation	Product	Ingredients
Menthol preparations	• ActivOn Topical Analgesic Ultra Strength Joint and Muscle • Icy Hot Extra Strength Medicated Patch • Ben Gay Ultra Strength Pain Relieving Patch • Absorbine Jr. Pain Relieving Liquid • Aspercreme Heat Pain Relieving Gel • Flexall Maximum Strength Relieving Gel	Menthol 4.127% Menthol 5% Menthol 5% Menthol 1.27% Menthol 10% Menthol 16%
Camphor preparations	JointFlex Arthritis Pain Relieving Cream	Camphor 3.1%
Capsaicin preparations	Capzasin Arthritis Pain Relief No Mess Applicator Zostrix Arthritis Pain Relief Cream Zostrix HP Arthritis Pain Relief Cream WellPatch Natural Capsaicin Pain Relief Patch	Capsaicin 0.15% Capsaicin 0.025% Capsaicin 0.075% Capsaicin 0.025%
Trolamine preparations	Aspercreme Analgesic Creme Rub Mobisyl Maximal Strength Arthritis Pain Relief Cream Sportscreme Deep Penetrating Pain Relieving Rub	Trolamine 10% Trolamine 10% Trolamine 10%
Combination preparations	• Tiger Muscle Rub • ActiveOn Topical Analgesic Ultra Strength Backache • Salonpas Pain Patch • Icy Hot Extra Strength Pain Relieving Chill Stick • Icy Hot Extra Strength Relieving Balm • Heet Pain Relieving Formula – Freeze It Advanced Therapy Pain Relief, Roll On	Methyl salicylate 15% Menthol 5% Camphor 3% Histamine dihydrochloride 0.025% Menthol 4.127% Camphor 3.15% Camphor 1.12% Menthol 5.7% Methyl salicylate 6.3% Methyl salicylate 30% Menthol 10% Methyl salicylate 29% Menthol 7.6% Camphor 3.6% Methyl salicylate 18% Oleoresin capsicum 0.25% Camphor 0.2% Menthol 3.5%

correlation was found between regular OTC analgesic use (at least monthly) and viewing of television (odds ratio [OR] 1.16, 95% CI: 1.08–1.24) (60). Playing video games and Internet use was not significantly associated with analgesic use. The authors note that this study did not evaluate the extent to which adolescents were exposed to advertisements during television viewing (60).

Self-administration of medications by children and adolescents can be influenced by multiple factors and is potentially dangerous. Huott and Storrow (61) surveyed 203 adolescents aged 13 to 18 years who presented to an emergency room or acute care clinic. The adolescents completed a 1-page survey assessing their knowledge of OTC medication toxicity. An informal survey of the investigators' colleagues and standard texts served as the reference point regarding medication toxicity (61). Survey results of the adolescents indicated that 63 percent considered aspirin, 57 percent acetaminophen, 24 percent iron, 22 percent camphor, and 17 to 21 percent methyl salicylate to be nonlethal, which was contradictory to the faculty's viewpoint (61). The results of this study emphasize that education regarding the toxicity of OTC medications needs further emphasis.

Although analgesic use is common among adolescents in general, the pattern of their use among student athletes in particular has not been clearly elucidated. Many student athletes experience muscle aches and pains as well as sports-related injuries; thus, they may self-medicate with OTC analgesic agents including NSAIDs. Evidence indicates that many adolescents are unaware of the potential toxicity or risk for side effects associated with nonprescription analgesic medications. Warner and colleagues distributed a self-administered questionnaire to 604 high school football athletes to compare users with nonusers of NSAIDs and discern differences in attitudes regarding daily use of NSAIDs (62). The study found that 75 percent had used NSAIDs in the previous 3 months while 15 percent considered themselves daily users of NSAIDs (62). After controlling for confounding variables, those who perceived that NSAIDs enhanced performance (adjusted odds ratio [AOR] 2.4; 95% CI 1.4–4.1), those who used prophylactic NSAIDs (AOR 2.5; 95% CI 1.5–4.3), and those who self-administered NSAIDs (AOR 2.2; 95% CI 1.01–4.9) were more likely to take NSAIDs on a daily basis (62).

Often in athletes, student as well as elite, studies focus on medications of abuse rather than common prescription and nonprescription medications. Alaranta and colleagues (63) used a questionnaire to determine the frequency of prescribed medications in a group of elite athletes. In 2002, a total of 446 athletes, supported by the U.S. National Olympic Committee, completed the survey and were matched to 1,503 controls obtained from a population-based study done by the National Public Health Institute (63). Among athletes, within the previous 7 days, 34.5 percent had used a prescription medication compared with approximately 25 percent of the controls (63). NSAIDs were among the most frequently prescribed medications (8.1%) in athletes, with an AOR of 3.63 (95% CI: 2.25–5.84) for use within the preceding 7 days (63). Adverse events were reported in 20 percent of NSAID users (63).

12.5 Conclusions

The idea of "no pain, no gain" is a common misperception that should be dispelled. Muscle soreness can be expected with strenuous activity or due to an unaccustomed activity, but significant pain is the body's response that rest should occur to allow for healing (6). Too often, athletes do not take the time off from training or competition to allow for adequate healing (64). By using analgesics, in particular NSAIDs, pain may subside but further damage can result from continued exercise. Also, NSAIDs, via their inhibition of prostaglandins, may impede the healing process and muscle regeneration after an acute injury. Although these agents are relatively safe, they are not without side effects and caution is warranted. There is only limited evidence (albeit conflicting) in DOMS that NSAIDs can provide a benefit as prophylactic therapy.

Overall, analgesic agents (including NSAIDs, acetaminophen, and topical OTC agents) can effectively relieve pain associated with acute or chronic musculoskeletal injury. Data regarding the ability of NSAIDs to improve muscle recovery and allow a faster return to activity remains controversial. This area of focus has not been adequately studied with acetaminophen and topical OTC analgesics. In considering an analgesic for alleviating pain, the lowest dose for the shortest time interval should be used. Risk for side effects should be considered and compared with the benefits of the medication. Long-term use for symptoms of sport-related injuries should be avoided, especially with NSAIDs, owing to their side-effect profile and concern for the risk of impeding the healing process. Data do not adequately support the use of prophylactic NSAIDs prior to sporting events, and such use should be avoided.

Acknowledgments

Adapted with permission from Feucht CL, Patel DR. Analgesics and anti-inflammatory medications in sports: use and abuse. Pediatr Clin North Am 2010;57;(3):751–74. The authors thank Kim Douglas and Amy Esman, Kalamazoo Center for Medical Studies, for assistance in the preparation of this article.

References

1. Almekinders L. Anti-inflammatory treatment of muscular injuries in sport, an update of recent studies. Sports Med 1999;28(6):383–88.
2. Garrett WE. Muscle strain injuries: clinical and basic aspects. Med Sci Sports Exerc 1990;22:436–43.
3. Mehallo C, Drezner J, Bytomski J. Practical management: nonsteroidal anti-inflammatory drug (NSAID) use in athletic injuries. Clin J Sport Med 2006;16:170–74.
4. Micheli L. Common painful sports injuries: assessment and treatment. Clin J Pain 1989;5 (Suppl 2):S51–S60.
5. Howatson G, van Someren K. The prevention and treatment of exercise-induced muscle damage. Sports Med 2008;38(6):483–503.
6. Smith B, Collina S. Pain medications in the locker room: to dispense or not. Curr Sports Med Rep 2007;6:367–70.
7. Almekinders LC, Gilbert JA. Healing of experimental muscle strains and the effects of non-steroidal anti-inflammatory medication. Am J Sports Med 1986;14:303–8.
8. Crisco JJ, Jokl P, Heinen GT, et al. A muscle contusion injury model: biome-chanics, physiology and histology. Am J Sports Med 1994;22:702–10.
9. Tidball JG. Inflammatory cell response to acute muscle injury. Med Sci Sports Exerc 1995;27:1022-32.
10. Kuipers H. Exercise-induced muscle damage. Int J Sports Med 1994;15:132–35.
11. Jarvinen TA, Jarvinen TL, Kaariainen M, et al. Muscle injuries biology and treatment. Am J Sports Med 2005;33:745–64.
12. Maroon J, Bost J, Borden M, et al. Natural anti-inflammatory agents for pain relief in athletes. Neurosurg Focus 2006;21(4):E11.

13. Herndon C, Hutchinson R, Berdine H, et al. Management of chronic nonmalignant pain with nonsteroidal anti-inflammatory drugs. Pharmacotherapy 2008;28(6):788–805.

14. Burke A, Smyth E, FitzGerald G. Analgesic-antipyretic and anti–inflammatory agents; pharmacotherapy of gout. In: Brunton L, Lazo J, Parker K, editors. Goodman and Gilman's, the pharmacological basis of therapeutics. 11th edition. New York: McGraw-Hill; 2006. p. 671–715.

15. Vane J, Botting R. Mechanism of action of nonsteroidal anti-inflammatory drugs. Am J Med 1998;104(3A):2S-8S.

16. Furst DE, Ulrich RW, Varkey-Altamirano C. Nonsteroidal anti–inflammatory drugs, disease-modifying antirheumatic drugs, nonopioid analgesics, drugs used in gout. In: Bertram GK, Susan BM, Anthony JT, eds. Katzung's basic and clinical pharmacology, 11th ed. New York: McGraw-Hill, 2009:621–42.

17. Smyth EM, FitzGerald GA. The eicosanoids: prostaglandins, thromboxanes, leukotrienes, related compounds. In: Bertram GK, Susan BM, Anthony JT, eds. Katzung's basic and clinical pharmacology, 11th ed. New York: McGraw-Hill, 2009:313–30.

18. Vane J, Botting R. The mechanism of action of aspirin. Thromb Res 2003;110:255–58.

19. Drug Facts and Comparisons [database on the Internet]. Facts and comparisons. Indianapolis (IN). 4.0; 2009. Nonsteroidal anti–inflammatory agents; [about 21 pages]. Accessed 2011 Jun 21. URL: http://0-online.factsandcomparisons.com.libcat.ferris.edu/MonoDispaspx?id5570727&book5DFC

20. Lexi-Comp, Inc (Lexi-Drugs®). Lexi-Comp. Accessed 2011 Jun 21.

21. Natural medicines comprehensive database [database on the Internet]. Stockton (CA): Therapeutic Research Faculty; c1995–2009. Antiplatelet. Accessed 2011 Jun 21. URL: http://www.naturaldatabase.com/(S(wqklte55rbhkbvzskfpaim45))/nd/Search.aspx?cs5MHSLA%7ECP&s5ND&pt59&Product5antiplatelet

22. Kirchain W, Allen R. Drug-induced liver disease. In: DiPiro JT, Talbert RL, Yee GC, Matzke GR, Wells BG, Posey LM, eds. Pharmacotherapy: A pathophysiologic approach, 7th ed. New York: McGraw-Hill, 2008:652.

23. Scheiman JM, Fendrick AM. Practical approaches to minimizing gastrointestinal and cardiovascular safety concerns with COX-2 inhibitors and NSAIDs. Arthritis Res Ther 2005;7(Suppl 4):S23–S29.

24. Golstein JL, Eisen GM, Burke TA, et al. Dyspepsia tolerability from the patients' perspective: a comparison of celecoxib with diclofenac. Aliment Pharmacol Ther 2002;16 (4):819–27.

25. Goldstein JL, Eisen GM, Burke TA, Peña BM, Lefkowith J, Geis GS. Comparison of upper gastrointestinal toxicity of rofecoxib and naproxen in patients with rheumatoid arthritis. N Engl J Med 2000;343:1520–28.

26. Laine L. Nonsteroidal anti-inflammatory drug gastropathy. Gastrointest Endosc Clin North Am 1996;6:489–504.

27. Gabriel SE, Jaakkimainen L, Bombardier C. Risk for serious gastrointestinal complications related to use of nonsteroidal anti–inflammatory drugs: a meta-analysis. Ann Intern Med 1991;115:787–96.

28. Ekström P, Carling L, Wetterhus S, Wingren PE, Anker-Hansen O, Lundegårdh G, et al. Prevention of peptic ulcer and dyspeptic symptoms with omeprazole in patients receiving continuous nonsteroidal anti–inflammatory drug therapy: a Nordic multicentre study. Scand J Gastroenterol 1996;31(8):753–58.

29. Hippisley-Cox J, Coupland C, Logan R. Risk of adverse gastrointestinal outcomes in patients taking cyclo-oxygenase-2 inhibitors or conventional non-steroidal anti–inflammatory drugs: population based nested case-control analysis. BMJ 2005;331:1310-6.

30. Bennett W, Turmelle Y, Shepherd R. Ibuprofen-induced liver injury in an adolescent athlete. Clin Pediatr 2009;48(1):84–86.

31. Rubenstein JH, Laine L. Systematic review: the hepatotoxicity of non-steroidal anti-inflammatory drugs. Aliment Pharmacol Ther 2004;20:373–80.

32. Rostom A, Goldkind L, Laine L. Nonsteroidal anti–inflammatory drugs and hepatic toxicity: a systematic review of randomized controlled trials in arthritis patients. Clin Gastroenterol Hepatol 2005;3:489–98.

33. Whelton A. Nephrotoxicity of nonsteroidal anti–inflammatory drugs: physiologic foundations and clinical implications. Am J Med 1999;106(Suppl 5B):S13–S24.

34. Clive DM, Stoff JS. Renal syndromes associated with nonsteroidal anti-inflammatory drugs. N Engl J Med 1984;310:563–72.

35. Henrich WL. Nephrotoxicity of nonsteroidal anti-inflammatory agents. Am J Kidney Dis 1983;2:478–84.

36. Nakahura T, Griswold W, Lemire J, Mendoza S, Reznik V. Nonsteroidal anti-inflammatory drug use in adolescents. J Adolesc Health 1998;23(5):307–10.

37. Solomon SD, McMurray JJ, Pfeffer MA, Wittes J, Fowler R, Finn P, et al. Cardiovascular risk associated with celecoxib in a clinical trial for colorectal adenoma prevention. N Engl J Med 2005;352(11):1071–80.

38. Bresalier RS, Sandler RS, Quan H, Bolognese JA, Oxenius B, Horgan K, et al. Cardiovascular events associated with rofecoxib in a colorectal adenoma chemoprevention trial. N Engl J Med 2005;352(11):1092–102.

39. McGettigan P, Henry D. Cardiovascular risk and inhibition of cyclooxygenase, a systematic review of the observational studies of selective and nonselective inhibitors of cyclooxygenase 2. JAMA 2006;296:1633–44.

40. COX-2 selective (includes Bextra, Celebrex, and Vioxx) and non-selective non-steroidal anti-inflammatory drugs (NSAIDs). U.S. Food and Drug Administration, Drug Safety and Availability. Accessed 2011 Jun 21. URL: http://www.fda.gov/Drugs/DrugSafety/PostmarketDrugSafetyInformationforPatientsandProviders/ucm103420.htm

41. Lanier A. Use of nonsteroidal anti–inflammatory drugs following exercise-induced muscle injury. Sports Med 2003;3:177–86.

42. Moore RA, Tramèr MR, Carroll D, Wiffen PJ, McQuay HJ. Quantitative systematic review of topically applied non-steroidal anti-inflammatory drugs. BMJ 1998;316(7128):333–38.

43. Peterson B, Rovati S. Diclofenac epolamine (Flector®) patch, evidence for topical activity. Clin Drug Investig 2009;29(1):1–9.

44. Zacher J, Altman R, Bellamy N, Brühlmann P, Da Silva J, Huskisson E, et al. Topical diclofenac and its role in pain and inflammation: an evidence-based review. Curr Med Res Opin 2008;24(4):925–50.

45. Drug Facts and Comparisons [database on the Internet]. Facts and comparisons. Indianapolis (IN). 4.0; 2009. Acetaminophen; [about 5 pages]. Accessed 2011 Jun 11. URL: http://0-online.factsandcomparisons.com.libcat.ferris.edu/MonoDisp.aspx?monoID5fandc-hcp10022&quick5acetaminophen&search5acetaminophen&disease5

46. Dalton J, Schweinle J. Randomized controlled noninferiority trial to compare extended release acetaminophen and ibuprofen for the treatment of ankle sprains. Ann Emerg Med 2006;48:615–23.

47. Woo WW, Man SY, Lam PK, Rainer TH. Randomized double-blind trial comparing oral paracetamol and oral nonsteroidal anti-inflammatory drugs for treating pain after musculoskeletal injury. Ann Emerg Med 2005;46(4):352–61.

48. Wright E. Musculoskeletal injuries and disorders. In: Berardi R, Ferreri S, Hume A, Kroon LA, Newton GD, Popovich NG, et al, eds. Handbook of nonprescription drugs, an interactive approach to self-care, 16th ed. Washington, DC: American Pharmacists Association, 2009:95–113.

49. Heng MC. Local necrosis and interstitial nephritis due to topical methyl salicylate and menthol. Cutis 1987;39(5):442–44.
50. Yip A, Chow W, Tai Y, Cheung KL. Adverse effect of local methylsalicylate ointment on warfarin anticoagulation: an unrecognized potential hazard. Postgrad Med J 1990;66 (775):367–69.
51. Joss J, LeBlond R. Potentiation of warfarin anticoagulation associated with topical methyl salicylate. Ann Pharmacother 2000;34(6):729–33.
52. Love J, Sammon M, Smereck J. Are one or two dangerous? Camphor exposure in toddlers. J Emerg Med 2004;27(1):49–54.
53. Gouin S, Patel H. Unusual cause of seizure. Pediatr Emerg Care 1996;12(4):298–300.
54. Patel T, Ishiuji Y, Yosipovitch G. Menthol: A refreshing look at this ancient compound. J Am Acad Dermatol 2007;57:873–78.
55. Vyklický L, Nováková-Tousová K, Benedikt J, Samad A, Touska F, Vlachová V. Calcium-dependent desensitization of vanilloid receptor TRPV1: a mechanism possibly involved in analgesia induced by topical application of capsaicin. Physiol Res 2008;57(Suppl 3): S59–S68.
56. Knotkova H, Pappagallo M, Szallasi A. Capsaicin (TRPV1 agonist) therapy for pain relief farewell or revival? Clin J Pain 2008;24:142–54.
57. Mason L, Moore A, Derry S, Edwards JE, McQuay HJ. Systematic review of topical capsaicin for the treatment of chronic pain. BMJ 2004;328(7446):991.
58. Drugstore. Topical analgesics. Accessed 2011 Jun 02. URL: http://www.drugstore.com/ search/search_results.asp?N50&Ntx5mode%2Bmatchallpartial&Ntk5All&srchtree55& Ntt5topical1analgesics
59. Chambers C, Reid G, McGrath P, Finley GA. Self-administration of over-the-counter medication for pain among adolescents. Arch Pediatr Adolesc Med 1997;151(5):449–55.
60. Van den Bulck J, Leemans L, Laekeman G. Television and adolescent use of over-the-counter analgesic agents. Ann Pharmacother 2005;39:58–62.
61. Huott M, Storrow A. A survey of adolescents' knowledge regarding toxicity of over-the-counter medications. Acad Emerg Med 1997;4:214–18.
62. Warner D, Schnepf G, Barrett M, Dian D, Swigonski NL. Prevalence, attitudes, and behaviors related to the use of nonsteroidal anti-inflammatory drugs (NSAIDs) in student athletes. J Adolesc Health 2002;30(3):150–53.
63. Alaranta A, Alaranta H, Heliövaara M, Airaksinen M, Helenius I. Ample use of physician-prescribed medications in Finnish elite athletes. Int J Sports Med 2006;27(11):919–25.
64. Alaranta A, Alaranta H, Helenius I. Use of prescription drugs in athletes. Sports Med 2008;38(6):449–63.

13 Concepts of rheumatoid disorders

Donald E. Greydanus, Mary D. Moore, and Cynthia L. Feucht

Rheumatoid diseases (RDs) are both common and rare conditions of adolescents; they present with a wide variety of features due to inflammation in joints, muscles, and other tissues. The hallmark of the RDs is the presence of a chronic inflammatory process that, if left uncontrolled, often leads to significant morbidity and even mortality. The most common of these autoimmune diseases are juvenile idiopathic arthritis (JIA) and systemic lupus erythematosus (SLE). JIA, SLE, and other related rheumatoid conditions are considered in this review. Medications for RDs can have significant adverse effects. Management of these conditions is complex; it must be individualized and coordinated with appropriate subspecialists.

13.1 Introduction

Rheumatic diseases are conditions involving inflammation and pain in connective tissues and supporting body structures: joints, ligaments, tendons, and muscles (1,2,3,4,5,6,7). The primary presentations involve joint pain, swelling, and stiffness (especially morning type) with resultant and variable disability complicated by underlying autoimmune dysfunction. RDs are also complicated by the involvement of other organs in the body. More than 100 RDs have been identified that involved nearly 50 million people in the United States (see ▶Tab. 13.1). RDs are a more common cause of limitation of activity than diabetes mellitus, cancer, and heart disease. Most RDs are more common in females, although some (such as gout) are seen more commonly in males. The most common rheumatic disorders are juvenile idiopathic arthritis and the spondyloarthropathies, which are seen in 0.5 to 2.0 per 1,000 children and adolescents.

13.1.1 Symptomatology

Rheumatoid diseases can present with a myriad of signs and symptoms in addition to those involving the joints and muscles. Any body system can be involved and there can be dermatologic conditions (rashes, skin or mucosal ulcers, alopecia), pain (joints, muscles, chest, abdomen, headaches, generalized), eye involvement (conjunctivitis, iritis), gastrointestinal problems (anorexia, dysphagia, weight loss), pulmonary disease (shortness of breath, hemoptysis), vasomotor instability, fatigue, fever, and others.

A careful medical history seeks to identify the cause of the pain, such as bone pain or neuropathic pain. Stiffness after rest (night sleep, long naps, long car rides, others) is a classic feature of RD inflammation and may be due to reduced hyaluronic acid in inflamed synovial fluid. RDs can change over time and thus meticulous, regular reevaluations over time are important. A variety of conditions must be considered if the youth presents with musculoskeletal complaints, including RDs, vasculitides, connective tissue infections, bone cancer (Ewing's sarcoma, osteogenic sarcoma – see chapter 7),

Tab. 13.1: Rheumatic and related disorders.

Juvenile idiopathic arthritis (JIA); juvenile rheumatoid arthritis (JRA)

Rheumatic Fever

Spondyloarthropathies
- Enthesitis-related arthritis
- Ankylosing spondylitis
- Reiter's syndrome (reactive arthritis)
- Psoriatic arthritis
- Arthritides of inflammatory bowel disease
- Unclassified (undifferentiated) types

Systemic lupus erythematosus

Scleroderma (systemic or localized forms)

Dermatomyositis

Hereditary syndromes with musculoskeletal manifestations
- Benign joint hypermobility syndrome (BJHS)
- Ehlers-Danlos syndrome
- Marfan's syndrome
- Marfanoid hypermobility syndrome
- Multiple epiphyseal dysplasias
- Osteogenesis imperfecta
- Williams syndrome

Inborn errors of metabolism
- homocystinuria, hyperlysinemia

Vasculitis
- Churg-Strauss disease
- Henoch-Schönlein purpura (HSP)
- Hypersensitivity (leukocytoclastic) vasculitis
- Kawasaki disease
- Polyarteritis Nodosa
- Sjögren's syndrome
- Takayasu's arteritis
- Wegener's granulomatosis

Infectious joint disease
- Bacterial arthritis/osteomyelitis
- Viral arthropathy

(Continued)

Tab. 13.1: Rheumatic and related disorders. (*Continued*)

- STD arthritis
- Lyme disease

Pain amplification syndromes
- Complex regional pain syndrome
- Joint hypermobility syndrome
- Reflex sympathetic dystrophy (RSD)
- Fibromyalgia

Sarcoidosis

Miscellaneous arthropathies

Traumatic arthritis

Congential hip dislocation

Legg-Calvé-Perthes disease

Osgood Schlatter disease

Patellofemoral syndromes

Slipped femoral epiphyhsis

Any poorly healed fracture or inadequately treated infection

Systemic disorders often complicated by arthritis
- Hemophilia
- Secondary gout and pseudogout
- Serum sickness
- Sickle cell disease
- Neoplastic disease
- Hypertrophic osteoarthropathy

Miscellaneous/rare
- Mixed connective tissue disease
- Weber-Christian disease
- Jaccoud's arthritis
- Behçet's syndrome
- Relapsing polychronritis

Others

Modified with permission from Greydanus DE: Rheumatoid disorders and other Miscellaneous disorders. In: Hofmann AD, Greydanus DE: (eds): Adolescent Medicine, 3rd ed. Stamford, CT: Appleton & Lange; 1997;20:433.

psychosomatic and/or chronic pain syndromes, peripheral neuropathies, primary muscle disorders, overuse injuries, and others. ▶Tab. 13.2 lists conditions to consider in youths who present with monoarthritis (acute versus chronic) and polyarthritis.

13.1.2 RD studies

A variety of laboratory and imaging studies are important, depending on the specific conditions being evaluated (8). There are signs of inflammation, such as an elevated erythrocyte sedimentation rate (ESR) or C-reactive protein (CRP). The finding of auto-antibodies in rheumatoid diseases can be very helpful in specific conditions and must be interpreted carefully. These include rheumatoid factor (RF), various antinuclear antibodies (ANAs), cyclic citrullinated peptide (CCP), and antineutrophil cytoplasmic antibody (ANCA).

For example, RF is commonly found in rheumatoid arthritis (RF-positive polyarticular juvenile idiopathic arthritis), Sjögren's syndrome, and hepatitis C–induced cryoglobulinemia. RF may occasionally be found in other conditions such as dermatomyositis, SLE, scleroderma, mixed connective tissue disease, and chronic bacterial infections. CCP is found in RF-positive polyarticular JIA.

Other tests include joint fluid examination, human leukocyte antigen (HLA) typing, complement analysis, and measurement of cryoglobulins. Imaging involves judicious use of computed tomography (CT) and magnetic resonance imaging (MRI), which have higher diagnostic yields than plain radiography and ultrasound. Consultation with rheumatology specialists is needed to successfully navigate the complex world of RDs and RD laboratory interpretation.

13.2 Juvenile idiopathic arthritis (JIA)

Different terms have been used over the past decades to refer to a heterogenous group of chronic inflammatory arthritides in childhood. These terms include JRA (juvenile rheumatoid arthritis), JCA (juvenile chronic arthritis), JA (juvenile arthritis), and, in this text, JIA–based on the ILAR system of classification (7). JIA involves the development of arthritis in which there is persistent (over 6 weeks) joint swelling and/or painful joint movement restriction versus arthralgia, in which there is joint pain with or without inflammation. The term *juvenile* refers to the onset of the condition before 16 years of age.

Three historic subtypes of JIA are recognized: pauciarticular, polyarticular (RF-positive and RF-negative), and systemic-onset (Still's disease). The ILAR classification for JIA also includes psoriatic arthritis, enthesitis-related arthritis, and undifferentiated arthritis. The workup must exclude other causes of arthritis (▶Tab. 13.2), including septic arthritis, reactive arthritis, postinfectious arthritis, Lyme arthritis, and other rheumatoid disorders.

JIA typically presents with stiffness after a prolonged rest (i.e., morning stiffness), with mild aching and variable joint swelling (9,10). Fortunately severe pain is not the norm. Those with pauciarticular JIA are at increased risk for the development of uveitis (iritis), which is usually insidious and typically found only on eye screening; some may present

Tab. 13.2: Conditions presenting as arthritis.

Acute monoarthritis

Enthesitis-related arthritis
• Hemophilia
• Leukemia

Neuroblastoma
• Oligoarthritis
• Psoriatic arthritis
• Reactive arthritis
• Septic arthritis

Trauma
Chronic monoarthritis

Enthesitis-related arthritis
• Episodic fever syndromes
• Hemophilia
• Hemangioma
• Juvenile idiopathic arthritis (JIA)

Juvenile psoriatic arthritis

Lyme arthritis
• Oligoarthritis
• Sarcoidosis

Synovial chondromatosis
• Tuberculosis
• Villonodular synovitis

Polyarthritis

Spondyloarthropathies
• Enthesitis-related arthritis
• Arthritis with inflammatory bowel disease

Juvenile idiopathic polyarthritis
Lyme disease (usually monoarticular)
Malignancies
Periodic fever syndromes
Polyarthritis related to infection
Psoriatic juvenile idiopathic arthritis
Reactive arthritis
Rheumatic fever (migratory joint involvement)
Sarcoidosis
Serum sickness, systemic juvenile idiopathic arthritis, SLE, vasculitis, viral arthritis
Systemic juvenile idiopathic arthritis
Systemic lupus erythematosus
Vasculitis
Viral arthritis

Modified with permission from: Patel DR, Moore MD: Concepts of rheumatology. In Handbook of Clinical Pediatrics: An Update for the Ambulatory Pediatrician. DE Greydanus, DR Patel, VN Reddy, AN Feinberg, HA Omar, eds. Hackensack: NJ: World Scientific; 2010:702.

with more overt eye symptoms, such as eye pain, redness, photophobia, and/or vision changes. Patients with polyarthritis are at less risk for chronic uveitis.

In pauciarticular JIA (oligoarthritis) there is a limp with nonpainful swelling of four or less joints within 6 months of disease onset and the onset is typically in individuals under 8 years of age. In polyarticular JIA, the joint swelling involves five or more joints within 6 months of disease onset; the age of onset is bimodal 1 to 6 years of age and 11 to 16 years of age. There are two types of polyarthritis JIA: RF-negative and RF-positive (i.e., two or more positive RF tests during the first 6 months after disease onset at least 3 months apart) (11).

In systemic-onset JIA there is arthritis in one or more joints with a variable of age onset; it occurs with or is preceded by a fever with high spikes lasting for 2 or more weeks that is daily (quotidian) for 3 days or more. In addition there is one or more of these features: recurrent rash (evanescent, erythematous), hepatosplenomegaly (one or both), generalized lymphadenopathy, and serositis (pericarditis and/or pleuritis and/or peritonitis).

Laboratory tests in JIA are either normal or only mildly elevated, the RF is negative in over 90 percent of JIA patients, and there is a low ANA titer in 70 to 90 percent. There is no test or combination of laboratory tests to conclusively distinguish JIA from other disorders. Laboratory testing is used to exclude other conditions such as septic arthritis or malignancy. Joint aspiration (▶Tab. 13.3) is useful in this differential process and includes a Gram's stain, culture, cell count, fluid glucose, and other tests in selective situations (i.e., fungal or acid-fast bacillus evaluation, cytology, crystal examination).

13.2.1 Differential diagnosis

A wide variety of disorders must be considered in the differential of common rheumatic conditions that can manifest as musculoskeletal pain. For example, benign hypermobility syndrome presents as intermittent pains at night more commonly in females with an age of onset of 3 to 10 years and often with a positive family history. There may be hyperextended metacarpophalangeal joints, elbows, or knees. The clinician should rule out Ehlers-Danlos syndrome and Marfan's syndrome. Benign nocturnal limb pains of childhood (growing pains of childhood) presents as cramping lower leg pain in the evenings or at night, with an age of onset between 3 and 10 years; the examination and laboratory tests are normal. SLE is discussed in the next section.

Acute rheumatic fever (ARF) or streptococcal infection–related arthritis presents as migratory arthritis 2 to 3 weeks after streptococcal pharyngitis, usually during the school-age years, with a distribution related to streptococcal infection risk. A persistent arthritis may indicate streptococcal infection–related arthritis or poststreptococcal reactive

Tab. 13.3: Synovial fluid analysis.

Normal	White blood count (WBC): 200–500	Synovial glucose ⅔ of serum	Sterile fluid
Inflammatory	WBC: 10,000 to 50,000	Synovial glucose is variable; can be very low	Sterile fluid
Septic	WBC: >50,000	Synovial glucose is very low	Positive culture from synovial fluid, blood, other
Hemorrhagic	WBC: 200–500	Synovial glucose is normal	Sterile fluid

arthritis (PSRA). Also, the streptococci can directly invade the joint, causing a bacterial arthritis distinct from the type of arthritis seen in ARF and PSRA. The characteristic rash is called erythema marginatum, and carditis is a serious complication; additional features of the revised Jones criteria for ARF include subcutaneous nodules and chorea. There is evidence of an antecedent streptococal infection. A review of the treatment of streptococcal pharyngitis is available. (See Tab. 2 in chapter 18 in Greydanus DE, Patel DR, Omar HA, Feucht C, Merrick J: Adolescent Medicine – Pharmacotherapeutics in General, Mental and Sexual Health. Berlin: de Gruyter; 2012.)

Malignancy includes osteosarcoma, leukemia, lymphoma, Ewing's tumor, rhabdomyosarcoma, and others (see chapter 7). The presentation includes painful joints, bone pain, and variable constitutional symptoms. The youth may be ill appearing with joint swelling, malignant effusions, an abnormal CBC, elevated ESR, and abnormalities noted by radiography and imaging studies.

Henoch-Schönlein purpura (HSP) is the second most common vasculitis in children and adolescents that presents with a purpuric rash and abdominal pain often triggered by an upper respiratory tract infection in school-age children with a median age of 4 years (2–11 years of age). There is nonspecific swelling of joints and hematuria as well as proteinuria; in addition, hypertension may occur. Management is supportive (i.e., hydration, nutrition, pain relief). Corticosteroids are used if necessary and severe disease may require the use of various other rheumatic disease medications, as reviewed later. Long-term outcome is dependent on the underlying renal involvement, and approximately 8 percent of patients develop end-stage renal disease (ESRD).

Spondyloarthropathies include arthritis with enthesitis, ankylosing spondylitis, reactive arthritis (Reiter's syndrome), psoriatic arthritis, and arthritides of inflammatory bowel disease. Arthritis with enthesitis presents with ankle pain, heel pain, Achilles' apophysitis, and back (lumbosacral) or hip stiffness. The pain is usually worse at the day's end and there is often a positive family history of spondyloarthropathy. There is inflammation and tenderness at sites of tendon insertion, and the condition is often diagnosed as overuse syndrome for many years before this diagnosis is made. Acute symptomatic uveitis may develop and the HLA-B27 antigen is often positive.

Ankylosing spondylitis (AS) presents with insidious chronic low (lumbar) back pain and stiffness in males usually 13 years of age and older. Painful iritis is common. There can be enthesitis and peripheral arthritis. Classic radiographic AS spinal changes may not be evident for years. One should observe for vertebral compression fractures. Laboratory data shows a positive HLA-B27 antigen, and negative ANA; the platelet count as well as ESR are elevated.

Reiter's syndrome (reactive arthritis) presents with painful joints with swelling following a genitourinary or gastrointestinal infection in a teenager 13 years of age or older. The classic triad is arthritis, urethritis, and uveitis (conjunctivitis); arthritis is usually acute, asymmetrical, and affecting the lower limb. Evidence of ankylosing spondylitis occurs in 10 percent, and there can be mouth ulcers as well. The HLA-B27 is typically positive whereas the ANA is usually negative.

Psoriatic arthritis presents with a psoriatic rash that may occur after the arthritis (mono- or polyarthitis) develops. The arthropathy can take a variety of forms and is more common in males. There may also be dactylitis, nail pitting or onycholysis, and a positive family history of psoriasis in a first-degree relative. The HLA-B27 is often positive. See chapter 2 for a discussion of psoriasis and its management.

Arthritides of inflammatory bowel disease (IBD) involve large-joint polyarthritis with chronic or recurrent abdominal pain, weight loss or lack of normal weight gain, malaise, positive HLA-B27, and negative ANA. It occurs in about one third of those with IBD and tends to resolve with control of the IBD (see chapter 5). There can be spinal disease, ankylosing spondylitis, mouth ulcers, skin lesions (pyoderma gangrenosa, erythema nodosum), and uveitis.

13.2.2 JIA complications

The natural history of children and adolescents with JIA is quite varied; fortunately most do well with early diagnosis and appropriate management by experts in rheumatoid diseases. Some, however, have chronic and recalcitrant disease. There can be joint destruction as well as, growth inhibition with resultant short stature, contractures, bone overgrowth, and cervical spine involvement with spinal cord compression including the cervical spine.

Eye involvement is noted in up to half of those with oligoarticular JIA, 10 percent of those with polyarticular disease, rarely in individuals with systemic-onset JIA. The most common eye condition is uveitis (also referred to as iritis or iridocyclitis), which is often painless and progressive. It can lead to many eye complications including secondary glaucoma, cataracts, band keratopathy, posterior synechiae with papillary complications, vision loss, and blindness. The severity of the arthropathy does not correlate with the risk of uveitis. Regular screening visits for eye disease are important for RD patients since the eye damage can be insidious and progressive, especially if undertreated.

Death from JIA arises as a result of complications from pharmacologic management, infections, traumatic injury to the cervical spine, or the rare macrophage activation syndrome (MAS). MAS is a form of hemophagocytic lymphohistiocytosis syndrome, which may be precipitated by viral infections or drugs. Those with MAS develop the rapid onset severe illness with fever, adenopathy, organomegaly, petchiae, pancytopenia, bleeding, rapidly lowering ESR, and very high ferritin levels. Supportive care is necessary, and there may be improvement with high-dose corticosteroids, cyclosporine, and tumor necrosis factor inhibitors (see sections 13.3.2,13.3.4, and 13.3.5). Mortality in MAS can exceed 30 percent.

13.2.3 JIA Management

Each youth with arthritis needs an individual plan managed by a clinician skilled in arthropathy management (4). Conservative measures can be helpful for pain such as use of moist heat, joint support (i.e., casting, splinting, canes, crutches), rest, and appropriate physical activity. Non-narcotics are also helpful for pain and narcotics used very judiciously for severe pain keeping in mind the problematic potential for addiction (see chapter 10 in Greydanus DE, Patel DR, Omar HA, Feucht C, Merrick J: Adolescent Medicine – Pharmacotherapeutics in General, Mental and Sexual Health, de Gruyter, Berlin, 2012). Attention to co-morbid sleep problems, mood disturbances, and anxiety conditions is very important. Many adolescents with rheumatoid disorders find help online via chat rooms and other types of support from local RD chapters. (See chapter 3 in Greydanus DE, Patel DR, Omar HA, Feucht C, Merrick J: Adolescent Medicine – Pharmacotherapeutics in General, Mental and Sexual Health. Berlin: de Gruyter; 2012.)

Non-pharmacologic treatments include relaxation therapy, physical therapy, occupational therapy, heat and cold applications, hydrotherapy, transcutaneous electrical nerve stimulation (TENS), and others. Also, corticosteroid intra-articular infections can be very useful in JIA management, especially in children and adolescents with involvement of only a few joints. Surgery – including arthroscopic surgery, bone fusion, osteotomy, and arthroplasty – may be helpful as well.

The use of nutritional supplements remains controversial and unproven. This includes proposed use of glucosamine and chondroitin sulfate, or SAM-e (S-adenosylmethionine), for osteoarthritis, SAM-e for fibromalgia, or dehydroepiandrosterone (DHEA) for SLE. Hyaluronic acid substitutes mimic a natural body substance that lubricates joints and some adults with osteoarthritis receive intra-articular injections in attempts to relieve pain and provide better joint motion. However, hyaluronic acid substitutes are not useful in inflammatory arthritis and are not approved by the U.S. Food and Drug Administration (FDA) in the pediatric population.

13.3 RD medication: general considerations

The specific medication used for arthropathy depends on the specific condition and the specific patient (12,13). Drugs used for rheumatoid disorders are generally used to control pain, reduce inflammation and joint damage and to limit both RD symptoms and functional decline. Medications may slow the disease course and limit or prevent more damage to joints or other body parts. Cure is not possible except in select situations, such as correct use of antibiotics in infectious arthritis or early use of antibiotics in Lyme disease.

13.3.1 Analgesics

Nonsteroidal anti-inflammatory drugs (NSAIDs) are the most commonly used medications for the management of inflammatory arthropathy, noninflammatory musculoskeletal disorders, and many other conditions. They have become very popular analgesics since their introduction in the 1960s (see the Preface). These medications together with their dosages are listed in ▶Tab. 13.4 and potential side effects are noted in ▶Tab. 13.5. These drugs do not affect the long-term outcome but can control pain, stiffness, swelling, and fever. ▶Tab. 13.6 lists components of common topical analgesics (see chapter 12). Despite the convenience of topical agents and their minimal systemic absorption, some youth do not like or tolerate the burning sensation or the texture of some topical medications.

IR, immediate-release; ER, extended-release; DR, delayed-release; NTE, not to exceed.

Traditional NSAIDs include ibuprofen, naproxen, acetylsalicylic acid, indomethacin, sulindac, tolmetin sodium, and others (see chapter 12). They nonselectively inhibit cyclooxygenase 1 and 2 (COX-1 and COX-2), which contributes to their adverse effects. For example, the COX-1 enzyme is expressed in various organ systems such asthe renal, gastrointestinal (GI), and hematologic (i.e., platelets) systems (▶Tab. 13.5). NSAIDs can lead to drowsiness, headache, and dizziness; these effects tend to stop with discontinuing the NSAID.

Tab. 13.4: Systemic analgesics and anti-inflammatory drugs (see chapter 12, Tabs. 12.1–12.4).

Generic name	Adult dosage	Pediatric dosage
Diclofenac sodium	100–200 mg daily (2–4 divided doses) ER given once or twice daily	2–3 mg/kg per day (2–4 divided doses)
Diclofenac potassium	100–200 mg daily (two to four divided doses)	2–3 mg/kg per day (two to four divided doses)
Diclofenac epolamine	180-mg patch every 12 hours	N/A
Etodolac	600–1,000 mg daily (two to three divided doses)	20–30 kg: 400 mg daily 31–45 kg: 600 mg daily 46–60 kg: 800 mg daily >60 kg: 1,000 mg daily Age 6–16 years Based on ER product
Fenoprofen calcium	200–600 mg three to four times day Max: 3,200 mg/day	N/A
Flurbiprofen	200–300 mg daily (two to four divided doses)	N/A
Ibuprofen	1,200–3,200 mg daily (three to four divided doses)	4–10 mg/kg per dose three to four times a day Max: 40 mg/kg per day
Indomethacin	50–200 mg daily (two to three divided doses)	1–2 mg/kg per day (2–4 divided doses) Max: 4 mg/kg per day, NTE: 150–200 mg/day Age >2 years
Ketoprofen	IR: 150–300 mg/day (three to four divided doses) ER: 100–200 mg daily	N/A
Ketorolac tromethamine	20 mg initially, 10 mg four times a day Max: 5-day duration	N/A
Meclofenamate sodium	200–400 mg daily (three or four divided doses)	N/A
Mefenamic acid	500 mg initially, 250 mg every 6 hours as needed (NTE: 1 week)	N/A
Meloxicam	7.5–15 mg daily	0.125 mg/kg per day Max: 7.5 mg daily Age ≥2 years
Nabumetone	500–2000 mg daily (1–2 divided doses)	N/A

(Continued)

Tab. 13.4: Systemic analgesics and anti-inflammatory drugs (see chapter 12, Tabs. 12.1–12.4). (*Continued*)

Generic name	Adult dosage	Pediatric dosage
Naproxen	Naproxen: 250–500 mg twice aday Naproxen sodium: 200–500 mg twice a day Naproxen DR: 375–500 mg twice a day	Analgesia: 5–7 mg/kg per dose every 8–12 hours Inflammatory disease: 10–15 mg/kg per day (two divided doses) Max: 1,000 mg/day Age >2 years
Oxaprozin	600–1,200 mg daily Max: 1,800 mg daily (in divided doses)	22–31 kg: 600mg daily 32–54 kg: 900 mg daily ≥55 kg: 1,200 mg daily Age 6–16 years
Piroxicam	10–20 mg daily	0.2–0.3 mg/kg per day Max: 15 mg daily
Sulindac	150–200 mg twice a day	2–4 mg/kg per day (two divided doses) Max: 6mg/kg per day, NTE: 400 mg/day
Tolmetin sodium	600–1,800 mg daily (three divided doses) Max: 2,000 mg daily	Analagesia: 5–7 mg/kg per dose every 6–8 hours Inflammatory disease: 15–30mg/kg per day (three to four divided doses) NTE: 1,800 mg/day Age ≥2 years
Celecoxib	100–400 mg daily (one or two divided doses)	10–25 kg: 50 mg twice a day >25 kg: 100 mg twice a day Age ≥2 years
Diflunisal	500–1,000 mg daily (two to three divided doses) Max: 1,500 mg daily	N/A
Magnesium salicylate	Novosal: 600 mg three to four times a day, maximum 4,800 mg daily Doan's: 934 mg every 6 hour as needed	N/A
Salsalate	3,000 mg daily (two to four divided doses)	N/A
Choline magnesium trisalicylate	500–1,500 mg two to three times a day	30–60mg/kg per day (three to four divided doses)

More recent selective COX-2 inhibitors (i.e., celecoxib, valdecoxib, rofecoxib) produce less GI adverse effects but increase the risk of cardiovascular toxicity. However, valdecoxib and rofecoxib were removed from the market owing to the increased risk of cardiovascular adverse effects in adults taking these agents. Celecoxib has been approved by the FDA for use in JIA.

Tab. 13.5: Adverse effects of nonsteroidal anti-inflammatory drugs (see section 13.3.1; see chapter 12).

Acute renal insufficiency

Anaphylaxis

Bone marrow suppression

Bronchospasm

Bruising

Dizziness

Fluid retention or peripheral edema

Gastritis

Gastrointestinal ulceration and bleeding

Headache

Hepatotoxicity

Hyperkalemia

Hypersensitivity reactions

Increased risk of cardiovascular thrombotic events, myocardial infarction and stroke

Indigestion, heartburn

Interstitial nephritis

Nausea, vomiting

Peptic ulcer

Photosensitivity

Rash

Tinnitus

Tab. 13.6: Over-the-counter topical counterirritant analgesic agents (see chapter 12, Tab. 12.7).

Active ingredients used alone	Active ingredients often used in combination	Combination product examples
Camphor	Turpentine oil	Camphor 3%, menthol 5% and methyl salicylate 15%
Menthol	Histamine dihydrochloride	Camphor 3.6%, oleoresin capsicum 0.25%, methyl salicylate 18%
Capsaicin	Ammonia water	Camphor 1.2%, menthol 5.7%, methyl salicylate 6.7%
Trolamine salicylate	Allyl isothiocyanate	Menthol 4.127%, histamine dihydrochloride 0.025%
	Methyl salicylate	Menthol 7.6%, methyl salicylate 29%
	Methyl nicotinate	Menthol 10%, methyl salicylate 30%

Acetylsalicyclic acid (aspirin, ASA) has a historic background as an analgesic but has been replaced by the traditional NSAIDs in JIA management. Concern is raised with the small but well-known risk of Reye's syndrome and other aspirin-related adverse effects (see chapter 12). Salicylates should be avoided in youths who also have active infection with varicella or influenza. Salicylates (particularly ASA) are the only NSAIDs that result in less platelet aggregation with clinical relevance; this effect can last for 4 to 6 days with as small a dose as 80 mg. Selective COX-2 inhibitors do not reversibly inhibit platelet aggregation. Salicylates are associated with an increased frequency of side effects and more toxicity results from an overdose compared with other NSAIDs.

The adverse effects of NSAIDs are due to a complex mix of various factors including the specific drug, duration of use, dose, degree of COX-1 inhibition, comorbid disorders, and use of other medications. NSAIDs should be avoided in youths with asthma if they are aspirin-sensitive. Use of misoprostol or proton pump inhibitors can decrease the GI toxicity of NSAIDs for patients generally including those at high risk of GI toxicity (i.e., history of GI disorders, additional use of cortocosteroids).

Dermatologic side effects range from urticaria to Stevens-Johnson syndrome. Chronic use of naproxen can lead to pseudoporphyria, a photosensitive rash especially seen in fair-complexioned persons; chronic scarring may result. Hepatotoxicity is possible with NSAIDs including increased liver transaminases (3% with chronic use including 5% with salicylates) and a rare liver toxicity that can be fatal. Renal toxicity may occur in some, including hyperkalemia, proteinuria, and even interstitial nephritis. Leukopenia may arise;it is typically mild and resolves when the NSAID is discontinued; however, it may be severe and permanent in rare situations. Aseptic meningitis can occur in patients on NSAIDs, particularly in those with SLE; reports have included the following NSAIDS: ibuprofen, naproxen, diclofenac, ketoprofen, tolmetin, sulindac, and rofecoxib.

NSAIDs approved by the FDA for use in children include aspirin, ibuprofen, naproxen, oxaprozin, etodolac SR, meloxicam, indomethacin, and celecoxib. Some persons note more benefit from one versus another NSAID and sometimes a trial-and-error method is needed to find the best agent for each person. An NSAID that can be given once or twice a day is best for young people, so as to minimize difficulties in school and improve compliance. Some NSAIDs are available in liquid form (i.e., ibuprofen, naproxen, meloxicam, indomethacin, and various salicylate preparations); some are also available for parenteral administration (ketorolac and indomethacin); and diclofenac is available in a topical gel and patch formulation. Those on chronic NSAID treatment should receive periodic (i.e., every 3 months) screening for renal, GI, and hematopoietic toxicity. Screening for GI toxicity is done by evaluating for melena and abdominal pain; a proton pump inhibitor may be added, as previously noted. Serum levels of NSAIDs are not clinically usefully except to monitor salicylate levels in those on chronic salicylate management.

13.3.2 Corticosteroids

Corticosteroids are strong anti-inflammatory agents that have been around for many decades (see chapter 1). These drugs (i.e., prednisone, cortisone, hydrocortisone, methylprednisolone, others) are commonly used for rheumatoid disorders because they reduce inflammation and powerfully suppress the immune system. They can be given orally, topically, intra-articularly, intramuscularly, or intravenously (4).

Tab. 13.7: Corticosteroid side effects.

Acute effects (usually reversible)

• Swelling (sodium and fluid retention)

• Increased appetite

• Weight gain ("moon facies"; Cushingoid appearance)

• Emotional lability

• Acne (steroid acne)

• Sleep disturbances

• Severe muscle weakness (rare)

• Psychosis (rare)

Effects from chronic use

• Striae

• Dyslipidemias

• Accelerated atherogenesis

• Osteoporosis

• Osteonecrosis of hips (2% for most; up to 25% in SLE)

• Excessive hair growth

• Growth failure

• Hypertension

• Damage to arteries

• Hyperglycemia

• Cataracts

• Pseudotumor cerebri

• Infections

They are potent drugs with great benefit but also have the potential for significant adverse effects (▶Tab. 13.7). Because of potentially severe adverse effects, oral or parenteral corticosteroids are often used only for refractory RDs and severe JIA complications (such as anemia, pericarditis, and others). The lowest effective dose should be used, as well as alternate-day dosing to reduce adverse effects. Doses vary and oral doses can range from 1 to 3 mg/kg per day.

Side effects include infections ranging from typical bacterial microbes to increased risk of *Mycobacterium tuberculosis* and various opportunistic infections. Patients on chronic corticosteroids should receive appropriate calcium and vitamin D supplementation and counseled about the importance of weight-bearing exercise. Annual bone density studies should be done and clinicians should consider the use of a bisphosphonate to prevent osteoporosis for those on chronic steroid therapy.

Intra-articular injections of corticosteroids are beneficial, especially in those with minimal joint involvement; they may ameliorate the need for regular systemic corticosteroid or chronic NSAID use. The amount of the steroid varies with the joint size and may control synovitis for several months after an injection. Large joints (i.e., sacroiliac or hip) require that the injection be performed under fluoroscopy or with ultrasound guidance. A short-acting sedative may be necessary for youths with severe anxiety about the procedure, and general anesthesia is needed if several joints are to be injected. Sometimes joint injection is difficult owing to infection, bone changes, or fibrosis; if severe synovial hypertrophy is present, dispersal of the injection throughout the joint may be compromised. There may also be minor atrophy along the needle tract area due to steroid leakage into adjacent tissue.

13.3.3 Disease-modifying antirheumatic drugs (DMARDS)

DMARDs are used in rheumatoid arthritis, ankylosing spondylitis, and other inflammatory arthropathies in an effort to control the inflammatory process. The result may be less swelling, joint destruction, and pain for these individuals. DMARDs do not reverse damage that has already occurred. They include methotrexate, hydroxychloroquine, intramuscular gold salts, sulfasalazine, D-penicillamine, and leflunomide (▶Tab. 13.8) (4,6,13,14,15,16,17). Methotrexate is the DMARD most often used by rheumatologists treating these disorders. For example, methotrexate is often begun in patients with polyarthritis, oligoarticular conditions refractory to other measures, and chronic uveitis that is severe and refractory to corticosteroids. Because of excess toxicity, gold salts are rarely used, if at all. Similarly, leflunomide is used infrequently in adolescent females owing to its long half-life and risk of teratogenesis.

Methotrexate in moderate doses may be combined with hydroxychloroquine, sulfasalazine, or biological response modifiers (see section 13.3.5) to control inflammation and joint destruction more that noted with use of a single agent. Exact combinations of medications and dosages should be determined in each patient by an experienced clinician. As noted with many chronic conditions, there is no "cookbook" approach that covers all situations. Leflunomide has similar benefit and toxicity to methotrexate; however, as noted, it has a long half-life and detoxification is required if a patient wishes to become pregnant.

13.3.4 Cytotoxic agents

Cytotoxic drugs are used infrequently for RD individuals with very severe disease that have failed other treatments. They include cyclophosphamide, chlorambucil, and azathioprine. They may be part of protocols involving autologous bone marrow transplantation. Other drugs that may be used for such refractive situations include immune-modulating agents such as cyclosporine and mycophenolate mofetil. These are less often utilized owing to the high incidence of adverse effects and the availability of alternative agents. Live vaccine administration should be avoided while an individual is on these drugs. Cytotoxic agents are briefly reviewed in ▶Tab. 13.9 but should be employed only by experts experienced in their use (18).

13.3.5 Biological response modifiers

Biologicals or biological response modifiers are a group of genetically engineered drugs designed to block identified pathways in the immune system that are involved in the inflammatory process (4,6,19). RDs represent complex dysfunction of the immune system; thus biologics are beneficial in the treatment of some with RDs, including those

Tab. 13.8: DMARDs for rheumatoid disorders.

Generic name	Adult dosage	Adverse effects	Monitoring
Methotrexate	10–15 per week; usually given IM or orally Folic acid 1 mg daily added	Anorexia, nausea, emesis, abdominal cramps, hepatotoxicity, hepatic fibrosis, bone marrow suppression, allergic pneumonitis, opportunistic infections. Teratogenic; abortifacient; avoid with renal insufficiency (CrCl <30mL/min); increased toxicity if given with NSAIDs, trimethoprim/ sulfamethoxazole	LFTs, hepatitis B and C serologies for those with risk factors for infection, CBC with platelets, Scr
Leflunomide	Initial: 100 mg/day for 3 days. Maintenance: 10 to 20 mg/day Folic acid 1 mg added daily	Diarrhea, nausea, reversible hair loss, rash, bone marrow suppression, hepatoxocity, interstitial lung disease, peripheral neuropathy, anaphylaxis, severe dermatologic reactions, weight loss. Teratogenic	LFTs, CBC with platelets Drug elimination procedure: leflunomide stopped and cholestyramine 8 g administered three times a eay for 11 days Must verify that plasma level is <0.02 mg/L
Hydroxy-chloroquine	400–600 mg/day; maintenance is 200–400 mg/day; also used as an antimalarial drug	Dermatologic reactions including skin and mucosal pigmentation (blue/black), nausea, epigastric pain, retinal damage, blurred vision, keratopathy, central nervous system toxicity, hemolysis with G6PD deficiency	Ophthalmic exams, CBC with platelets, G6PD
Gold salts Gold sodium thiomalate (Solganol; Myochrysine)	IM: 10 mg as an initial dose, followed by 25 mg on week 2, then 25–50 mg weekly until 1 g total dose is achieved Maintenance: 25–50 mg every 2–4 weeks	Nausea, diarrhea, stomatitis, decreased appetite, exfoliative dermatitis, proteinuria, hepatitis, interstitial pneumonitis, enterocolitis, blood dyscrasias with bone	CBC with platelets, urinalysis

(Continued)

Tab. 13.8: DMARDs for rheumatoid disorders. (*Continued*)

Generic name	Adult dosage	Adverse effects	Monitoring
		marrow suppression "Nitroid" reaction: flushing, fainting, sweating, and dizziness within 30 minutes of injection	
Sulfasalazine	500 mg daily increasing to a maximum daily dose of 3,000 mg (in two divided doses) May consider adding folic acid 1 mg daily; also used for inflammatory bowel disease	Nausea, anorexia (enteric coated form may reduce these), rash, headache, hepatitis, bone marrow suppression, hemolytic anemia with G6PD deficiency, oligospermia (reversible), aplastic anemia, hypersensitivity reactions, renal toxicity	CBC with platelets, LFTs, urinalysis, G6PD
D-penicillamine	Initial: 125–250 mg/day increased by 125–250 mg/day at 1–3 month intervals Maintenance: 500–750 mg/day May consider addition of pyridoxine 25 mg/day Also used to treat Wilson's disease, cystinuria, arsenic poisoning	Aplastic anemia, lupus-like syndrome, pruritis/rash, proteinuria, membranous glomerunephritis, elastosis performans serpiginosa, myasthenic syndrome, bone marrow suppression, drug fever, mouth ulcers, GI distress, altered taste, neuropathy, intrahepatic cholestasis Contraindicated during pregnancy To be avoided in renal insufficiency Not to be used concomitantly with gold therapy, antimalarial, and cytotoxic agents Not to be coadministered with antacids, iron, or food	CBC with platelets, urinalysis, LFTs

CBC, complete blood count; LFT, liver function test; Scr, serum creatinine; CrCl, creatinine clearance; IM, intramuscular; G6PD, glucose 6 dehydrogenase deficiency.

Tab. 13.9: Cytotoxic and immune-modulating agents for rheumatoid disorders.

Generic name	Adult dosage	Adverse effects	Monitoring
Cyclo-phosphamide	1–3.5 mg/kg per day Nitrogen mustard alkylating agent Indications: SLE, JIA, nephrotic syndrome, neoplasms, others Cytotoxic agent	Nausea, emesis, anorexia, lethargy, diarrhea, rash, hair loss, weakness, bone marrow suppression, hemorrhagic cystitis, hematuria, proteinuria, amenorrhea, nail and skin pigmentation, fertility impairment, anaphylaxis Teratogenic Dosage adjustment required for hepatic and renal dysfunction Metabolized by CYP 450 system: potential for drug interactions	CBC with platelets, urinalysis, Scr, LFTs, bilirubin
Chlorambucil	0.1 to 0.2 mg/kg per day (4–10 mg/ day on average) Nitrogen mustard alkylating agent Indication: treatment of various cancers Cytotoxic agent	Agitation, confusion, peripheral neuropathy, bone marrow suppression, tremor, hypersensitivity reactions, interstitial pnemonitis, hepatotoxicity, fertility impairment, sterility Low emetogenic potential Teratogenic Dosage must be adjusted in renal insufficiency	CBC with platelets, Scr
Azathioprine	Variable; 1 mg/kg per day orally for 6–8 weeks; may be increased by 0.5 mg/kg per day every 4 weeks up to a maximum of 2.5 mg/kg per day Antagonizes purine metabolism Indications: RA and organ transplant rejection	Nausea, emesis, fatigue, hair loss, fever, bone marrow suppression (especially with TPMT deficiency), acute pancreatitis, hepatotoxicity, increased neoplasm risk, increased risk of serious infections, fertility impairment Teratogenic	CBC with platelets, LFTs, thiopurine S-methyltransferase (TPMT)

(Continued)

Tab. 13.9: Cytotoxic and immune-modulating agents for rheumatoid disorders. (*Continued*)

Generic name	Adult dosage	Adverse effects	Monitoring
Cyclosporine	Variable; initial: 2.5 mg/ kg per day orally divided into two doses up to a maximum of 4 mg/kg per day (Neoral and Gengraf only) Inhibits production and release of interleukin 2; immuno-suppressive agent Indications: psoriasis, to prevent organ transplant rejection, RA All cyclosporine products not interchangeable	Acne, nausea, abdominal pain, headache, tremor, dizziness, increased hair growth, nephrotoxicity, hepatotoxicity, hypertension, malignancy, increased risk of serious infections, encephalopathy Avoided in patients with renal impairment, uncontrolled hypertension, and malignancy Concomitant use of other nephrotoxic agents to be avoided Metabolized by and inhibitor of CYP 450 enzyme system	Scr, electrolytes, LFTs, CBC with platelets, blood pressure
Mycophenolate	Variable; 1 g orally twice a day Inhibits guanosine nucleotide synthesis pathway Indications: prevent organ transplant rejection	Anorexia, nausea, emesis, weakness, cough, headache, back pain, rash, increased infection risk, reactivation of latent viral infections, possible increased risk for lymphoma and other cancers, leukopenia, pure red cell aplasia, others Teratogenic Multiple drug interactions including decreased efficacy of oral contraceptives	CBC with platelets

CBC, complete blood count; LFT, liver function test; SLE, systemic lupus erythematosus; JIA, juvenile idiopathic arthriitis; RA, rheumtoid arthritis; TPMT, thiopurine methyltransferase or thiopurine S-methyltransferase; Scr, serum creatinine

involving inflammatory joint disease and bowel disease. However, their immune blocking mechanism can lead to an increase in infections (including reactivation of latent tuberculosis and hepatitis B) as well as certain types of cancer (including lymphoma). These drugs may be given via home injection or infusion in clinics. Biologicals include such drugs as etanercept, infliximab, abatacept, rituximab, adalimumab, certolizumab pegol, golimumab, and tocilizumab (▶Tab. 13.10). These agents are extremely expensive in the U.S. health care system and long-term safety is still a concern, with the possible increased risk of malignancies like lymphoma and demyelinating disorders.

Biological response modifiers may be used alone or in combination with other DMARDs (most commonly methotrexate) and are often utilized for those with moderate to severe disease or who have failed previous trials of other DMARDs. Combination therapy using more than one agent is not recommended owing to the high risk for adverse effects and lack of additive benefit. Antibody production against the agent may occur, which may lower the response to therapy. Patients receiving biological agents may receive vaccines but should avoid live vaccines. Guidelines for RA and JIA have been published by the American College of Rheumatology (2008 and 2011, respectively) (3,5). Guideline recommendations in determining drug therapy focus on the duration of disease, disease activity, and presence or absence of features indicative of poor prognosis. These medications should be used only by experts in RDs and their management.

Tab. 13.10: Biological response modifiers for RDs.

Generic name	Adult dosage	Adverse effects	Monitoring
Etanercept	25 mg SQ twice a week or 50 mg SQ once a week Indications: RA, JIA, psoriatic arthritis, ankylosing spondylitis (AS), others	Inhibits tumor necrosis factor (TNF) Side effects: increase risk of serious infection, reactivation of latent TB and hepatitis B, neoplasm (rare lymphoma), injection site reactions, allergic reactions, pancytopenia, new or worsening heart failure, hepatotoxicity	Tuberculin skin test, CBC, LFTs, Scr, hepatitis B and C serology for those with risk factors for infection
Infliximab	IV infusion: 3 mg/kg at 0, 2, and 6 weeks, then every 8 weeks Indications: RA, JIA, inflammatory bowel disease, psoriasis, AS May premedicate with H2 blocker, acetaminophen and/or corticosteroids	Anti-TNF monoclonal antibody. Inhibits tumor necrosis factor (TNF) Often used in combination with methotrexate Side effects similar to etanercept including increased risk for autoantibody formation and demyelinating disease	Tuberculin skin test, CBC, LFTs, Scr, hepatitis B and C serology for those with risk factors for infection
Abatacept	IV infusion: 500 to 1,000 mg at 0, 2, and 4 weeks, then monthly (dosage based on body weight)	Fusion protein that inhibits costimulation of T cells Nausea, headache, cough, dizziness, infusion-related reactions, serious infections,	Tuberculin skin test, hepatitis B C serology for those with risk factors for infection

(Continued)

Tab. 13.10: Biological response modifiers for RDs. (*Continued*)

Generic name	Adult dosage	Adverse effects	Monitoring
	Indications: RA, JIA	reactivation of latent TB and hepatitis B, antibody formation, malignancy	
Rituximab	IV infusion: 1,000 mg on days 1 and 15 in combination with methotrexate Premedication with corticosteroid recommended Indications: RA and non-Hodgkin's lymphoma	Monoclonal antibody selectively binds to CD20 Severe infusion-related reactions (occasionally fatal), anaphylactic reaction, rash, weakness, nausea, cough, hematologic toxicity, hyper- or hypotension, arrhythmias, tumor lysis syndrome, serious viral infections, reactivation of hepatitis B, fatal mucocutaneous reactions	CBC with platelets, hepatitis B and C serology for those with risk factors for infection
Adalimumab	40 mg subcutaneously every other week Indications: RA, JIA, Crohn's disease, AS, psoriasis	Anti-TNF monoclonal antibody; inhibits tumor necrosis factor (TNF). Side effects similar to other TNF inhibitors (see above).	Tuberculin skin test, CBC, LFTs, Scr, hepatitis B and C serology for those with risk factors for infection
Anakinra	100 mg/day subcutaneously Indication: RA	Antagonizes the interleukin-1 receptor Nausea, diarrhea, headache, serious infections (predominantly bacterial), injection-site reactions, neutropenia, antibody formation, hypersensitivity reactions Dose adjusted when CrCl <30 mL/min	CBC with platelets, Scr
Certolizumab pegol	400mg (2 SQ injections of 200 mg) at weeks 0, 2, and 4 and then 200 mg every other week Indications: Crohn disease, RA	Selective inhibitor of TNF-α Headache, fatigue, hypertension, back pain, rash, upper respiratory tract infections Same class warnings as noted with other TNF-α inhibitors (see above); risk of malignancy similar to placebo in clinical trials	Tuberculin skin test, CBC, LFTs, Scr, hepatitis B and C serology for those with risk factors for infection

(*Continued*)

Tab. 13.10: Biological response modifiers for RDs. (*Continued*)

Generic name	Adult dosage	Adverse effects	Monitoring
		Conjugated with polyethylene glycol to extend duration	
Golimumab	50 mg SQ once monthly Indications: RA, psoriatic arthritis, AS	Monoclonal antibody that binds to TNF-α Dizziness, hypertension, upper respiratory tract infections, injection-site reactions Same class warnings as noted with other TNF-α inhibitors (see above)	Tuberculin skin test, CBC, LFTs, Scr, hepatitis B and C serology for those with risk factors for infection
Tocilizumab	4 mg/kg IV infusion every 4 weeks; may increase to 8 mg/kg; maximum single dose of 800 mg Indications: RA, JIA Indicated after inadequate response to one or more TNF-α inhibitors	Interleukin-6 receptor monoclonal antibody Increased risk of serious infections, latent viral reactivation, bone marrow suppression, anaphylaxis, bowel perforation, increased LFTs, increased risk of malignancy, hypertension, increased LFTs, hyperlipidemia, antibody formation, infusion reaction Not to be initiated if ANC <2000/mm^3, platelets <100,000/mm^3, or AST/ALT >1.5 times the upper limit of normal Dosage modifications required for increased LFTs, neutropenia and thrombocytopenia (see manufacturer recommendations) May increase metabolism of drugs that are CYP 450 substrates.	Tuberculin skin test, Hepatitis B and C serology for those with risk factors for infection, CBC with platelets, LFTs, fasting lipid profile, blood pressure

RA, rheumatoid arthritis; JIA, juvenile idiopathic arthritis; TB, tuberculosis; CBC, complete blood count; LFT, liver function test; Scr, serum creatinine; IV, intravenous; SQ, subcutaneously; AST, aspartate transaminase; ALT, serum glutamic-pyruvic transaminase; ANC, absolute neurtrophil count.

13.4 Management of spondyloarthropathies

Management of these conditions with enthesitis/inflammation is similar to that used for JIA. Treatment is based on pain control with NSAIDs as well as rest and exercise. Depending on the specific condition, exercise is recommended to protect back flexibility and inserts to protect heels and plantar fascia. The addition of doxycycline for an acute exacerbation of reactive arthritis may be helpful by reducing the number of days of the acute episode. The judicious use of additional drugs for chronic or recalcitrant spondyloarthropathy include methotrexate, sulfasalazine, chronic NSAIDs, low-dose prednisone, and even the newer biological agents. Corticosteroid injection into involved joints can be very helpful. The treatment of associated or underlying conditions, such as psoriasis (chapter 2) or inflammatory bowel disease (chapter 5), is important.

13.5 Management miscellaneous RD and related disorders

▶Tab. 31.11 provides a list of various RDs, related conditions, and comments on overall pharmacologic management (4,20,21). SLE is discussed in section 13.6.

13.6 Systemic lupus erythematosus (SLE)

Systemic lupus erythematosus (SLE) is the second most common rheumatoid disease in adolescence; JIA is the first (1,2,3,4,5,6, ,22,23,24,25,26,27). SLE is found in 15 to 50 in 100,000 and has a female-to-male ratio of 8:1. SLE is more common in Hispanic, Asian, and African American patients.

Tab. 13.11: Miscellaneous RDs and related conditions.

Name	Comments	Pharmacologic treatment
Dermatomyositis	Rare autoimmune disorder involving the skin and striated muscles. Myopathic and neuropathic muscle weakness. Complement-mediated microangiopathy with muscle fiber destruction. Red or violaceous dermatitis in butterfly pattern; neck and shoulder pattern seen also. May see heliotrophe rash over eyelids with periorbital edema. Positive Gottron sign/papules. Variable lab work.	RD medications including corticosteroids and good skin care. Sun exposure to be avoided daily high-SPF sunscreen used. Physical therapy and occupational therapy for optimal muscle function. Use of steroids can include high-dose pulse methylprednisolone (maximum dose of 1 g/day for 3 days). Other meds can include methotrexate, hydroxychloroquine, IV immunoglobulin, mycophenolate mofetil, or cyclosporine. If on

(Continued)

Tab. 13.11: Miscellaneous RDs and related conditions. (*Continued*)

Name	Comments	Pharmacologic treatment
		long-term steroids: calcium and vitamin D supplementation.
Fibromyalgia	Seen in 3%–5% of older teen females. Present with chronic, diffuse pain of various body sites, with sleep disturbance, emotional lability, long history of chronic complaints, fatigue. Often, positive family history for fibromalgia and/or irritable bowel syndrome. Exam notes tender points over the back and anterior chest wall. Lab tests usually normal. Can use official criteria with major and minor criteria.	Variable treatments based on presenting concerns. Management focuses on pain control (avoid narcotics), improved sleep, reduced stress (psychotherapy as needed), judicious use of psychopharmacologic agents (low-dose amitryptyline, nortriptyline, fluoxetine, sertraline, anxiolytics, anticonvulsants). Pregabalin is an anticonvulsant that is FDA-approved for adults with neuropathic pain. Also physical therapy and active exercise program will help.
Hypersensitivity vasculitis	Diverse group of vasculitides with deposits of immune complexes in capillaries, venules, and sometimes arterioles. Antigen stimulation can be due to many factors – infections, drugs, others. Can include serum sickness, Henoch-Schönlein syndrome, mixed cryoglobulinemia.	Treatment of the specific syndrome. Removal of the offending antigen if possible. Antihistamine treatment for urticaria and immunosuppressive medications as needed, such immunosuppressive drugs for progressive renal disease.
Granulomatosis of (allergic angiitis and granulomatosis of) Churg and Strauss	Rare systemic vasculitis (fibrinoid necrosis of small to medium-sized vesssels) mostly in the skin, lungs, and peripheral nerves. Any organ can be involved. Eosinophilia and asthma often noted. Increased IGE and various allergies may be seen.	Supportive care and corticosteroids are key treatment principles. Cyclophosphamide may reduce relapse incidence. Others include methotrexate, azathioprine, infliximab, or IFN-α (21).
Joint hypermobility syndrome (JHS)	12% have hyperextensible joints; most prevalent in dancers, gymnasts, instrumental musicians; JHS diagnosis based on showing joint hyperextension in testing of five joint maneuvers. out Marfan's or Ehlers Danlos	Limit activities that cause pain, physical therapy (strengthening, bracing, pain control), analgesics (NSAIDs), avoid narcotics. Hypermobility tends to improve over time.

(*Continued*)

Tab. 13.11: Miscellaneous RDs and related conditions. (*Continued*)

Name	Comments	Pharmacologic treatment
	syndrome must be ruled out; joint laxity can lead to arthralgias, dislocations, transient joint effusions, and pain syndromes such as fibromyalgia. Higher incidence of mitral valve prolapse seen.	
Kawasaki disease	Acute systemic vasculitis developing mostly in children under age 5 (most under age 2), with highest rates noted in Japan. Etiology unknown. Can develop fever with polymorphous rash (classic: groin/buttocks), bilateral conjunctivitis (nonpurulent), oral changes (dry lips with cracking, bleeding, peeling, strawberry tongue), cervical lymphadenopathy, extremity changes (palmar redness, swollen hands/feet, dequamation. A variety of other features including coronary aneurysms detected on echocardiograms.	IV immune globulin (IVIG): 2 g/kg over 12 hours; can be repeated. Aspirin (80–100 mg/kg per day reduced to 3–5 mg/kg per day in children when fever subsides. Aspirin is a good anti-inflammatory and antiplatelet agent. Follow up with echocardiograms. Anticoagulation is prescribed in the presence of abnormal coronary arteries. Other medications used in resistant situations include IV methylprednisolone, plasmapheresis, cyclophosphamide, and infliximab.
Mixed connective tissue disease	Overlap syndrome with features of SLE, systemic slcerosis, arthritis, and mysoitis. Teens usually present with Raynaud's, puffy hands, and arthritis. Less renal disease seen than in children with SLE. Pulmonary hypertension (with anticardiolipin antibodies) and infections are the most common causes of death. Antibodies to extractable nuclear antigen ribonucleoprotein (anti-RNP) and against U1–70 kD small nuclear ribonucleoproteins (smRNP) are seen. May evolve into more classic RD or systemic sclerosis.	Supportive, corticosteroids; other RD drugs as necessary.
Osteoporosis	Decreased bone mass can develop in many conditions,	Careful use of drugs that can induce osteomalacia or

(*Continued*)

Tab. 13.11: Miscellaneous RDs and related conditions. (*Continued*)

Name	Comments	Pharmacologic treatment
	including use of steroids for RDs. It can be seen with chronic amenorrhea, eating disorders, renal disorders, GI disorders, metabolic disorders, chronic use of other drugs (as anticonvulsants), and others. Osteomalacia can arise in renal disease, vitamin D deficiency states, and inborn errors of vitamin D metabolism.	osteoporosis; followed by bone marrow measurements (DEXA). Dietary counseling and supplemental use of calcium and vitamin D. Judicious use of bisphosphonates (i.e., alendronate or risedronate).
Panarteritis nodosa (PAN)	Uncommon in adolescents; necrotizing fasciculitis of medium-sized vessels involving many tissues: kidneys, lungs, skin, joints, intestinal tract, peripheral nerves. Cutaneous PAN involves mainly skin. Lab results depend on what organs are involved but show signs of inflammation. Streptococcal screen require.	Supportive care; use of corticosteroids (oral and IV pulse) and other RD drugs depend on specific involvement. These include cyclophosphamide (IV or oral), methotrexate, azathioprine, dapsone, cyclosporine, and anti-TNF agents. Antibiotic prophylaxis is provided if there is an infectious trigger for the PAN.
Raynaud's phenomenon	Episodes of vasospasm stimulated by cold or stress. Fingers can turn white, then a dusky blue, and, with rewarming, bright red. Primary form has no underlying disorders. Nail fold changes include telangietasias. Some develop evidence of RDs over time. Some 10% of those with dermatomyositis , SLE, and adult RD develop Raynaud's phenomenon.	Patients should avoid cold exposure and use warm clothes; also avoid or manage emotional stress and avoid tobacco, since it can stimulate episodes. Severe situations require use of calcium channel blockers (nifedipine SR [30–60 mg/day] or amlodipine [2.5–10 mg/day]). Other drugs include losartan, bosentan, sildenafil, prazosin. ACE inhibitors (captopril or enalapril) are used for hypertension with renal disease. Disorders associated with Raynaud's must be treated. Methotrexate or mycophenolate mofetil used for skin involvement. Cyclophosphamide for pulmonary alveolitis.
Reflex sympathetic dystrophy (RSD) (complex regional pain syndrome	Trauma (even mild)-induced extremity that is very painful ("pins and needles"), mottled,	Pain control, prompt mobilization of affected extremity in acute episode, analgesics (NSAIDs),

(Continued)

Tab. 13.11: Miscellaneous RDs and related conditions. (*Continued*)

Name	Comments	Pharmacologic treatment
type I) (Old names: causalgia, Sudeck's atrophy, reflex neurovascular dystrophy)	swollen, cool. Overlying skin has increased sweating; sometimes is dry. Often confused with inflammatory arthritis. Lab work is usually normal. Bone scan or thermography can be helpful. May be secondary to underlying diabetes or degenerative cervical spine disease in adults.	physical therapy, biofeedback, counseling (cognitive behavioral therapy; chapter 8). Most resolve over time. Severe disorder can lead to contractures and disability. Low-dose amitriptyline (10–50 mg orally ½ hour before bedtime). Trial of anticonvulsant (as gabapentin). Give analgesic prior to a nerve block (sympathetic or epidural).
Secondary gout	Abnormal purine metabolism with hyperuricemia, urate crystal deposition in cartilage or joints, leading to arthritis. Mainly seen in adults. Seen in youths with neoplasms, blood dyscrasias, adverse effects of some drugs. Initial attack is in one joint; later attacks can occur with many joints: first metatarsophalangeal joint, ankle, midfoot, or knee.	Management of acute attack: NSAIDs (indomethacin), colchicine, steroids. Chronic hyperuricemia: Offending drugs must be removed and antihyperuricemia drugs (allopurinol, probenecid) used.
Systemic vasculitis	Group of idiopathic disorders with different clinical manifestations and involvement of different sizes of vessels. Common vasculitides of adolescents include Kawasaki disease and Henoch-Schönlein purpura.	Supportive, steroids, other RD medications depending on specific issues.
Takayasu's arteritis	Inflammation of the aorta and major branches. Called "pulseless" disease. Most patients are postpubertal females, especially of Asian (Japanese) descent. There is anorexia, fatigue, poor weight gain, growth inhibition, hypertension. There can be acute hypertensive encephalopathy with seizures, cerebral ischemia, congestive heart failure due to renal and systemic arterial occlusion.	High-dose corticosteroids, methotrexate, azathioprine; cyclophosphamide, mycophenolate mofetil, anti TNF-α therapy. Hypertension treated. Vascular surgery if possible. Poor prognosis.

Tab. 13.11: Miscellaneous RDs and related conditions. (*Continued*)

Name	Comments	Pharmacologic treatment
	Increased ESR and gamma globulin seen. Blood vessel studies reveal the abnormality.	
Weber-Christian disease (relapsing nodular nonsuppurative panniculitis)	Rare idiopathic disorder or collection of disorders with systemic vasculitis and successive crops of tender red nodules in subcutaneous fat of breasts, trunk, or thighs. Nodules appear over months to years and undergo fat liquefaction with release of oily material.	Supportive; corticosteroids.
Wegener's granulomatosis	Necrotizing, granulomatous angiitis involving upper and lower respiratory tract (90%), kidneys (>75%), joints (60%), and other organs. Fever and polyarthritis followed by lung or upper airway involvement. Extensive symptomatology. Varied neurologic features up to 50%. Lab data reflect inflammation; increased serum antineutrophil cytoplasmic antibody. Biopsy is diagnostic. *Limited Wegener's* refers to lesions in the orbi and respiratory tract but not the kidneys or vascular system.	High, rapid mortality rate in untreated individuals. Steroids, cyclophosphamide, other cytotoxic agents (i.e., azathioprine), and other RD drugs (i.e., methotrexate). Antibiotics may be helpful. Subglottic stenosis usually does not improve with use of systemic drugs; use frequent intratracheal dilation and injection of long-acting glucocorticoids; this may prevent the need for tracheostomy (21).
Systemic sclerosis (diffuse scleroderma)	Localized form involves linear scleroderma or morphea in the skin. Systemic form: rare in teens with multisystemic inflammatory changes. Most also develop Raynaud's phenomenon. Variant is the CREST syndrome.	Physical therapy to maintain joint function and keep the skin soft. Methotrexate may be helpful. Other RD medications (i.e., methotrexate plus steroids) are helpful depending on specific issues. Use steroids cautiously in systemic sclerosis to avoid triggering a renal crisis. Superficial morphea: topical steroids or ultraviolet (UV) therapy.

SPF, sun protective factor; FDA, Food and Drug Administration; IFN, interferons; NSAIDs, nonsteroidal antiflammatory drugs; RD, rheumatoid drugs; CREST, Calcinosis, Raynaud's syndrome, Esophageal dysmotility, Sclerodactyly, Telangiectasia.

13.6.1 Clinical features

Common features include arthritis, arthralgia, fever, fatigue, headache, and weight loss. SLE can have many other clinical features; specific diagnosis is based on the presence of 4 of 11 specific classification criteria (▶Tab. 13.12) including rash, arthritis, nephritis, serositis, neurologic or hematologic abnormalities, and specific serologic markers (▶Tab. 13.13).

Classic features include the SLE butterfly malar rash, alopecia, cutaneous vasculitis (livedo reticularis, palpable purpura), generalized photosensitivity, and others. SLE renal disease is noted in 50 to 70 percent and ranges from minimal mesangial proliferation to diffuse proliferative glomerulonephritis based on kidney biopsy. SLE inflammatory lesions can develop in the CNS, with resultant seizures, stroke, psychosis, and even coma.

SLE arthritis can resemble JIA or more commonly be seen as small joint swelling and stiffness in hands or feet; it is usually nondisfiguring and usually overshadowed by other SLE features. The term *Jaccoud's arthritis* refers to distinctive and reversible hand involvement see in SLE. The etiology of this autoimmune disease is unknown, although there are a number of drugs that can induce an SLE reaction (▶Tab. 13.14).

The presence of anti-dsDNA and various antibodies to cytoplasmic antigens is more specific and sensitive than a positive ANA test. The combination of depressed complement with elevated anti-dsDNA is 100 percent specific for SLE; these titers are also useful to monitor disease activity as well as prediction for an acute episode. One third of these patients have antiphospholipid antibodies or other lupus anticoagulants (▶Tab. 13.13).

13.6.2 Management

Specific management is based on organ involvement and response to medication. All patients are advised to use sunscreen with a high sun protective factor (SPF). Arthritis and mucocutaneous involvement is treated with NSAIDs and hydroxychloroquine. Systemic steroids are used for visceral disease including severe hematologic complications. Steroids can be started at 2 mg/kg per day of prednisone up to 60 to 80 mg/day. Alternative-day dosing is used when possible to reduce steroid side effects (▶Tab. 13.7). Some 25 percent of those on steroids develop avascular necrosis of the hips.

Severe disease (i.e., progressive renal or pulmonary insufficiency, systemic vasculitis, or CNS disease) requires larger doses of steroid: intravenous pulse methylprednisolone at 30 mg/kg up to 1,000 mg. Immunosuppressive medications are used for refractory SLE disease. Other medications used to treat SLE include methotrexate, azathioprine, cyclophosphamide, cyclosporine, intravenous gamma blobulin, and others (26). Anti-CD20 monoclonal antibodies are used to treat SLE hemolytic anemia and thrombocytopenia.

Diffuse proliferative glomerulonephritis is treated with monthly intravenous cyclophosphamide, since steroids are often not enough to prevent significant renal progression. Methotrexate, azathioprine, and cyclosporine are also used and can be used to lower steroid doses (26). Autologous bone marrow transplantation is used for refractory SLE disease. Those patients with antiphospholipid antibodies or lupus anticoagulant are at increased risk for arterial and venous thromboses with resultant strokes, thrombophlebitis, and miscarriages. If contraception is requested, estrogen-based contraceptives are contraindicated.

Tab. 13.12: Diagnostic criteria for SLE.

Criterion	Comment
1. Facial butterfly rash	Flat or raised malar erythema with or without edema. May develop vesicles, crusting, or ulcerations. Present in half of all cases. Nonspecific for SLE.
2. Discoid lupus	Scaly erythematous plaques predominating on face and scalp with or without scarring, atrophy, pigmentary changes, and telangiectasia. May be an isolated cutaneous disorder or part of a systemic disease. Other skin lesions that may be seen with SLE include urticaria; tender nodules on palms, fingertips, and soles; digit gangrene; and periungal erythema.
3. Photosensitivity	Includes sun exposure–induced urticarial plaques on the skin.
4. Oral or nasopharyngeal ulceration	May result in epistaxis or perforation of the septum.
5. Nephritis or nephrotic syndrome	Renal involvement occurs in half of cases, including persistent proteinuria, hematuria, or cellular casts (glomerular or tubular).
6. Joint swelling	Polyarthritis (two or more peripheral joints) similar to juvenile rheumatoid arthritis but without joint destruction. Present in nine of ten cases.
7. Pleuritis or pericarditis	Also may develop peritonitis, myocarditis, endocarditis (Libman-Sacks),or parenchymal lung disease. Cardiac tamponade is rare.
8. Psychosis or convulsions	Other CNS manifestations that may be seen include mononeuritis, cranial nerve neuropathy, chorea, myelopathy, aseptic meningitis, and cerebrovascular accidents.
9. Hemolytic anemia, leukopenia, lymphopenia, and/or thrombocytopenia	Coombs test will be positive if hemolytic anemia is present. Splenomegaly is also seen.
10. Positive immunoserology	The LE cell is positive in 50% of SLE patients; not currently widely used. Other tests include anti-DNA antibody to native DNA in abnormal titer, anti-Sm antibody to Sm nuclear antigen, persistent false-positive serologic test for syphilis (with negative FTA test).
11. Antinuclear antibody	Fluorescence or equivalent assay.

Established by the American Rheumatism Association or American College of Rheumatology in 1971 and revised in 1982. The presence of four or more of the criteria (serially or simultaneously) is associated with a positive pathologic diagnosis in nine of ten cases.

Tab. 13.13: Laboratory features of SLE.

Positive ANA (good as screening test; lacks specificity)
Antibodies to double-stranded DNA (anti-dsDNA) and cytoplasmic antigens
Low C3 and C4 levels
Leukopenia
Low platelet count
Coombs-positive hemolytic anemia
Anti-phospholipid antibodies
Other lupus anticoagulants

Tab. 13.14: Drugs that can induce SLE reactions.

Hydralazine	Captopril
Propylthiouracil	Isoniazide
Chlorpramazine	Quinidine
Alpha methyldopa	Beta blockers
Lithium	Penicillamine
Sulfasalazine	Procainamide
Antibiotics	Oral contraceptives
Anticonvulsants a. Diphenylhydantoin b. Ethosuximide c. Trimethadone	

(See chapter 19 in Greydanus DE, Patel DR, Omar HA, Feucht C, Merrick J: Adolescent Medicine – Pharmacotherapeutics in General, Mental and Sexual Health. Berlin: de Gruyter; 2012.) These youth may be placed on low dose aspirin. Life-long anticoagulation is needed for those with a significant thrombotic event. Death in SLE patients occurs due to infection, renal failure, pulmonary hemorrhage, severe CNS disease, and early myocardial infarction. The degree of renal involvement directly affects morbidity and mortality.

13.7 Conclusions

Rheumatoid diseases (RDs) comprise a wide variety of complex autoimmune disorders (4,28,29,30,31,32,33). The hallmark of the RD is the presence of a chronic inflammatory process that, if left uncontrolled, often leads to significant morbidity and even mortality. The most common RD is juvenile idiopathic arthritis (JIA), and SLE is the second most common. Management includes nonpharmacologic measures (such as physical therapy, occupational therapy, splints, braces, assistive devices) and pharmacologic measures, as reviewed in this chapter. A wide range of pharmacologic agents are available to the specialist in rheumatology, including analgesics (NSAIDs), corticosteroids, DMARDs (disease-modifying antirheumatic drugs), and biological response modifiers. Concepts of other RDs as well as SLE are also presented.

References

1. Cassidy JT, Petty RE, eds. Textbook of pediatric rheumatology, 5th ed. Philadelphia, PA: Saunders Elsevier, 2005.
2. Junnila JL, Cartwright VW. Chronic musculoskeletal pain in children: Part II. Rheumatic causes. Am Fam Physician 2006;74:293–300.
3. Klippel JH, Crofford LJ, Stone JH, Weyand CM, eds. Primer on the rheumatic diseases, 12th ed. Atlanta, GA: Arthritis Foundation, 2001.
4. Moore MD. Rheumatic diseases, In: Greydanus DE, Patel DR, Pratt HD, eds. Essential adolescent medicine. New York: McGraw Hill, 2006:201–34.
5. National Institute of Arthritis and Musculoskeletal and Skin Diseases. Arthritis and rheumatic diseases. Bethesda, MD: National Institutes Health Publication, 08-4999, 2008.
6. Patel DR, Moore MD. Concepts of rheumatology. In: Greydanus, Patel DR, Reddy VN, Feinberg An, Omar HA, eds. Handbook of clinical pediatrics: An update for the ambulatory pediatrician. Singapore: World Scientific, 2010:697–713.
7. Petty RE, Southwood TR, Manners P, Baum J, Glass DN, Goldenberg J, et al. International League of Associations for Rheumatology classification of juvenile idiopathic arthritis, second revision, Edmonton, 2001. J Rheumatol 2004;31(2):390–92.
8. Agarwal M, Sawhney S. Laboratory tests in pediatric rheumatology. Indian J Pediatr 2010;77(9):1011–16.
9. Hilderson D, Corstijens F, Moons P, Wouters C, Westhovens R. Adolescents with juvenile idiopathic arthritis: who cares after the age of 16? Clin Exp Rheumatol 2010;28 (5):790–97.
10. Martini A, Lovell DJ. Juvenile idiopathic arthritis: state of the art and future perspectives. Ann Rheum Dis 2010;69(7):1260–63.
11. Singh S, Mehra S. Approach to polyarthritis. Indian J Pediatr 2010; 77(9):1005–10.
12. Hashkes PJ, Laxer RM.: Medical treatment of juvenile idiopathic arthritis. JAMA 2005;294(13):1671–84.
13. Hayward K, Wallace CA. Recent developments in anti-rheumatic drugs in pediatrics: Treatment of juvenile idiopathic arthritis. Arthritis Res Ther 2009;11(1):216–20.
14. Beresford MW, Baildam EM. New advances in the management of juvenile idiopathic arthritis-1: non-biological therapy. Arch Dis Child Educ Pract Ed 2009;94(5):144–50.
15. Holzinger D, Frosch M, Föll D. Methotrexate in the therapy of juvenile idiopathic arthritis. Z Rheumatol 2010;69(6):496–504.
16. Ruperto N, Martini A. Pediatric rheumatology: JIA, treatment and possible risk of malignancies. Nat Rev Rheumatology 2011;7(1):6–7.
17. Neovius M, Simard JF, Askling J. ARTIS study group. Ann Rheum Dis 2011;70(4):624–29.
18. Quartier P. Current treatments for juvenile idiopathic arthritis. Joint Bone Spine 2010;77 (6):511–16.
19. Lamot L, Bukovac LT, Vidovic M, Frieta M, Harjacek M. The head to head comparison of etanercept and infliximab in treating children with juvenile idiopathic arthritis. Clin Exp Rheumatol 2011;29(1): 131–39.
20. Kimura Y, Walco GA. Treatment of chronic pain in pediatric rheumatic disease. Nature Clin Pract Rheumatol 2007;3:210–18.
21. Light MJ, Blaisdell CJ, Homnick DN, Schechter MS, Weinberger MM, eds. Pediatric pulmonology. Elk Grove Village, IL: American Academy of Pediatrics, 2011.
22. Pineles D, Valente A, Warren B, Peterson MG, Lehman TJ, Moorthy LN. Worldwide incidence and prevalence of pediatric onset systemic lupus erythematosus. Lupus 2011 Jul 18. [Epub ahead of print]

23. Mikita N, Ikeda T, Ishiquro M, Furukawa F. Recent advances in cytokines in cutaneous and systemic lupus erythematosus. J Dermatol 2011 July 18. [Epub ahead of print]
24. Manson JJ, Rahman A. Systemic lupus erythematosus. Orphanet J Rare Dis 2006;1(6):22–26.
25. Kalunian K, Joan TM. New directions in the treatment of systemic lupus erythematosus. Curr Med Res Opin 2009;25(6):1501–14.
26. Szer IS, Kimura Y, Malleson PN, Southwood TR, eds. Arthritis in children and aolescents: Juvenile idiopathic arthritis. Oxford: Oxford University Press, 2006.
27. Aringer M, Hiepe F. Systemic lupus erythematosus. Z Rheumatol 2011;70(4):313–23.
28. Wright E. Musculoskeletal injuries and disorders. In: Berardi R, ed. Handbook of nonprescription drugs, an interactive approach to self-care. Washington DC: American Pharmacists Association, 2009:95–113.
29. Drugstore. Topical analgesics. Accessed 2011 Jun 02. URL: http://www.drugstore.com/search/search_results.asp?N50&Ntx5mode%2Bmatchallpartial&Ntk5All&srchtree5 5&Ntt5topical1analgesics. Accessed July 5, 2011.
30. Facts and comparisons. Drug information full monographs. Wolters Kluwer Health, Incorporated. Accessed 2011 Jun 02. URL: http://0-online.factsandcomparisons.com.libcat.ferris.edu/index.aspx.
31. Pediatric Lexi-drugs. Lexi-Comp, Inc. 2011. Accessed 2011 Jun 02. URL: http://www.lexi.com/
32. Drugs for rheumatoid arthritis. Treatment guidelines. Med Letter 2009;7(81):37–46.
33. Beukelman T, Patkar NM, Saag KG, Tolleson-Rinehart S, Cron RQ, DeWitt EM, et al. 2011 American college of rheumatology recommendations for the treatment of juvenile idiopathic arthritis: initiation and safety monitoring of therapeutic agents for the treatment of arthritis and systemic features. Arthritis Care Res 2011;63(4):465–82.

14 Concepts of metabolic disorders

Donald E. Greydanus and Cynthia L. Feucht

Inborn errors of metabolism (IEMs), or metabolic disorders, are complex conditions involving abnormalities in the biochemical and metabolic pathways necessary for healthy human existence. They are often caused by partial or total deficiency of key enzymes and usually present in infancy or early childhood. Some may not be identified until adolescence or even during the adult years. This discussion reviews some of the IEMs that can become evident in the adolescent years, such as adrenoleukodystrophy, glycogen storage diseases, lysosomal storage diseases, urea cycle disorders, and others. Management focuses on symptomatic treatment and, when available as well as affordable, enzyme replacement therapies. Gene therapy and stem cell transplantation are options under current research, in addition to finding more replacement enzymes.

14.1 Introduction

Inborn errors of metabolism (IEMs), or metabolic disorders, are unusual, complex conditions involving abnormalities in the biochemical and metabolic pathways necessary for human life. Although often identified in infancy or childhood, some of these conditions may not be diagnosed until adolescence or adulthood. The initial term *inborn errors of metabolism* was introduced by Sir Archibald Garrod in 1902 and referred to cystinuria, albinism, alkaptonuria, and benign pentosuria (1). Phenylketonuria (PKU) was identified in 1934 by Ivar Asbjørn Følling; by the second half of the twentieth century, over 500 IEMs had been identified (2). ▶Tab. 14.1 presents a partial list of IEMs (2).

IEMs are complex conditions that are usually genetic, typically inherited in an autosomal recessive manner, although a few are X-linked recessive conditions (i.e., Fabry's disease, ornithine carbamylase deficiency, or pyruvate dehydrogenase deficiency). Autosomal dominance is noted in Marfan's syndrome, familial hypercholesterolemia, and acute intermittent porphyria. Some IEMs are caused by mitochondrial genome mutations and there can be enzyme deficiencies or problems with cellular transporters.

14.2 Incidence

The incidence of IEMs varies to a considerable extent depending on the specific condition. For example, congenital hypothyroidism is noted in 1 of 4,500 cases, congenital adrenal hyperplasia in 1 of 10,000 cases, medium-chain acyl CoA dehydrogenase (MCAD) phenylketonuria in 1 of 15,000 cases, and galactosemia in 1 of 30,000 cases. A number of IEMs are much rarer – such as fatty acid oxidation disorders, organic acidemias, homocystinuria, maple syrup urine disease (MSUD), and others – and noted in 1 of 100,000 cases (2). Some IEMs are seen in increased incidence

Tab. 14.1: Inborn errors of metabolism (2).

---

1. Aminoacidurias (disorders of amino acid metabolism)

    a. Homocystinuria

    b. Maple syrup urine disease

    c. Nonketotic hyperglycemia

    d. PKU (phenylketonuria)

    e. Tyrosinemia

2. Carbohydrate metabolism disorders

    a. Galactosemia

    b. Glycogen storage diseases

3. Fatty acid oxidation disorders

    a. Short-chain acyl coenzyme A (CoA) dehyrogenase (SCAD)

    b. Medium-chain acyl CoA dehyrogenase (MCAD)

    c. Long-chain acyl CoA dehyrogenase (LCAD)

    d. Very long-chain acyl CoA dehyrogenase (VLCAD)

4. Lipid storage disorders

    a. Gaucher's disease

    b. Metachromatic leukodystrophy

    c. Tay-Sachs disease

5. Lysosomal disorders

    a. Combined defects

    b. Glycoproteinosis

    c. I-cell disease

    d. Sphingolipidosis

    e. Mucopolysaccharidoses (MPS)

    • MPS I (Hurler-Scheie disease)

    • MPS II (Hunter's disease)

    • MPS III (Sanfilippo disease)

    • MPS IV (Morquio's disease)

    • MPS VI

    • MPS VII

6. Mitochondrial metabolisms disorders

    a. Glutaric aciduria

    b. MELAS (**m**itochondrial **m**yopathy, **e**ncephalopathy, **l**actic **a**cidosis, and **s**troke-like episodes)

    c. Pyruvate dehydrogenase deficiency

7. Metal metabolism disorders

    a. Hemochromatosis

    b. Menkes disease

    c. Wilson's disease

(Continued)

Tab. 14.1: Inborn errors of metabolism (2). (*Continued*)

8. Organic acidemias (organic acid metabolism disorders)

   a. Methylmalonic acidemia

   b. Propionic acidemia

9. Peroxisomal disorders

   a. Adrenoleukodystrophy

   b. Adult Refsum's disease

   c. Chondrodysplasia punctata

   d. Zellweger's syndrome

10. Purine transport metabolism disorder

   a. Lesch-Nyhan syndrome

11. Steroid pathway disorders

   a. Congenital adrenal hyperplasia

   b. Smith-Lemli-Opitz syndrome

12. Transport disorders

   a. Cystinosis

   b. Hypercholesterolemia

13. Urea cycle disorders

   a. Arginosuccinate deficiency

   b. Carbamoyl phosphate synthetase deficiency

   c. Ornithine transcarbamylase deficiency

14. Miscellaneous

   a. Hemoglobinopathies

   b. Hypothyroidism

among certain populations, such as Tay-Sachs disease in the Ashkenazi Jewish population or maple syrup urine disease (MSUD) in Pennsylvania Mennonites. Consanguinity is a factor in some of these conditions.

14.3 Presentation

IEMs may present with *metabolic* syndromes (acute acidotic or hypoglycemia crises), *hepatic* syndromes (liver disease with abnormal liver function tests), *cardiac* syndromes (acute cardiac myopathy or cardiovascular collapse), or *neurologic* syndromes (altered mental status or neurological functioning). The neurologic syndromes can have acute or chronic presentations and involve seizures, sensory dysfunction, coma, changes of tone, intellectual deterioration, behavioral dysfunction, psychosis, and others. In the metabolic presentations, there can be acidosis, hypoglycemia, or hyperammonemia (i.e., urea cycle defects). There can also be progressive, chronic cellular storage disorders with variable presentations.

Some cases – such as metachromatic leukodystrophy, Tay-Sachs disease, Gaucher's disease, lysosomal storage disorders, and others – can present later in childhood (2). There can be progressive neurologic deterioration, and some conditions lead to mental subnormality that appears in adolescence or adulthood (▶Tab. 14.2) (3). A wide variety of features can be seen including dysmorphic phenotypes as well as abnormalities in different organ systems, such as the gastrointestinal, dermatologic, hematologic, and other systems.

Unique odors can be present:, burnt sugar or maple syrup as in MSUD; fruity in acidemias (propionic or methylmalonic); mousy (musty) in PKU, cheese-like ("sweaty socks") in isovaleric acidemia, malt-like in methionine malabsorption, fish-like in trimethylaminuria or carnitine excess, cat urine–like in 3-methylcrotonic acidemia or 3-hydroxy-3-methyl glutaric aciduria, or cabbage-like in tyrosinemia (2).

Thus a careful evaluation along with a high index of clinical suspicion is necessary to make the correct diagnosis, often in consultations with experts in genetics, metabolic disorders, and others. The diagnosis may be delayed for many years if the presentation is nonspecific or mild, often due to a partial enzyme deficiency.

14.3.1 Mental subnormality

As noted, IEMs can result in variable levels of intellectual and developmental disability (IDD), and severe to profound IDD is usually diagnosed in early childhood. Routine metabolic screening is usually not helpful in a youth with IDD unless clues are found in the evaluation, such as new-onset psychiatric or neurologic features (4,5). Selective testing for metabolic disorders may be helpful, including laboratory work such as blood studies (i.e., lactate, quantitative amino acids, aldolase, creatine kinase, acylcarnitine, lipid profile), urine studies (i.e., quantitative amino acids, organic acids, myoglobin), imaging (magnetic resonance imaging of the brain, echocardiography), muscle and/or skin biopsies, and genetic studies.

Tab. 14.2: Adult (adolescent-onset) metabolic disorders with mental retardation.

1. Amino acid disorder
   a. Homocystinuria
2. Lipid storage disorders
   a. Juvenile metachromatic leukodystrophy
   b. Adult metachromatic leukodystrophy
   c. Mannosidosis
   d. Niemann-Pick disease type C
   e. GM1 gangliosidosis
   f. GM2 gangliosidosis
3. Mucopolysaccharidoses
   a. Sanfillipo gisease type B
   b. Sanfillipo gisease type D
4. Peroxisomal disorder
   a. X-linked adrenoleukodystrophy
5. Urea cycle disorders
   a. Ornithine transcarbamylase deficiency

Chromosomal abnormalities are the most common identifiable causes found in evaluations for IDD in adolescents; aneuploidy is the most common defect, followed by abnormal X-linked genes, as in fragile-X syndrome or X-linked adrenoleukodystrophy (3). Over 200 genes causing X-linked mental retardation have been identified (3).

Finding a specific cause for an adolescent's mental retardation can be beneficial to both the family and youth, with closure being brought to the many years if searching to find a reason for the IDD. The youth and his or her normal-IQ siblings may have worries regarding their reproductive futures and may request a full genetic evaluation.

14.3.2 Phenylketonuria (PKU)

This discussion presents comments about a number of IEMs that can present in the adolescent or even adult years. Sometimes the paucity of symptoms hides the diagnosis for many years, often because of a partial and not absolute deficiency of the responsible enzyme or enzymes. For example, PKU is usually identified in infancy and is caused by a defect of phenylalanine hydroxylase, which converts phenylalanine to tyrosine. A plasma amino acid screen reveals very high levels of phenylalanine and the urine contains phenylpyruvic acid. Although the individual may be normal at birth, the toxic levels of phenylalanine result in an infant with emesis, irritability, and eventual neurologic injury with mental retardation; the urine has a musty or mousy odor. PKU can also lead to generalized hypopigmentation, leading to the classic blond and fair-skinned PKU child owing to the blockage of phenylalanine to tyrosine.

A newborn screen identifies the PKU and allows treatment, which has traditionally consisted of restricting dietary intake of phenylalanine for the life of the individual so that plasma phenylalanine is at a safe level (i.e., not too high or not too low). Medication is now also available – sapropterin dihydrochloride (Kuvan), which is a synthesized normal cofactor for phenylalanine hydroxylase (tetrahydrobiopterin [BH4]) and boosts phenylalanine levels residual enzyme activity in those with mild PKU mutations.

Thus the clinician will usually encounter an adolescent with PKU who has been diagnosed in infancy and is on the proper diet management and perhaps sapropterin if a mild PKU condition is present (▶Tab. 14.3). If this youth goes off the diet plan, neurologic injury may develop and include concentration problems, cognitive impairment, psychosocial problems, and even psychosis.

14.3.3 Maple Syrup Urine Disease (MSUD)

MSUD is a disorder of branched-chain amino acid metabolism caused by deficiency of four different enzymes and leading to the oxidative decarboxylation of ketoacids. It is usually diagnosed in infancy and the plasma amino acid screen reveals an increase in allo-isoleucine (pathognomonic for MSUD), isoleucine, leucine, and valine. The infant develops an acute metabolic crisis with metabolic acidosis and massive ketonuria. A variety of symptoms develop, including feeding difficulties, lethargy, emesis, abnormal breathing, seizures, opisthotonos, rigidity, cerebral edema, mental retardation, and death. The maple syrup smell of the urine led to the name of this disease, which was first identified in 1934 (2).

Treatment is early diagnosis with a lifetime dietary restriction of branched-chain amino acids and a diet that is low in isoleucine, leucine, and valine; the levels of

Tab. 14.3: Medications for inborn errors of metabolism.

Medication	Indication	Adult dosage	Side effects	Comments
Penicillamine	Cystinuria	Initial: 250 mg/day Usual dose: 2g/day (1–4g/day) Also administer pyridoxine 25 day/day	Aplastic anemia, pruritus/rash, hypersensitivity reactions, proteinuria, membraneous glomerulopathy, increased skin friability, myasthenic syndrome, neurological toxicity, bone marrow suppression, drug fever, mouth ulcers, GI distress, anorexia, altered taste, neuropathy, intrahepatic cholestasis. Avoid during pregnancy and lactation. Avoid interruption in therapy due to risk of sensitivity reactions with reinstitution. Avoid in renal insufficiency.	The greater the fluid intake the lower the dose required. Administer 1 hour before or 2 hours after meals. Administer at least 1 hour apart from other drugs, food, or milk.
Pyridoxine (vitamin B6)	Homocystinuria	Usual: 300–600 mg/day Range: 25–600 mg/day	Sensory neuropathic syndromes, ataxia, paresthesias, unstable gait, photoallergic reactions.	May be given in conjunction with vitamin B12 and folate. Drug interactions with levodopa and phenytoin.
Betaine	Homocystinuria	3 g orally twice daily	GI distress, nausea.	Dissolve in 4–6 ounces of water and administer immediately. Monitor plasma homocysteine levels.
Glycine	Isovaleric acidemia	150 mg/kg per day (orally)	Nausea, vomiting.	Avoid in anuric patients.
Biotin	Multiple carboxylase deficiency	Usual dose: 10–40 mg daily	GI upset.	Anticonvulsants may impair biotin absorption.

Lorenzo's oil	Adrenoleukodystrophy	Pediatric: 2–3 mL/kg per day (based on one study)	Thrombocytopenia, purpura, petechiae, bleeding, GI upset, gingivitis, increased LFTs.	Dietary supplement: no standard regulation in the United States. Triglyceride mixture of glycerol trierucate and glycerol trioleate in 1:4 ratio. May reduce risk of developing cerebral disease.
Pyrimethamine	GM2 gangliosidosis	25–100 mg/day (based on one open-label phase I/II clinical trial in adults) Consider addition of daily folinic acid supplement	Folic acid deficiency, hemolytic anemia (with G6PD deficiency), severe hypersensitivity reactions, anorexia, vomiting, atrophic glossitis, bone marrow suppression, hyperphenylalaninemia. May be carcinogenic. Use with caution in renal and hepatic impairment.	Increased incidence of adverse events with escalating dose in trial. Administer with food to minimize vomiting. Drug interactions with myelosuppressive agents and antifolate drugs.
Genistein	Sanfilippo syndrome	5 mg/kg per day in divided doses Dosage based on two open-label trials	Constipation, nausea, bloating, diarrhea, insomnia, rash.	Studies utilized a genistein-rich soy isoflavone extract. No adverse effects reported in the two trials. Supplements are not regulated by the FDA. Isoflavone content can vary among the different forms of soy.
Sapropterin (Kuvan)	Phenylketonuria (mild)	Initial: 10 mg/kg per day	Abdominal pain, headache, diarrhea, nausea, vomiting, cough, pharyngolaryngeal pain, rhinorrhea,	Used in conjunction with a phenylalanine-restricted diet. Phenylalanine blood levels must be

(Continued)

Tab. 14.3: Medications for inborn errors of metabolism. (*Continued*)

Medication	Indication	Adult dosage	Side effects	Comments
		Maintenance: 5–20 mg/kg per day	bruising, neutropenia. Use with caution in hepatic and renal impairment (not evaluated).	monitored to determine response to therapy. Administered with food to increase absorption. Tablets must be dissolved and administered immediately in 4–8 oz water/apple juice and take within 15 min. *Drug interactions with levodopa , antifolate drugs and PDE-5 inhibitors

References: Facts and Comparisons. Drug information full monographs. Wolters Kluwer Health, Incorporated. Available at: http://0-online.factsandcomparisons.com.libcat.ferris.edu/index.aspx. Accessed August 15, 2011.

AltMedDex System (electronic version). Thomson Reuters, Greenwood Village, Colorado, USA. Available at http://www.thomsonhc.com. Accessed August 17, 2011.

DRUGDEX System (electronic version). Thomson Reuters, Greenwood, Village, Colorado, USA. Available at http://www.thomsonhc.com. Accessed August 17, 2011.

Delgadillo V, O'Callaghan M, Artuch R, Montero R, Pineda M. Genistein supplementation in patients affected by sanfilippo disease. J Inherit Metab Dis. 2011; May 10 [Epub ahead of print].

Piotrowska E, Jakobkiewicz-Banecka J, Tylki-Symanska A, Liberek A, Mary naik A, et al. Genistein-rich soy isoflavone extract in substrate reduction therapy for sanfilippo syndrome: an open-label, pilot study in 10 pediatric patients. Curr Ther Res 2008;69(2):166–79.

Natural Medicines Comprehensive Database. Evidence-based monographs. Therapeutics Research Faculty, Stockton, CA, USA. Available at http://0-naturaldatabase.therapeuticresearch.com.libcat.ferris.edu/home.aspx?cs=MHSLA~CP&s=ND. Accessed August 19, 2011.

Testai F, Gorelick F. Inherited metabolic disorders and stroke part 2, homocystinuria, organic acidurias and urea cycle disorders. Arch Neurol 2010;67 (2):148–53.

Clarke J, Mahuran D, Sathe S, Kolodny E, Rigat B, Raiman J, et al. An open-label phase I/II clinical trial of pyrimethamine for the treatment of patients affected with chronic GM2 gangliosidosis (Tay-Sachs or Sandhoff variants). Mol Genet Metab 2011;102(1):6–12.

these amino acids should be at the "Goldilocks level" – not to low and not to high for normal growth and development. As with PKU, the clinician normally encounters an adolescent with MSUD who has been diagnosed in infancy and is getting the proper dietary management. Rare situations do arise in which a mild mutation of one of the four MSUD enzymes allows a later presentation and perhaps more elusive symptoms. A minority of PKU patients are also thiamine-responsive.

14.3.4 Adrenoleukodystrophy (ALD)

ALD (Schilder's disease) is an X-linked recessive disorder due to dysfunction of beta oxidation of very long chain fatty acids (VLCFAs). It is the most common peroxisomal disorder; peroxisomes are organelles present in all cells except red blood cells, with many roles in key enzymes including the oxidation of VLCFAs. ALD is the result of mutations in the gene that encodes ALDP; it affects 1 in 21,000 males. If female hetero-zygotes are included, the overall frequency is 1 in 16,800. Females who carry the gene can develop features of ALD that are usually milder than those noted in males. The ALDP protein is involved in the breakdown of VLCFAs (12–18 carbons in length) found in normal diet. Lack of this protein leads to high levels of VLCFAs with damage to the peripheral nervous system, brain, and adrenal gland.

Evaluation reveals increased levels of VLCFAs (especially C26:0), and MRI can iden-tifies evidence of demyelination; cultured skin fibroblasts show the dysfunction of beta-oxidation of VLCFAs. Technology for the prenatal diagnosis of ALD is available and useful for preventing disease transmission.

The onset is usually between 3 and 10 years of age, and the disease may begin with ADHD-like or behavioral symptoms. Youths with this neurodegenerative, demyelinat-ing disorder develop a myriad of symptoms, including dementia, epilepsy, sensory loss (vision [optic atrophy] and hearing), spastic quadriplegia with ataxia, joint pains, dys-phagia, and others. Adrenal insufficiency may develop with hypoglycemia and salt-wasting episodes as well as hyperpigmentation similar to that seen in Addison's disease (6). Death will occur if this is not treated.

Management of ALD is based on the dietary restriction of VLCFAs and ingestion of shorter-chain fatty acids. However, restriction of VLCFAs does not stop cerebral deterioration once it develops. Correction of the adrenal insufficiency is important. Adding Lorenzo's oil (4:1 combination of glycerol trioleate and glycerol trierucate) can lower VLCFA levels in half of these patients; however, it does not lead to a sig-nificant improvement or prevent the overall disease (▶Tab. 14.3). Research is focus-ing on bone marrow transplantation in boys with childhood onset and also stem cell gene therapy (7,8). Hematopoietic stem cell transplantation can stabilize or even reverse cerebral demyelination if it is performed early but after differentiation of mild from severe disease can be made. The development of modern gene therapy viral vectors is under way; it seeks to allow the targeting of the leukodystrophy dis-ease gene into oligodendrocytes or astrocytes in order to treat various forms of leukodystrophies (8).

Another variant, adrenomyeloneuropathy (AMN), may develop in adolescents or adults with urinary dysfunction and spastic paraparesis due to distal axonopathy, mostly of the spinal cord. AMN may also be seen in females who are heterozygotes for ALD. AMN patients can also develop adrenal insufficiency, and this may be the cause of adrenal insufficiency in one out of three individuals with Addison's disease. Features also noted include psychosis, mania, and depression.

14.3.5 Metachromatic leukodystrophy (MLD)

Adolescents may develop the juvenile or adult form of MLD, which is an autosomal recessive lysosomal storage disease due to a deficiency of the enzyme arylsulfatase A. This can be identified in white blood cells or cultured skin fibroblasts; there is also increased sulfatide in the urine (9). There is intralysosomal storage of sulfatides (sphingolipid cerebroside 3-sulfates), which are found in high amounts in myelin and neurons (10).

Symptoms are due to demyelination and neurodegeneration; these include ataxia, painful joints, pain with swallowing, peripheral neuropathy, spasticity, personality changes (social withdrawal, obsessive features), deterioration in schoolwork, and others. There is also a heterozygous state. Research is focusing on hematopoietic stem cell gene therapy and intracerebral gene transfer (brain gene therapy) (10).

14.3.6 Refsum's disease

Classic or adult Refsum's disease is a rare disorder due to impaired alpha-oxidation of branched-chain fatty acids, leading to increase of phytanic acids and its derivatives in plasma and various tissues. It is also called heredopathia atactica polyneuritiformis. It should not be confused with infantile Refsum's disease, which is a peroxisomal disorder seen in infants. Adult Refsum's disease can present in the school-age child or adolescent with retinopathy, night blindness, cataracts, peripheral neuropathy, ataxia, anosmia, and sensorineural hearing loss. Skin changes may arise that resemble eczema or ichthyosis. Treatment includes placing the individuals on a phytanic acid–restricted diet that includes avoidance of fats from ruminant animals and some fish. Plasmapheresis has also been tried in some situations.

14.3.7 Glycogen storage disease type I

Glycogen storage disease type I (GSD I or von Gierke's disease) is the most common of the several types of glycogen storage diseases and is due to deficiency of the enzyme glucose-6-phosphatase, leading to hypoglycemia, lactic acidosis, hyperlipidemia, and hyperuricemia. It is an autosomal recessive condition with three subtypes: GSD Ia (mutations of G6PC), GSD Ib (mutations of G6PT1), and GSD Ic (other mutations).

Growth failure and developmental delay (including mental retardation) occurs in children in chronically poor metabolic control (11). Other problems include recurrent episodes of metabolic acidosis, neutropenia, impaired platelet aggregation (with epistaxis), and hepatomegaly. Additional problems may arise in adolescents and adults, such as depression, pancreatitis, hyperuricemic gout, hepatic adenomas, chronic renal failure, and premature atherosclerosis (12). Hepatic adenomas are found in most of the affected adults; they can bleed or undergo malignant transformation. Proteinuria develops with renal hypertension, renal stones, and eventual development of focal segmental glomerulonephritis.

Treatment involves prevention of hypoglycemia, metabolic acidosis, hyperlipidemia, and increased uric acid levels. Dietary control is important in this respect; an inexpensive way to help is with the use of cornstarch, which provides gradually digested glucose. Allopurinol may be needed to manage hyperuricemia (▶Tab. 14.4) and statin medications may be used to treat hyperlipidemia. Liver transplantation has been used in selected cases.

14.3.8 Glycogen storage disease type II

Glycogen storage disease type II (GSD II, Pompe disease, or acid maltase deficiency) is due toa deficiency in the acid alpha-glucosidase (GAA) enzyme; it is inherited in an autosomal recessive manner. Laboratory data include increased serum creatine kinase and urinary oligosaccharides along with a complete or partial deficiency of GAA. The *infantile* type presents in utero or infancy with failure to thrive. The *late-onset* type (childhood, juvenile, or adult) presents with respiratory dysfunction with proximal muscle weakness without cardiac disease. Death typically occurs in the adolescent to young adult years in the juvenile form. The adult form typically presents after age 20 (up to the sixties). GSD II (not GSD I) is also a lysosomal storage disease and most individuals with late-onset disease show characteristic muscle biopsy changes.

Management includes attention to specific dysfunctions such as respiratory insufficiency, cardiomyopathy (in the infantile type), physical therapy for muscle weakness, surgery for contractures, wheelchair use if necessary, and ventilator support as needed. Enzyme replacement therapy (ERT) is available with alglucosidase alfa, which is given intravenously and tends to work best with the adult or milder form of disease.

14.3.9 Gaucher's disease

This is a rare autosomal recessive disorder due to a deficiency of the enzyme glucocerebrosidase (acid β-glucosidase) resulting in lipid accumulation in cells (especially white blood cells) and various organs (i.e., brain, bone marrow, kidneys, lungs, liver, and spleen) (13). It is the most common of the lysosomal storage diseases and is due to a defective gene located on chromosome 1. Gaucher disease is increased in incidence in the Ashkenazi Jewish population; low enzyme activity is noted in leukocytes or cultured skin fibroblasts. Bone marrow aspiration reveals "Gaucher storage cells" (onionskin morphology in histiocytes).

Four types are identified, with type 2 usually dying during the first few years of age from failure to thrive and neurologic features such as ataxia, spasticity, dementia, seizures, myoclonus, and supranuclear ophthalmoplegia. Those with type 4 usually die within a few weeks of birth. Type 3 is a variant that is common in Scandinavian countries, with type 3a resulting in death in the adolescent or young adult years.

Type 1 (nonneuropathic) is the most common form of Gaucher's disease; it is relatively mild and may not be diagnosed because its features are subclinical. It is the most common lysosomal storage disease and there is an increased incidence in the Ashkenazi Jewish population. Most diagnosed type 1 patients present in the adolescent or early adult years. Painless hepatosplenomegaly develops, leading to abdominal distention and thrombocytopenia with excessive bleeding as well as anemia. The bone marrow expands because of the abnormal cells, with bone remodeling and chronic bone

Tab. 14.4: Medications for inborn errors of metabolism.

Medication	Indication	Adult dosage	Side effects	Comments
Penicillamine	Wilson's disease	0.75–1.5g/day Maximum: 2 g/day Also administer: pyridoxine 25 mg/day	Same as in ▶Tab. 14.3. Avoid interruption in therapy owing to risk of sensitivity reactions with reinstitution. Avoid in renal insufficiency.	Optimal dosage determined by measurement of urinary copper excretion and free copper in serum. Administer 1 hour before or 2 hours after meals. Administer at least 1 hour apart from other drugs, food or milk Therapy protects against relapse during pregnancy: reduce dose to 750 mg/day.
Trientine	Wilson's disease	Initial: 750–1,250 mg daily in two to four divided doses Maximum dose: 2 g daily	Hypersensitivity reactions, iron deficiency anemia, anorexia, dyspepsia, epigastric pain, muscle spasm, systemic lupus erythematosus, dystonia, myasthenia gravis.	Take on an empty stomach at least 1 hour before or 2 hours after a meal Administer at least 1 hour apart from all other medicines. Do not give mineral supplements. If contact with capsule contents, wash with water owing to risk of contact dermatitis.
Sodium phenylbutyrate	Urea cycle disorder Orinthine	Powder (>20 kg): 9.9–13g/m² per day in four to six equally divided doses	Menstrual dysfunction, altered taste, body odor, decreased appetite, GI upset, fatigue, sedation, depression, headache, increased LFTs, metabolic abnormalities (acidosis,	Mix powder with solid or liquid foods; avoid acidic beverages. Level teaspoon provides 3.2 g of powder and 3 g of sodium

transcarbamylase deficiency		Tablets (>20 kg): 9.9–13g/m² per day in three equally divided doses	hyperchloremia, hypophosphatemia, hyperuricemia), hypoalbuminemia, bone marrow suppression.	phenylbutyrate. Level tablespoon provides 9.1 g of powder and 8.6 g of sodium phenylbutyrate.
Arginine	Urea cycle disorder	Initial: 200 mg/kg IV over 90–120 min Maintenance: 200 mg/kg per day IV continuous infusion Maximum dose: 30 g	Extravasation, skin necrosis, hypersensitivity reactions, anaphylaxis. Excessive rate can lead to local irritation, flushing, nausea, vomiting, headache.	Hyaluronidase may be used empirically for extravasation.
Phenylacetate and sodium benzoate	Hyperammonemia associated with urea cycle disorder	Initial: 5.5g/m² IV over 90–120 min Maintenance: 5.5g/m2 IV over 24 hours	Extravastation, skin necrosis, injection-site reactions, pyrexia, nausea, vomiting, hyperglycemia, hypokalemia, convulsions, mental impairment, brain edema, agitation, hypotension. Use caution in patients with hepatic or renal impairment.	Use in conjunction with caloric supplementation and dietary protein restriction. Dilute prior to infusion. Administer through a central line. Do not administer repeat loading doses. Drug interactions with penicillin, probenecid, and valproic acid.
Carnitine	Organic acidemia	Oral solution initial: 1g per day Oral solution maintenance: 1–3g/day	Nausea, vomiting, abdominal cramps, diarrhea, body odor, seizures. Decreasing dose can reduce drug-related body odor or GI symptoms.	Solution may be given alone or placed in drink/liquid food. Space doses evenly apart. Administer during or after meals.

(Continued)

Tab. 14.4: Medications for inborn errors of metabolism. (*Continued*)

Medication	Indication	Adult dosage	Side effects	Comments
Allopurinol	Hyperuricemia	Tablets: 990 mg two to three times a day >300 mg/day in divided doses	Acute gouty attacks, sedation, headache, rash, severe hypersensitivity reactions, increased LFTs, nausea, diarrhea, peripheral neuropathy, bone marrow suppression.	Consume slowly to maximize tolerance. Adjust dose according to serum uric acid levels. Dosage adjustment required with renal insufficiency. Administer after meals. Prophylactic colchicine may be needed when initiating treatment to prevent acute gouty attacks. Multiple drug interactions.

Reference: Facts and Comparisons. Drug information full monographs. Wolters Kluwer Health, Incorporated. Available at: http://0-online. factsandcomparisons.com.libcat.ferris.edu/index.aspx. Accessed August 15, 2011.

pain, which may severe, generally occurs at night, and may be misdiagnosed as growing pains. Pathologic fractures and avascular necrosis of the hips may arise. Pulmonary infiltration may develop, leading to restrictive lung disease in adulthood.

ERT (intravenous recombinant glucocerebrosidase [imiglucerase; veraglucerase alfa]) is used for type 1 and most of type 3 Gaucher's patients. Bone marrow transplantation can cure nonneurologic features of Gaucher's but carries a high risk of complications. Other potential treatment options include splenectomy, blood transfusions, joint replacement, antibiotics, antiepileptics, bisphosphonates, and liver transplantation. Splenectomy is now a less frequent procedure for these patients because it can lead to deteriorating bone disease. Research is also evaluating such therapies as substrate reduction therapy (for type 2), gene therapy, and pharmacologic chaperoning with drugs that work at a molecular level – such as miglustat and isofagomine tartrate.

14.3.10 Nieman-Pick disease (NPD)

This is a rare, fatal, autosomal recessive lysosomal storage disease due to a deficiency of acid sphingomyelinase. NPD is classified as a lipid storage disease (sphingolipidosis), with high levels of lipids accumulating in tissues such as brain, bone marrow, lungs, spleen, and liver. Types A (infantile) and B NPD are due to mutations in the SMPD1 gene, whereas type C is due to mutations in NPC1 and NPC2 (14). NPD A and B are increased in the Ashkenazi Jewish population.

Type A is a severe degenerative disease in infants, whereas type B disease can present in mid- to late childhood or later with a progressively enlarged spleen. Cirrhosis and pulmonary insufficiency can also develop. Bone marrow examination reveals characteristic "foamy" storage cells, and enzyme deficiency can be seen in white blood cells ("sea blue" histiocytes) or cultured skin fibroblasts.

Treatment remains limited at this time, and those with type B and C disease may live to their teenage or adult years (15). Organ transplantation has been attempted for type B NPD, with limited efficacy. Research is focusing on such drugs as miglustat (Zavesca) for type C NPD with progressive neurologic impairment. Research is also evaluating enzyme replacement and gene therapy.

14.3.11 Late-onset GM1 gangliosidosis

This is an autosomal recessive lysosomal storage disease due to the deficiency of lysosomal hydralase, acid β-galactosidase (beta-galactosidase enzyme), leading to the accumulation of GM1 ganglioside, oligosaccharides, and the mucopolysaccharide keratin sulfate (and derivates) (16). Over 100 mutations have been reported in the beta-galactosidase gene (GLB1) (17). The enzyme deficiency leads to GM1 gangliosidosis and mucopolysaccharidosis type IVB (Morquio disease type B).

Three types of GM1 gangliosidosis are noted: *infantile* (type 1), *juvenile* (type 2), and *adult* (type 3). It is lethal in types 1 and 2. In the adult type onset occurs between 3 and 30 years of age. Features include early neurologic development with the gradual development of dementia, muscle atrophy, angiokeratomas, corneal clouding, extrapyramidal features, dystonia, and parkinsonian features. Intellectual disability may be seen in an adolescent with this GM1 gangliosidosis. There is no specific treatment for this disorder at this time. Research is focusing on bone marrow transplantation, stem cell transplantation, gene therapy, and enzyme replacement.

14.3.12 Late-onset GM2 gangliosidosis

This disorder is due to a deficiency of β-hexosaminidase A or A and B with a typical presentation in childhood between 2 and 10 years of age in an autosomal recessive pattern. Symptoms include ataxia, seizures, spasticity, dystonia, choreoathetosis, muscle wasting, blindness with retinal pigmentary features, pes cavus, psychomotor dysfunction, and others.

GM2 gangliosidosis may also develop in the adolescent years with severe mental health disorders – psychotic depression, paranoia, or acute schizophrenia. Enzyme deficiency is noted in serum, white blood cells, or cultured skin fibroblasts. The GM2 gangliosidoses include Tay-Sachs disease, AB variant; and Sandhoff disease. These are generally fatal by early childhood. Treatment options are limited and research is looking at such options as pyrimethamine (▶Tab. 14.3), leukovorin, enzyme replacement therapy, and gene therapy (18).

14.3.13 Fabry disease

Fabry disease (angiokeratoma corporis diffusum) is a rare X-linked recessive lysosomal storage disease. It is a sphingolipidosis due to the deficiency of α-galactosidase and usually presents in later childhood or around puberty in a male with episodes of severe burning pain in the feet and hands, which may be misdiagnosed as "growing pains." The pain is out of proportion to the examination and there may be a history of hypohydrosis and periodic fevers. Joint pain similar to pauciarticular arthritis develops, as does abdominal pain, which may resemble inflammatory bowel disease (19). Laboratory tests reveal α-galactosidase deficiency (blood, white blood cells, cultured skin fibroblasts) and increased urinary excretion of ceramide trihexoside; urine examination reveals birefringent lipid globules ("Maltese crosses"). Fabry disease is often difficult to diagnose in females, although heterozygous females may have pain episodes similar to those in males.

By ages 15 to 20 years, males develop angiokeratomata over the buccal mucosa, umbilicus, and genital areas (bathing suit area). These angiokeratomas are small red/purple papules with a vascular appearance and may bleed but without additional symptoms. There can be periodic gastrointestinal distress with postprandial discomfort, constipation, or diarrhea. Adolescent males also develop cardiac arrhythmias, and slit-lamp examination reveals corneal verticillata. Transition to later adolescence and adulthood can lead to peripheral neuropathy (with pain episodes as well as loss of vibration sense and somatosensation), hypertrophic cardiomyopathy, proteinuria, renal disease, transient ischemic attacks, and cerebrovascular accidents. Males can experience renal failure in their twenties to forties.

Treatment includes the use of various supportive medications such as antiepileptic drugs (i.e., gabapentin or carbamazepine), angiotensin converting enzyme (ACE) inhibitors (for renal protection), aspirin or clopidogrel bisulfate (for stroke prophylaxis), NSAIDs, and other analgesics. Infusion of enzyme replacement therapy (agalsidase alpha, agalsidase beta) is a very expensive treatment modality that allows the patient to develop normal metabolism, prevents worsening of the disease, and may lead to symptom reversal (20).

14.3.14 Alpha-mannosidosis

This is a rare autosomal recessive lysosomal storage disease caused by a deficiency of the enzyme alpha-D mannosidase; it can include mild to severe clinical subtypes (21). Deficient enzyme is noted in peripheral white blood cells or fibroblasts. MAN2B1 is a gene associated with this disorder. A severe type leads to death prenatally or in early infancy, whereas a moderate type leads to a variety of features before age 10, such as progressively skeletal abnormalities and myopathy.

The mild form may be identified in adolescence or adulthood without skeletal or muscle features. However, the mild subtype can include CNS disease (cerebellar dysfunction with ataxia), immunodeficiency, intellectual disability (mild to moderate), hearing impairment, psychiatric symptoms, skeletal abnormalities, and others. Disease progression can lead to hepatosplenomegaly, destructive arthritis, corneal opacities, and metabolic myopathy.

Management of alpha-mannosidosis involves carefully addressing specific issues as they arise, including treating infections, hydrocephalus, hearing loss, and others. Genetic counseling for this autosomal recessive disorder is needed. Research is focusing on gene therapy, bone marrow or peripheral blood stem cell transplantation, and enzyme replacement therapy.

14.3.15 Late-onset urea cycle disorders

A urea cycle disorder or urea cycle defect results from a deficiency of one or more enzymes in the human urea cycle that takes ammonia out of the blood. Nitrogen is a waste product of protein, converted to urea, and removed from the body via the urine.

A number of urea cycle disorders are noted, including deficiencies of these enzymes: N-acetylglutamate synthetase (with increased ammonia), carbamoyl phosphate synthetase I (with increased ammonia), argininosuccinic acid synthetase (increased citrulline–citrullinemia), arginase (increased arginine-argininemia), argininosuccinase acid lyase (increased argininosuccinic acid and citrulline-argininosuccinic aciduria), and ornithine transcarbamylase (with increased ornithine, uracil, and orotic acid; see below). Except for the X-linked recessive ornithine transcarbamylase deficiency (see below), these are autosomal recessive disorders.

Urea cycle disorders are generally identified in infancy or early childhood. However, some are diagnosed in adolescents or adults, probably owing to less severe degrees of enzyme deficiency. In late-onset urea cycle disorders there can be episodes of hyperammonemia caused by viral illnesses, lethargy, high-protein diets, childbirth, and even the consumption of valproic acid (22). There is also increased glutamine in urea cycle defects, along with alanine or asparagine as well as other amino acids depending on the specific defect. These defects can lead to lethargy, emesis, symptoms of psychiatric illness, cerebrovascular accident–like symptoms, coma, and death (23). Some female carriers are asymptomatic until later in adulthood when exposed to metabolic challenge (such as pregnancy).

Management involves providing required protein in the diet without inducing hyperammonemia. Supplementation is provided with amino acid formulas as well as intravenous arginine hydrochloride (except in argininemia) (▶Tab. 14.4), along with vitamins, minerals, trace elements, and calcium depending on the specific deficiency (24). Some medications can lower ammonia levels and increase long-term survival via an alternative pathway. Drugs that reduce ureagenesis include sodium phenylacetate and sodium benzoate (▶Tab. 14.4); they conjugate with nitrogen-containing amino acids to allow increased excretion of nitrogen in urine (25). Hemodialysis is needed for refractory situations and liver transplantation has been used in select cases. Improved newborn screening for urea cycle defects and other inborn errors of metabolism will allow early treatment and improved outcomes in these disorders.

14.3.16 Ornithine transcarbamylase deficiency

This rare X-linked recessive disorder is the most common of the urea cycle conditions and is due to deficiency of the enzyme ornithine transcarbamylase, leading to an increase in serum ammonia, uracil, and orotic acid (26). Some males die shortly after birth; half or more die by age 5 years. Some are not diagnosed until adolescence or at variable times in adulthood (27,28). A variety of symptoms can arise, including developmental delay, mental retardation, brittle hair, liver dysfunction, poor school performance, mood swings, encephalitis, and others. Some female carriers may not develop symptoms until they are subjected to metabolic stress induced by starvation, malnutrition, pregnancy, surgery, or others.

Since the individual cannot process a high nitrogen load, treatment involves a low-protein diet to reduce nitrogen intake and reduce excessive body protein breakdown, especially during acute illnesses, with hydration and appropriate nutrition. Medications such as sodium phenylbutyrate (▶Tab. 14.4) or sodium benzoate may (▶Tab. 14.4) be helpful in this regard (29). For example, sodium benzoate combines with glycine to produce hippurate and remove an ammonium group (▶Tab. 14.3). Supplemental amino acids such as leucine, isoleucine, valine, citrulline, and arginine (▶Tab. 14.4) are helpful. Biotin may benefical, since it can stimulate ornithine transcarbamylase and may reduce ammonia levels (▶Tab. 14.3). Liver transplantation has been used in some patients.

14.3.17 Alkaptonuria

This is a rare autosomal recessive disorder of phenylalanine and tyrosine metabolism due to a defect in the enzyme homogentisate 1,2-dioxygenase, a liver enzyme that catalyzes oxidation of homogentisic acid, which is the third step of tyrosine metabolism. Increased levels of homogentisic acid are noted in the blood as well as urine; non–freshly voided urine will oxidize to a brown/black-blue color. Alkaptonuria was the first IEM to be identified, by professor Sir Archibald E. Garrod in 1902, and it is found in greater frequency in Slovakia (1).

Although alkaptonuria is usually without symptoms in childhood and adolescence, extensive pigmentation may develop in adolescence, young adulthood, or later with the deposition of pigment (bluish or brownish) in the ears, sclerae, heart valves, and other organs (ochronosis). Valvular heart disease (aortic and mitral calcification and regurgitation), hip or spinal damage, and ochronotic arthritis may develop that is similar to symptoms of rheumatoid arthritis or osteoarthritis in adults. Renal stones may also develop.

Treatment includes joint or heart valve replacement and treatment of coronary artery disease, which may occur prematurely. There is no specific treatment for the defect of this disorder. Dietary restrictions of phenylalanine and tyrosine are recommended, as well as increased doses of vitamin C. Research is evaluating the effectivenss of nitisinone, which inhibits an enzyme generating homogentisic acid (30).

14.3.18 Sanfillipo disease

Mucopolysaccharidoses (MPS) are a group of metabolic disorders due to the lack of or defects in various lysosomal enzymes used to metabolize glycosaminoglycans. A variety of MPSs are noted (▶Tab. 14.2). Sanfillipo disease is a rare autosomal recessive lysosomal storage disease also called mucopolysaccharidosis III (MPS-III); it is due to a deficiency in one of the enzymes required for the metabolism of glycosaminoglycan heparan sulfate that is found in extracellular tissue and on the cell surface og glycoproteins.

Four types are identified: *MPS-III A* (deficiency of heparan N-sulfatase located on 17q25.3), *MPS-III B* (deficiency of N-acetyl-alpha-D-glucosaminidase located on 17q21), *MPS-III C* (deficiency of acetyl-CoA:alpha-glucosaminide acetyltransferase located on 8p11-q13), and *MPS-III D* (deficiency of N-acetylglucosamine-G-sulfate sulfatase located on 12q14). These four types are difficult to separate on clinical grounds and the specific diagnosis is made with assay of the specific deficient enzyme in tissues via gene sequencing; prenatal diagnosis can be also accomplished.

Sanfillipo disease usually presents in young childhood but may not be seen until later in childhood or adolescence. A variety of behavioral and developmental problems can develop, including intellectual decline (31). There can be hyperactivity, sleep disorders, aggressive behaviors, and others. Some MPS features (i.e., coarse hair, stiff joints, hirsutism) may present later. Mental retardation may be seen in adolescents with types B and D disease and some conditions present in adolescence with psychosis. Eventually other features also develop, including hepatosplenomegaly, diarrhea, carious teeth, osteonecrosis of the hips, progressive scoliosis, immobility (with need for a wheelchair), swallowing problems, and epilepsy (32). Most of these patients do not live beyond their early twenties.

Treatment mainly involves dealing with the specific complications that arise; bone marrow transplantation may be beneficial in early disease. Pharmacologic treatment of behavioral or psychiatric problems is usually not helpful. Replacement of the deficient enzymes does not penetrate the blood-brain barrier and neurologicl features of MPS are not improved. Research is focusing on gene therapy, development of replacement enzymes to penetrate the blood-brain barrier, improvement of defective enzymes, and the use of stem cell therapy. Improved neonatal screening would allow very early diagnosis, which would improve outcome and management plans. Research is also evaluating the potential benefit of the flavonoid genistein (▶Tab. 14.3).

14.3.19 Homocystinuria

This is an autosomal recessive aminoaciduria due to a dysfunction in methionine metabolism because of cystathionine beta synthase deficiency (33,34). It is a defect of sulfur-containing amino acids (i.e., cysteine, methionine), with increased levels of homocysteine being found in serum and urine. Homocystinuria eventually leads to a multisystemic condition affecting the cardiovascular system, CNS, connective tissue, and muscles. At least 150 different mutations have been seen in the cystathionine beta synthase gene (33).

A classic feature is the development of a marfanoid appearance, ocular lens dislocation, and developmental delay (mental retardation). The marfanoid habitus can include increased height, thin physique, dolichostenomelia, pes cavus, genu valgum, pectus excavatum (or carinatum), ectopia lentis, lens subluxation, myopia, glaucoma, and/or optic atrophy. The lens dislocation is usually downward versus an upward dislocation, as in Marfan's syndrome. Homocystinuria is part of a differential diagnosis for tall stature in adolescents, which includes Marfan's syndrome, hyperthyroidism, obesity, Kleinfelter's syndrome, cerebral gigantism, pituitary gigantism, XYY syndrome, constitutional tall stature, and others. Patients with homocystinuria have tight joints, not the loose joints or aortic root dilatation or dissection as noted with Marfan's syndrome.

There can be the development of atheromas of many arteries and intravascular thromboses due to increased homocystine in the blood, which can lead to death in young adulthood or even earlier. Variable mental illness can develop as well. The adolescent with homocystinuria may have scoliosis, epilepsy, and mental subnormality (60%); the cognitive dysfunction may be due to S-adenosylhomocysteine accumulation in the CNS and/or repeated strokes. There can also be osteoporosis, vertebral collapse, and scoliosis.

Approximately half of those with homocystinuria improve with high doses of pyridoxine (vitamin B6) (▶Tab. 14.3) and are called vitamin B6 responders; others can be placed on a low-methionine diet. Treatment options also include a high-cystine diet, use of trimethylglycine, a folic acid supplement, and even cystine. Betaine (N, N,N-trimethylglycine) can be used to lower homocystine levels because it stimulates conversion of homocysteine to methonine (▶Tab. 14.3); it is used with a low-protein diet (low in methionine). Folate is added if the serum homocysteine level is increased with identified methylenetetrahydrofolate reductase (MTHFR) gene mutation.

14.3.20 Cystinuria

This is caused by a defective kidney amino acid transporter protein as a result of which the kidney is not able to reabsorb basic, positively charged amino acids in filtration. It is an autosomal recessive disorder affecting 1 in 10,000 persons. It may be subclinical and may not present until adolescence or adulthood. The urine shows a marked increase in amino acids that are not absorbed, such as cysteine, ornithine, lysine, arginine, and to some extent histidine. A urinalysis shows hexagonal cystine crystals precipitating into the urine. Cystine stones develop in the kidney, leading to symptomatic nephrolithiasis. Management is with hydration, urine alkalinization (with citrate supplementation), and dietary changes to lower salt and protein intake. Chelation therapy may be needed with such agents as penicillamine (▶Tab. 14.3). Surgery may be needed to remove renal stones.

14.3.21 Wilson's Disease

Wilson's disease (WD; hepatolenticular degeneration) is an autosomal recessive condition due to a dysfunction in copper metabolism that leads to impaired biliary excretion of copper with copper accumulation in various tissues (i.e., liver, brain, cornea) and neurodegeneration (35). Copper is toxic to these tissues. The genetic defect is on chromosome arm 13q and it affects the copper-transporting adenosine triphosphatase (ATPase) gene (ATP7B) in the liver (36).

WD was first noted in 1912; half of these patients develop symptoms by midadolescence, although the copper accumulation in tissues starts in infancy. It is unusual for symptoms to appear before 6 years of age. The urinary copper level is increased (>100 μg/24 h) and a liver biopsy shows increased copper deposits. Ceruloplasmin is the protein that binds copper and serum ceruloplasmin is typically low in WD; the serum copper is also low. The serum ceruloplasmin can be normal in up to 20 percent of homozygotes for WD and low in 10 percent of homozygotes who do not have the overt disease symptomatology.

The classic disease triad is due to copper deposits and includes hepatic disease, neuropsychiatric symptoms (parkinsonian symptoms, schizophrenia, bipolar disorders), and Kayser-Fleisher rings (corneal copper deposits with golden discoloration in the membrane of Descemet at the limbic regions). However, manifestations of WD can be protean and the diagnosis difficult (37). There can be dystonia, dystonic posturing, incoordination, arm "wing-beating," dysphagia, dysarthria (nearly all), and even anarthria. The clinical and histologic picture of WD can be identical to that of chronic active hepatitis.

Adolescents with unexplained recurrent liver disease and neurologic symptoms should be evaluated for WD (36). The differential diagnosis includes cystic fibrosis, α_1-antitrypsin deficiency, sclerosing cholangitis (usually due to inflammatory bowel disease), chronic active hepatitis, and childhood cirrhosis. Menkes disease is an X-linked copper excretion disorder in boys due to a different copper transporter than WD in the Golgi apparatus; it starts in early infancy and leads to seizures, hypothermia, hypotonia, "wire-like" hair (pili torti), spasticity, failure to thrive, skin looseness, bladder diverticula, and death usually before age 3 years. There are no Keyser-Fleischer rings in Menkes disease and copper chelation does not benefit these patients.

WD is fatal without effective therapy. The adolescent with WD should be on a low-copper diet and avoid such foods as dried fruits, nuts, shellfish, liver, mushrooms, chocolate, and cocoa. Treatment involves early diagnosis and copper chelation with D-penicillamine or trientine (►Tab. 14.4). Penicillamine is the most frequently used chelation agent for WD.

Usually the clinician begins with a low dosage of 250 mg/day, since rapid loss of copper from tissues may lead to neurologic dysfunction or an acute hemolytic crisis. One can raise the dosage by 250 mg per week up to 1,000 to 1,200 mg/day. Adverse effects include gastric irritation, which reduces compliance with the D-penicillamine. Pyridoxine is added to avoid the development of phosphate deficiency. Other potential side effects include proteinuria, nephrotic syndrome, bone marrow suppression, fever, pemphigus, lymphadenopathy, and collagen disease–like symptoms. The addition of corticosteroids may improve many of these side effects.

About 6 months to a year after treatment, daily urinary copper excretion should be one third or less of values seen before staring chelation. If this is not seen, noncompliance with the D-penicillamine may be the reason. If the treatment is successful, the Kayser-Fleischer corneal rings disappear in 1 to 2 years. Progress is greatly improved if an early diagnosis is made and effective chelation occurs; some patients may even become asymptomatic. Chelation is also given to asymptomatic patients, since treatment can prevent the onset of symptoms. Zinc acetate can be used after successful chelation or in the individual with asymptomatic WD disease. Mutational analysis is used to screen family members of one with a known WD causative mutation; haplotype analysis is also used in genetic screening (35).

14.4 Conclusions

Inborn errors of metabolism (IEMs) are rare, complex, and often poorly understood disorders that typically involve deficiencies of enzymes needed for the healthy maintenance of normal biochemical and metabolic pathways and life itself. There are hundreds of IEMs; their volume, complexity, and rarity results in limited understanding by clinicians and the high expense of their treatment.

Although many are identified in utero or early infancy, some present in later childhood, adolescence, or even at various times in the adult years. A confusing myriad of features can be noted, also adding to the complexities of accurate as well as timely diagnosis and successful management. IEMs present society with considerable challenges, including how much care and research will be allotted for such often rare, complicated, and costly disorders of human physiology.

This discussion focuses on some of the known IEMs presenting in the adolescent years, such as adrenoleukodystrophy, glycogen storage diseases, lysosomal storage diseases, urea cycle disorders, and others. Management is often symptomatic or nonspecific, dealing with the numerous problems that can arise over the lifetimes of these individuals. Enzyme replacement therapy is provided if available and affordable since it is very expensive. Research is also looking at gene therapies, stem cell transplantation, and bone marrow transplantation.

References

1. Garrod AE. The incidence of alkaptonuria: a study in chemical individuality. Lancet 1902;2:1616-20.
2. Kamboj MK. Inborn errors of metabolism. In: Patel DR, Greydanus DE, Omar HA, Merrick J, eds. Neurodevelopmental disabilities: Clinical care for children and young adults. Dordrecht: Springer, 2011:53–67.
3. Greydanus DE, Pratt HD. Syndromes and disorders associated with mental retardation. Indian J Pediatr 2005;72(10):859–64.
4. Curry CJ, Stevenson RE, Aughton D. American College of Medical Genetics: Evaluation of mental retardation: Recommendations of a consensus conference. Am J Med Genet 1997;72:468–77.
5. Shevell M. Practice parameter: Evaluation of the child with global developmental delay: Report of the Quality Standards Subcommittee of the American Academy of Neurology and the Practice Committee of the Child Neurology Society. Neurology 2003;60:367–80.

6. Hsieh S, White PC. Presentation of primary adrenal insufficiency in childhood. J Clin Endocrinol Metab 2011;96(6):E925–28.

7. Salzman A. Adrenoleukodystrophy patient perspective: turning despair into a gene therapy. Hum Gene Ther 2011;22(6):647–48.

8. Biffi A, Aubourg P, Carter N. Gene therapy for leukodystrophies. Hum Mol Genet 2011; 20:R42–53.

9. Hayashi T, Nakamura M, Ichiba M, Matsuda M, Kato M, Shiokawa N, et al. Adult-type metachromatic leukodystrophy with compound heterozygous ARSA mutations: A case report and phenotypic comparison with a previously reported case. Psychiatr Clin Neurosci 2011;65(1):105–8.

10. Sevin C, Cartier-Lacave N, Aubourg P. Gene therapy in metachromatic leukodystrophy. Int J Clin Pharmacol 2009;47(Suppl 1):S128–31.

11. Storch E, Keeley M, Merlo L, Jacob M, Correia C, Weinstein D. Psychosocial functioning in youth with glycogen storage disease type I. J Pediatr Psychol 2008; 33(7):728–38.

12. Talente GM, Coleman RA, Alter C, Baker L, Brown BI, Cannon RA, et al. Glycogen storage disease in adults. Ann Int Med 1994;120(3):218–26.

13. Grabowski GA. Phenotype, diagnosis, and treatment of Gaucher's disease. Lancet 2008; 372:1263-71.

14. Xiong H, Bao XH, Zhang YH, Xu YN, Qin J, Shi HP, et al. Nieman-Pick disease type C: analysis of 7 patients. World J Pediatr 2011;8(7):10–15.

15. Sévin M, Lesca G, Bauman N, Millat G, Lyon-Caen O, Vanier MT, et al. The adult form of Niemann-Pick disease type C. Brain 2007;130(Pt 1):120–33.

16. Brunetti-Pierri N, Scaglia F. GM1 gangliosidosis: review of clinical, molecular, and therapeutic aspects. Mol Genet Metab 2008;94(4):391–96.

17. Caciotti A, Garman SC, Rivera-Colón Y, Procopio E, Catarzi S, Ferri L, et al. GM1 gangliosidosis and Morquio B disease: An update on genetic alterations and clinical findings. Biochim Biophys Acta 2011;12(7):782–90.

18. Tsuji D, Akeboshi H, Matsuoka K, Yasuoka H, Miyasaki E, Kasahara Y, et al. Highly phosphomannosylated enzyme replacement therapy for GM2 gangliosidosis. Ann Neurol 2011;69(4):691–701.

19. Marchesoni CL, Roa N, Pardal AM, Neumann P, Caceres G, Martinez P, et al. Misdiagnosis in Fabry disease. J Pediatr 2010;156(5):828–31.

20. Hoffmann B, Beck M, Sunder-Plassmann G, Borsini W, Ricci R, Mehta A. Nature and prevalence of pain in Fabry Disease and Its response to enzyme replacement therapy. A retrospective analysis from the Fabry Outcome Survey. Clin J Pain 2007;23(6):535–42.

21. Malm D, Nilssen O. Alpha-mannosidosis. Orphanet J Rare Dis 2008;3(1):21–24.

22. Summar ML, Barr F, Dawling S, Smith W, Lee B, Singh RH, et al. Unmasked adult-onset urea cycle disorders in the critical care setting. Crit Care Clin 2005;21(Suppl 4):S1–8.

23. Gropman A, Batshaw M. Cognitive outcome in urea cycle disorders. Mol Genet Metab 2004;81(Suppl 1):58–62.

24. Scaglia F. New insights in nutritional management and amino acid supplementation in urea cycle disorders. Mol Genet Metab 2010;100(Suppl 1):572–76.

25. Enns GM, Berry SA, Berry GT, Rhead WJ, Brusilow SW, Hamosh A. Survival after treatment with phenylacetate and benzoate for urea-cycle disorders. N Engl J Med 2007;356 (22):2282–92.

26. Tuchman M, Jaleel N, Morizono H, Sheehy L, Lynch MG. Mutations and polymorphisms in the human ornithine transcarbamylase gene. Hum. Mutat 2002;19(2): 93–107.

27. Rohininath T, Costello DJ, Lynch T, Monavari A, Tuchman M, Treacy EP. Fatal presentation of ornithine transcarbamylase deficiency n a 62-year old man and family studies. J Inherit Metab Dis 2004;27(2):285–88.

28. Brajon D, Carassou P, Pruna L, Feillet F, Kaminsky P. Ornithine transcarbamylase deficiency in an adult. Rev Med Interne 2010;31(10):709–11.
29. Marini JC, Lanpher BC, Scaglia F, O'Brien WE, Sun Q, Garlick PJ, et al. Phenylbutyrate improves nitrogen disposal via alternative pathway without eliciting an increase in protein breakdown and catabolism in control and ornithine transcarbamylase deficient patients. Am J Clin Nutr 2011;93(6):1248–54.
30. Suwannarat P, O'Brien K, Perry MB, Sebring N, Bernardini I, Kaiser-Kupfer MI, et al. Use of nitisinone in patients with alkaptonuria. Metab Clin Exp 2005;54(6):719–28.
31. Valstar MJ, Marchal JP, Grootenhuis M, Colland V, Wijburg FA. Cognitive development in patients with Mucopolysaccharidosis type III (Sanfilippo syndrome). Orphanet J Rare Dis 2011;6:43–46.
32. White KK, Karol LA, White DR, Hale S. Musculoskeletal manifestations of Sanfilippo syndrome (mucopolysaccharidosis type III). J Pediatr Orthop 2011;31(5):594–98.
33. Mudd SH. Hypermethioninemias of genetic and non-genetic origin: A review. Am J Med Genet C Semin Med Genet 2011;157(1):3–32.
34. Maillot F, Kraus JP, Lee PJ. Environmental influences on familial discordance of phenotype in people with homocystinuria: a case report. J Med Case Reports 2008;2(1): 113–16.
35. Ferenci P. Wilson's disease. Clin Gastroenterol Hepatol 2005;3(8):726–33.
36. Hancu A, Mihai MC, Axelerad AD. Wilson's disease: A challenging diagnosis. Clinical manifestations and diagnostic procedures in 12 patients. Rev Med Chir Soc Med Nat Iasi 2011;115(1):58–63.
37. Pfeiffer RF. Wilson's disease. Handb Clin Neurol 2011;100:681–709.

15 The kidney

Alfonso D. Torres and Donald E. Greydanus

The renal system is a critically important and complex organ system needed for normal growth and health. This chapter reviews major issues in this regard including urinary tract infections, proteinuria, hematuria, and glomerulonephritis. This discussion considers the nephrotic syndrome, minimal changes disease (MCD), collapsing focal segmental glomerulosclerosis, IgA nephropathy, poststreptococcal glomerulonephritis, Henoch-Schönlein purpura (HSP) nephritis, hemolytic-uremic syndrome, lupus nephritis, and other renal disorders in adolescents. Concepts of diagnosis and management are presented. Consultation with colleagues in nephrology is recommended for adolescents with complex and refractory renal conditions.

15.1 Introduction

Urinary tract infections are common conditions in adolescent females. Glomerular diseases represent the most characteristic abnormalities affecting the kidney in adolescents. The clinical manifestations range from asymptomatic, incidental findings during a routine medical assessment, such as proteinuria or microscopic hematuria, to life-threatening condition with rapid deterioration of multiple organ function including acute kidney injury. The clinical evaluation rests in a comprehensive history, physical examination, and other investigations aimed to assess renal function and the presence of extrarenal disease. Asymptomatic urine abnormalities are the most frequent conditions reported. The incidence is related to community or national practices for routine urinalysis. In the United States a urinalysis is requested for adolescents who enroll in organized sports at the high school or at college level and for individuals who join the Armed Forces. In Japan and other Asian countries urinalysis is routinely performed at school.

15.1.1 Some definitions

The definition of microscopic hematuria in children is three or more red blood cells (RBCs) per high-power field in the centrifuged sediment from 10 mL of freshly voided midstream urine with the RBCs usually dysmorphic. In the adult the upper normal limit of RBCs in the urine is two per high-power field in the spun urinary sediment.

Proteinuria can detected by the ubiquitous use of the dipstick or the use of sulfosalicylic acid test and be semiquantitatively assessed by methods such as the ratio of urine protein concentration in milligrams per deciliter to urine creatinine concentration in milligrams per deciliter, with the accepted normal value of less than 0.2 for older children, adolescents and adults; this is also done by 24-hour urine collection for the determination of urine protein, with values of $150/1.73m^2$ per milligram in 24 hours accepted as upper normal values in boys and in girls. The presence of proteinuria and hematuria, particularly with dysmorphic RBCs and casts, is an indication of glomerular involvement. Macroscopic hematuria or gross hematuria (usually brown or red in color) with proteinuria and no clots, which is sometimes recurrent, is seen in adolescents with IgA nephropathy.

The nephrotic syndrome is defined as heavy proteinuria causing hypoalbuminemia; in the adult the proteinuria is greater than 3.5 g/day; in the child it is 50 mg/kg per day of protein excretion in association with edema, hypercholesterolemia, and lipiduria. The nephrotic syndrome is usually characterized by sudden onset of oliguria, hematuria, red cell casts moderated proteinuria, oliguria hypertension and edema, usually preceded by an infection; in general it is self-limited.

Rapid progressive glomerulonephritis is characterized by rapid deterioration of renal function in a matter of days or weeks associated with moderate nonsevere proteinuria, usually less than 3g/day; the blood pressure may be normal or moderately elevated. Often extrarenal manifestations of vasculitis are also observed. The renal biopsy usually demonstrated crescentic glomerulonephritis in a high percentage of the glomeruli. Rapid therapeutic intervention is needed to preserve renal function. Chronic glomerulonephritis is characterized by decreased renal function, hypertension, proteinuria of variable severity, and usually small kidneys.

Clinical symptoms of an underlying acute or chronic renal parenchymal disorder, when present, usually relate to the dominant physiologic disturbance. For instance, adolescents with chronic reflux nephropathy and moderately severe hypertension may complain of blood pressure–related headaches or visual disturbances. By contrast, patients with acute nephritis may experience flank pain, while those with the severe anemia characteristic of nephronophthisis/medullary cystic disease may be most concerned about their fatigue and diminished mental performance. In many youths, the clinical course of the kidney disease is silent until the process is sufficiently advanced to produce findings such as diminished growth, edema, uremia, oliguria, hypertension, or colic from urolithiasis. Therefore many of those cases with initially silent clinical courses may be discovered only at routine health screening examinations.

Many serious renal disorders that present in childhood may, for the adolescent, progress to become the problems of chronic or even end-stage renal disease, dialysis, and transplantation. Other disorders do not appear until the teenage years, with diagnostic and early treatment issues as the principal clinical concerns. The importance of chronic renal insufficiency in adolescents is reflected in the finding that between 25 and 27 percent of chronic renal failure in pediatric patients is reported in adolescents between 13 and 17 years of age. This section primarily focuses on those renal disorders that may arise and require evaluation during the teenage years. However, we start with a discussion of urinary tract infections.

15.2 Urinary tract infection

15.2.1 Epidemiology

Urinary tract infections (UTIs) are common infections identified throughout the life span, particularly for females. Infection of the bladder (cystitis) is three to five times more common in the female versus the male and typically develops as a primary infection in a healthy individual (1,2,3). The incidence decreases during the first 10 years of life and gradually increases over time, especially in the female. ▶Tab. 15.1 lists as risk factors for UTI occurrence; these include vesicoureteral reflux (VCR), voiding dysfunction, constipation (a cause of voiding dysfunction), and others. Five percent or more of females who are 5 to 18 years of age develop a UTI with an incidence of 2 percent in adolescent females; over 20 percent of females experience

Tab. 15.1: Factors contributing to the risk of UTI.

Females	Anatomic short urethra
	Poor perineal hygiene
	Coital irritation, change of coital patterns, new sexual partner ("honeymoon cystitis")
	Vulvovaginitis
	Vaginal or rectal colonization with pathogenic bacterial serogroups (e.g., *Escherichia coli*)
	Pregnancy (abnormal ureteral peristalsis)
	Bladder contamination secondary to douching
	Vaginal foreign body
	Diaphragm and/or spermicide use (controversial for disease)
Males	Urethral strictures (extremely rare in girls who have not had prior surgery, trauma, or radiation)
	Posterior urethral valves
	Phimosis
	Meatal stenosis
	Sexual practices exposing the urethra to fecal flora
	UTI is increased in uncircumcised versus circumcised males
Males or females	Urologic abnormality with stasis and/or obstruction (dysfunctional bladder [neurogenic or other], ectopic ureter, nephrolithiasis, etc.)
	Vesicoureteral reflux
	Urethral instrumentation (catheters, foreign bodies, masturbatory)
	Urethral trauma Other foci of infection (direct extension from kidney, prostate, vagina, or hematogenous spread from distant site)
	Lowered host resistance to infection (including due to HIV infection)
	Multiple antibiotic usage and development of resistant organisms
	Infrequent or incomplete voiding
	Voluntary urinary retention
	Chronic illnesses such as diabetes

Reprinted with permission from Greydanus DE, Torres, AD, Wan JH: Genitourinary and renal disorders. In DE Greydanus, DR Patel, DH Pratt, eds. Essential Adolescent Medicine. New York: McGraw Hill; 2006:330.

at least one UTI during their reproductive years. Approximately 30 percent of females have recurrent UTIs. The incidence of UTI in males is highest in the first year of life and after 55 years of age (due to prostatic hypertrophy); it is at its lowest during the young adult years.

15.2.2 Etiology

The main uropathogens of cystitis in adolescents are Enterobacteriaceae (particularly *Escherichia coli*) and coagulase-negative staphylococci, although others may be causative as well (see ▶Tab. 15.2) (4). A number of factors place the individual at risk for UTIs, as noted in ▶Tab. 15.1. This includes coital behavior in females that may result in incomplete bladder emptying. Approximately 20 percent of females with bacteriuria have vesicoureteral reflux (VUR). The virulence of the *E. coli* strain can be enhanced by pili or fimbriae (*E. coli* types 1 and 2) on the outer surface of the bacterium that increase its adherence to epithelial cells, leading to more invasive infections. Virulence factor genes are associated with persistence or recurrence of infections.

Urogenital abnormalities increase the incidence of infection, leading to an upper urinary tract infection (pyelonephritis) due to *E. coli*, drug-resistant enteric pathogens, and others – especially in individuals with chronic or recurrent diseases. Recurrent infection may represent a relapse (with the same organism as before) versus a reinfection with a different organism. Multiple antibiotic usage may lead to infection with two or more pathogenic strains. A relapse may be due to incomplete treatment of an initial infection and/or complication of underlying urolithiasis or structural urogenital abnormality.

15.2.3 Diagnosis

Clinical manifestations of UTIs can range from being asymptomatic to fulminant systemic infections. Typical symptoms of a simple cystitis or lower urinary tract infection are listed in ▶Tab. 15.3. Pain on urination (dysuria) along with other UTI symptoms suggests a lower UTI; suprapubic pain may be present These features may also be present in the acute urethral syndrome and urethritis. Dysuria may also occur in individuals

Tab. 15.2: Etiologic agents in UTIs.

Escherichia coli (*E. coli*: 80%–90%)
Staphylococcus saprophyticus (15%)
Enterobacter aerogenes
Enterococcus species
Klebsiella pneumoniae
Proteus mirabilis
Pseudomonas aeruginosa
Serratia marcescens
Gastrointestinal pathogens (i.e., *Salmonella, Shigella, Campylobacter*)
Adenovirus (types 11 and 21)
Rare: *Staphylococcus aureus* (consider other source of infection), group B *Streptococcus*
Mycobacterium tuberculosis, Haemophilus influenzae type B
Nosocomial infection (yeasts [*Candida albicans*], *Staphylococcus aureus*, gram-negative rods)
Human papovavirus BK

Tab. 15.3: Urinary tract symptoms.

Dysuria
Urinary frequency
Hesitancy
Urgency
Nocturia
Urination produces small amount of urine (can be turbid or bloody)
Low abdominal pain including suprapubic pain
Low-grade temperature elevation
Hematuria (gross or microscopic)

with vaginitis, although there is usually less urinary frequency and urgency along with the presence of vulvovaginal inflammation. Examination may reveal phimosis in males, labial adhesions in females, or evidence of sexual abuse or trauma in both. There may be a dimple over the back or other defects noted with neurogenic bladder and spinal cord involvement.

Frequency and urgency can result from viral cystitis and also from irritation induced by the consumption of chocolate, caffeine, or carbonated beverages. Chemical irritation can occur from female hygiene products. Bedwetting in a previously toilet trained child and/or foul-smelling urine in a developmentally disabled child or adolescent may suggest a UTI as well. Acute hemorrhagic cystitis due to *E. coli*, adenovirus (types 11 and 21), or human papovavirus BK may occur. Adenovirus-induced hemorrhagic cystitis is more commonly seen in boys, is self-limiting, and usually resolves in 4 days or so. Interstitial cystitis is noted in adolescent females with UTI-like symptoms, including bladder/pelvic pain, that are improved with voiding but with negative urine cultures. Cystoscopy reveals bladder distention with mucosal ulcers. This is an idiopathic condition with no specific beneficial treatment.

Sometimes distinguishing a lower from an upper UTI (acute pyelonephritis [involvement of the renal parenchyma]) can be difficult because the symptoms may be similar. In pyelonephritis there may be fever, chills, and variable costovertebral tenderness. Confusion may occur with other causes of abdominal pain, such as appendicitis, cholecystitis, hepatitis, and others. The risk of developing pyelonephritis increases in those with functional or structural urinary tract abnormalities. These cases usually involve an ascending infection from the urethra to the bladder and upper urinary tract; rarely, the infection may be blood-borne. Potential complications of pyelonephritis include renal scarring (pyelonephritic scarring), renal abscess, septic shock, hypertension, proteinuria with or without focal segmental glomerulosclerosis (FSGS), pregnancy-related complications, renal impairment, and end-stage renal failure.

Laboratory

Classic supportive laboratory data include pyuria of over 10 white blood cels (WBCs) per high-power field of spun urine sediment, a positive Gram's stain with one or more bacteria per high-power field of uncentrifuged urine, and/or a positive urine culture with antibiotic sensitivities to identify the etiologic microbe and the most effective antibiotic treatment based on results of sensitivity testing. A urine dipstick typically includes tests of leukocyte esterase (LE) and nitrite for WBCs and gram-negative bacteria respectively. Sensitivity of the LE test is 76 to 85 percent and sensitivity of the nitrite reaction is variable, from 29 to 70 percent.

It should be noted that negative results from symptomatic patients require cautious interpretation, since false-negative results can be common while gram-positive and nonbacterial infections can be missed. A positive nitrite test performed on a freshly voided urine specimen is highly suggestive of a UTI, whereas negative microscopy for bacteria with a negative LE test has high a negative predictive value for a UTI. A negative Gram's stain of urine for bacteria with the presence of fewer than 10 WBCs per cubic millimeter essentially rules out a UTI.

Traditionally a bacterial colony count of greater than 10^5 colony forming units (CFUs) per milliliter of a specific bacterium from a clean-voided specimen defines the etiologic agent, allowing effective treatment for cystitis or pyelonephritis. This correlates with actual infection in 80 percent, with a false-positive rate of 20 percent; two positive cultures of the same microbe correlate with true infection in 95 percent. Youths with symptoms of cystitis or even pyelonephritis can have colony counts as low as 10^4/mL, whereas counts as low as 102/mL may be noteworthy in situations of urethritis or when the urine was gathered via suprapubic aspiration or catheterization. Symptomatic urethritis may have counts between 102 and 105, especially in males.

A negative urine culture in sexually active adolescents with symptoms suggestive of a UTI should prompt evaluation for urethral infection with such sexually transmitted disease (STD) agents such as *Chlamydia trachomatis*, *Neisseria gonorrhoeae*, *Trichomonas vaginalis*, or herpes simplex virus. The growth of mixed cultures, even with high counts, usually suggests contamination of the specimen. Approximately 70 percent of individuals with a significant culture have infections localized to the bladder, whereas 30 percent will have dual infection in the lower and upper urinary tracts. An elevated WBC count (leukocytosis, neutrophilia), elevated erythrocyte sedimentation rate, and elevated C-reactive protein may be seen in pyelonephritis.

Recurrent or complex UTIs

A single episode of a UTI in a male or repeated UTIs in female adolescents (i.e., two to three episodes of cystitis over 1–2 years) would warrant further investigation for underlying factors. Renal ultrasonography may reveal a urogenital abnormality such as hydronephrosis, renal cysts, or renal calculi. A computed tomography (CT) scan and intravenous urography can reveal renal calculi with a negative sonography. Voiding cystourethrography (isotope or contrast) can detect vesicoureteral reflux (VCU) as well as bladder and/or urethral abnormalities. Renal magnetic resonance imaging (MRI) is an effective tool for the diagnosis and follow-up of acute pyelonephritis. In subclinical or overt pyelonephritis, a technetium [99]m-dimercaptosuccinic acid (DMSA) renal scan can detect infectious foci in the renal parenchyma and/or renal scarring from previous renal infection. A CT scan or ultrasound can identify a renal abscess.

15.2.4 Management

Successful treatment of a UTI involves knowledge of the specific causative agent based on culture and sensitivity results (1, 2, 3, ,5,6). Prompt treatment reduces risks for recurrence and complications. Adolescent females with acute, uncomplicated cystitis can usually be adequately treated with a 3-day course of oral trimethoprim/sulfamethoxazole, trimethoprim, or a fluoroquinolone (see ▶Tab. 15.4). Treatment of urinary tract infections can also include use of oral analgesics (as NSAIDs) and urinary analgesics such as phenazopyridine hydrochloride. This urinary analgesic is given at 200 mg three times a day for 2 days and may partially relieve urinary burning, frequency, or urgency. Adverse effects include headaches, gastric irritation, and rash; the urine may turn orange or red and there can be staining of clothes or contact lenses.

Research suggests that fluoroquinolones (e.g., ciprofloxacin) may induce cartilage damage in children, but they have been effective against *Pseudomonas* infection. Oral cefixime and parenteral ceftriaxone can be effective against gram-negative microbes except for *Pseudomonas*. Aminoglycosides can have nephrotoxic and ototoxic effects but can be effective against *Pseudomonas*.

Ampicillin and cephalosporins alter periurethral and fecal flora, with the resultant encouragement of multidrug resistance. Recent studies note the emergence of extended-spectrum beta-lactamase–producing *E. coli*, leading to the increased resistance to beta-lactam antibiotics (i.e., amoxicillin-clavulanic acid, trimethoprim/sulfamethoxazole, quinolones) in addition to the ineffectiveness of cephalosporins and vancomycin against enterococci. Additional antibiotics include nitrofurantoin, fosfomycin (single dose in cystitis), daptomycin, linezolid, and others. Nitrofurantoin does not achieve effective renal tissue levels.

A longer course of antibiotics may be necessary with complicating factors, such as diabetes mellitus, pregnancy, use of a diaphragm, or history of frequent UTIs (6,7,8, 9,10). Cystitis in the male is treated for 7 to 10 days and mild cases of pyelonephritis may be managed on an ambulatory basis with 7 to 10 days of oral antibiotics. Those with severe disease and/or situations complicated by urosepsis, severe illness, or others may need hospitalization with intravenous antibiotic coverage, which can include third-generation cephalosporins; an alternative treatment is ampicillin plus gentamicin or an antipseudomonal penicillin. After the patient is improved, antibiotic switch therapy can be used in switching from intravenous to oral antibiotics in selective situations.

Tab. 15.4: Antibiotic treatment of simple UTIs.

Ciprofloxacin: 250 mg twice daily for 3 days* (used off label for patients who are prepubescent)

Levofloxacin 250 mg once a day for 3 days

Nitrofurantoin: 50–100 mg four times daily for 7 days

Trimethoprim/sulfamethoxazole double strength (160 mg/800 mg): Twice daily for 3 days

Trimethroprim: 100 mg twice daily for 3 days

Others: See section 15.2.4

Recurrent UTI management

The female with recurrent cystitis despite the absence of any genitourinary abnormality may see less infections if on antibiotic prophylaxis for 4 to 6 months (11,12,13). Examples include taking these antibiotics and doses at night: nitrofurantoin 50 to 100 mg, trimethoprim 100 mg, or trimethoprim/sulfamethoxazole (80 mg/400 mg) – half a tablet. If coital activity seems to be a factor, she can take an antibiotic immediately after coitus; examples include 100 mg of nitrofurantoin, ½ tablet (or 1 tablet) of trimethoprim/sulfamethoxazole (double strength), or 250 mg of ciprofloxacin.

Avoidance of coitus may also be helpful. Other measures that may be beneficial include proper perineal hygiene (particularly postdefecation) and postcoital voiding. If use of a diaphragm and spermicide is an underlying factor, a different form of birth control may be helpful. Recent research is looking at the efficacy of intravesical instillation of hyaluronic acid and chondroitin sulfate in adult females with recurrent UTIs (14). Cranberry juice has not been shown to prevent recurrent UTIs (15). In males, circumcision may help if phimosis is a precipitating factor.

15.3 Bacteriuria

Epidemiologic studies note that 3 to 5 percent of adolescent females without UTI symptoms have more than 105 CFU/mL of a specific bacterial microbe on repeat urine cultures. Evaluation reveals a normal upper urinary tract, bladder function, and normal vesicoureteral reflux (VUR) studies. The impact of this is unclear, although some do eventually clear themselves of the bacteria. Antibiotic coverage can transiently clear the bacteria, but the bacteriuria recurs when the antibiotics are stopped. Distinguishing between asymptomatic bacteriuria and a UTI can be difficult in some situations. Progressive renal injury is usually not seen in adolescents or young adults with histories of childhood bacteriuria.

There is increased risk of bacteriuria recurrence (asymptomatic or symptomatic) during pregnancy, and individuals who are not treated in childhood with antibiotics may develop reduced renal adaptation to later pregnancy (16). Although it is controversial, the treatment of adolescent females with asymptomatic bacteriuria and normal studies is not recommended in the absence of pregnancy and may be problematic because of possible alteration of the urinary flora from low-virulence to higher-virulence microbes. The workup should rule out incontinence (day or night) and perineal discomfort. If the patient has postcoital cystitis, treatment may be warranted. Also if she becomes pregnant, antibiotic treatment is recommended because of the increased risk for pyelonephritis, miscarriage, and fetal infection.

15.4 Proteinuria

Clinically asymptomatic proteinuria is a frequent finding in adolescents and young adults. The vast majority of patients with asymptomatic proteinuria will be found to have orthostatic (postural) or intermittent proteinuria. Orthostatic proteinuria has a good prognosis and intermittent proteinuria is carefully followed up to ensure that it does not become persistent. Also, proteinuria is a common hallmark of many renal diseases; unless it is sufficiently severe as to cause nephrotic syndrome, clinical findings may be scant. The situation may become more clouded, since fever, strenuous exercise, dehydration, extreme cold, and, possibly emotional stress can increase the rate of protein excretion both in normal individuals and patients with kidney disease–associated proteinuria.

False-positive dipstick results for urinary protein should be considered in all asymptomatic patients with unexplained proteinuria; such results may be due to highly buffered urine from alkaline medications or storage and urinary contamination by quaternary ammonium cleaning agents, a urinary pH greater than 7.0, leaving dipstick in the urine too long (i.e., washing out the buffer), and use of phenazopyridine (for some dipstick brands). Also urinary proteins other than albumin are not readily detected by standard dipstick testing. Thus gamma globulins, Bence-Jones proteins, hemoglobin, lysozyme, and others may produce negative results. Detection of nonalbumin urinary proteins can be routinely accomplished using sulfosalicylic acid and most specifically by protein electrophoresis in urine. A positive dipstick for proteinuria is an indication for the quantification of proteinuria.

15.4.1 Quantification of proteinuria

The traditional method for quantifying proteinuria has been the 24-hour urine collection, expressed as g/L or g/24 hour. Normal values range between 30 and 150 mg/24 hours in adults and around 100 mg/m^2 per day in children. A more practical alternative is the measurement of the protein:creatinine ratio expressed as gram of protein per gram of creatinine in a randomly collected urine sample. It has an excellent correlation with the 24-hour urine collection. Normal values are below 0.2 after 5 years of age.

15.4.2 Orthostatic proteinuria

Orthostatic proteinuria is a condition generally described as the presence of abnormally high rates of protein excretion occurring in the upright position only. When unassociated with any other urinary abnormality (e.g., hematuria), long-term follow-up studies have demonstrated that the risk of underlying significant renal disease is not increased for the normal population. Since the majority of adolescents evaluated for protein in the urine will be found to have intermittent or orthostatic proteinuria, the clinician's first task is to screen out those patients with a benign diagnosis.

Normal males excrete 20 to 26 mg/kg per day of creatinine, whereas normal females excrete 14 to 22 mg/kg per day. The upper limit of normal protein excretion is approximately 100 mg/m^2 every 24 hours (150–200 mg every 24 hours). The diagnosis of orthostatic proteinuria is based on first-morning recumbent urine protein testing by dipstick that is negative or trace, increased values during daytime activity, and less than 1,000 mg of protein every24 hours (some authors suggest an upper limit of 2,000 mg every 24 hours). A number of different algorithms for the diagnosis of orthostatic proteinuria have been proposed. A useful approach is described below; it can be applied to the adolescent found to have proteinuria and no historical or physical finding suggestive of underlying renal or urologic disease; this method allows one to demonstrate the orthostatic component of the proteinuria.

In this method a 24-hour "split" urine collection is recommended. The test requires two clean containers, usually provided by the laboratory performing the test. On the day of the test, the first voided urine specimen is discarded and the time is noted. All the urines voided the rest of the day are collected in one container and labeled "daytime urine collection." Before retiring to bed, the adolescent should rest, reclining for 1 to 2 hours. Just before going to bed, the teen should urinate, place the urine in the daytime urine collection container, note the time, and then retire to bed for the night. The following morning, the teen should urinate, if possible by the bedside. The urine is collected in the second container and labeled "nighttime urine collection." Both containers are taken to the laboratory for determination of volume and for protein and creatinine content; also, the ratio of grams of protein to grams of creatinine in each container is established. The normal urine protein:creatinine excretion ratio is below 0.2; an elevated protein excretion during the day in the presence of normal protein excretion during the night establishes the presence of orthostatic or postural proteinuria (17).

The general consensus among nephrologists is that orthostatic proteinuria has a good prognosis and that renal biopsy is not necessary; it seems prudent to follow these patients at yearly or 2-year intervals. Indications for renal biopsy vary according to the considerations of the ethnicity, age, and geographic characteristics of the population studied. The most common indications for renal biopsy are listed in ▶Tab. 15.5 (18).

Rapid deterioration of renal function requires an emergency renal biopsy to exclude or confirm crescentic glomerulonephritis. Isolated microscopic hematuria in which all other studies are normal requires follow-up but the need for prompt renal biopsy is less clear. Few contraindications for renal biopsy exist; they include uncontrolled bleeding diathesis, uncontrolled hypertension, uncooperative patient, renal neoplasm, and renal infection with multiple cysts; a solitary kidney is a relative contraindication. Contraindications for renal biopsy are noted in ▶Tab. 15.6.

Tab. 15.5: Indications for renal biopsy (18).

Nephrotic syndrome: in prepubertal children only if the clinical presentation is atypical for minimal change disease (MCD); renal biopsy is indicated in adolescents and adult patients because causes of nephrotic syndrome other than MCD are common.
In acute kidney injury after obstruction, reduced renal perfusion, acute tubular necrosis, acute poststreptococcal glomerulonephritis have been ruled out.
Systemic disease with renal dysfunction: small-vessel vasculitis, antiglomerular basement membrane disease, systemic lupus erythematosus. Those with diabetes only if atypical features are present.
Isolated microscopic hematuria only in unusual circumstances
Nonnephrotic-range proteinuria >1g/day
Unexplained chronic kidney disease, may be diagnostic: IgA nephropathy, Nephronophthisis.
Familial renal disease: biopsy of one affected member may be diagnostic and minimize clinical investigation of other affected members.
Renal transplant dysfunction: indicated if ureteral obstruction, infection, vascular thrombosis, and calcineurin toxicity are not present.

Tab. 15.6: Contraindications to renal biopsy (18).

Kidney status	Patient status
Multiple cysts	Uncontrolled bleeding diathesis
Solitary kidney (relative contraindication)	Uncontrolled blood pressure
Acute pyelonephritis/perinephric abscess	Uremia
Renal neoplasm	Obesity; uncooperative patient

15.4.3 Laboratory studies

Adolescents with persistent proteinuria, particularly associated with one or more of the renal factors listed above, should be considered for referral to a subspecialist for further evaluation and possible renal biopsy. Although many tests for underlying renal disease may be performed by the primary care physician, tests beyond quantitative protein excretion measurements and basic renal function studies are often best done in the context of a formal nephrology evaluation. Once the proteinuria has been characterized as a nonorthostatic, persistent proteinuria (see section 15.4.2) and appropriate measures taken, serial quantitative changes of protein excretion may be approximated without the need of repeated 24-hour urine collections.

The technique for this estimate uses a random daytime specimen of urine in which protein and creatinine concentrations are measured. The protein concentration divided by the creatinine concentration (in the same units, e.g., mg/dL, g/L) multiplied by the factor 0.63 gives the result in grams of protein excreted (i.e., g/m^2 per 24 hours). This method of long-term reevaluation is an attractive alternative to the task of 24-hour urine collections, one often dreaded by adolescents who are attending school or working.

Urinalysis is an important aspect of the evaluation of any patient with proteinuria; unfortunately the microscopic evaluation of the urinary sediment is becoming an infrequent exercise for many physicians. A simple estimation of renal function can be obtained by measuring blood urea nitrogen (BUN), creatinine, electrolytes, and CO_2 in serum. Adolescents with nonorthostatic proteinuria require a renal ultrasound evaluation to detect structural abnormalities, such as number of renal units, cystic diseases, renal asymmetry, or hydronephrosis. These basic studies can be perform by the primary care physician; however, adolescents with nonorthostatic proteinuria must be referred to a nephrologist for further evaluation and management.

15.5 Nephrotic syndrome

15.5.1 Etiology

Over the last decade, advances in knowledge of the structure and function of the filtering mechanism of the glomerulus have facilitated the understanding of familial and secondary forms of severe proteinuria manifesting as the nephrotic syndrome, a generic term describing the concomitant presence of proteinuria (greater than 50 mg/kg per day)

Tab. 15.7: Frequent glomerulopathies in adolescents.

Minimal change disease (MCD)	Mesangioproliferative glomerulonephritis
Focal segmental glomerulosclerosis (FSGS)	Poststreptococcal glomerulonephritis
Membranous nephropathy (MN)	Goodpasture's disease
Membranoproliferative glomerulonephritis (MPGN)	ANCA-associated vasculitis
Dense deposit disease (DDD)	Lupus nephritis

in children or a urine albumin:creatinine ratio greater than 2 mg of protein per milligram of creatinine, hypoalbuminemia of 25 g of albumin per liter, edema, and hypercholesterolemia secondary to hypoalbuminemia.

In brief, the glomerular filtering barrier is made up of a fenestrated endothelium, the endothelial surface layer, glomerular basement membrane, a slit diaphragm between interdigitating foot processes, and the subpodocyte space. Disruptions of the filtration barrier will results in loss of the permiselectivity and loss of protein in the urine, which can be severe, leading to the development of the nephrotic syndrome (19). There is evidence supporting the relative importance of each component of the filtering barrier in maintaining its integrity. Identification of mutations in a number of the genes causing familial forms of FSGS has resulted in significant advances (20).

There are multiple causes of nephrotic syndrome, including genetic causes, secondary causes that are immunologically mediated or secondary to infections or metabolic disease, and idiopathic causes. The traditional classification of the nephrotic syndrome has been based in the histopathologic alterations of the glomerulus as describe in the International Study of Kidney Disease in Children (ISKDC). Glomerulopathies are now considered (see ▶Tab. 15.7).

15.5.2 Minimal Change disease (MCD)

In children less than 10 years of age the nephrotic syndrome has a sudden onset with edema of the face and lower extremities, nephrotic range proteinuria, and hypoalbuminemia. On renal biopsy, the findings are that of normal histology by light microscopic examination and by immunofluorescence (IF). The abnormal findings are only detected by electron microscopic (EM) examination, demonstrating generalized foot processes effacement, thus the designation minimal change disease (MCD).

In individuals below of 10 years of age, MCD is observed in 80 to 90 percent of those with idiopathic nephrotic syndrome. MCD is seen in up to 50 percent of those older than 10 years and between 10 and 15 percent of nondiabetic adults who present with a sudden onset of idiopathic nephrotic syndrome. Based on this knowledge, a renal biopsy is not indicated in children below 10 years of age with the nephrotic syndrome. These children usually respond well to treatment with corticosteroids (21). On the other hand, in nondiabetic adults with a sudden onset of nephrotic syndrome, a renal biopsy (unless contraindicated) is necessary to determine the underlying pathologic lesion. In the majority of cases of MCD, there is no identifiable etiology. Recently the expression of CD80 on the podocytes and urinary excretion of CD80 in the urine in MCD has been reported (22).

The initial treatment of MCD is with corticosteroids in pediatric, adolescent, and as well adult patients (23). The initial dose of prednisone for the adolescent patient likely to have MCD is 60 mg/m² per day until the proteinuria disappears, usually by 2 weeks. Prednisone is continued at the same daily dose for 6 weeks , at which time the patient is switched to alternated-day, same-dose prednisone for another 6 weeks. Prednisone is then tapered by 15 mg/m² every 2 weeks.

Relapse occurs in up to 60 percent of these patients within the year of initiation of treatment and 30 to 40 percent will have frequent relapses (i.e., four or more relapses in 1 year). The treatment of a relapse consist of administration of prednisone at 60 mg/m² per day divided into three doses for 3 to 5 days until the proteinuria disappears; thereafter, the prednisone is decreased to 40 mg/m² per day divided into three doses every other day for 1 month and then discontinued. There are some other regimens for the treatment of frequent relapses and steroid-dependent treatment. Experience indicates that a longer duration of initial prednisone treatment decreases the number of relapses and in the long term results in less exposure to prednisone (24,25). When a patient continues to have frequent relapses or is steroid-dependent, he or she is at an increased risk for steroids side effects and may require the use of different medications before the steroid toxicity manifests itself.

The conventional treatment of MCD in the adult is the same as the treatment in children or adolescents. The initial dose of prednisone is 1 mg/kg per day with a maximal dose of 80 mg/day. The response to prednisone may be delayed up to 3 to 4 months of treatment and 25 percent will fail to respond. The dose of prednisone is decreased by half after remission, as observed by the disappearance of protein in the urine as shown by dipstick. Then prednisone treatment is continued for 4 to 6 more weeks. Relapses are less frequent in the adult than in the pediatric or adolescent patient. ▶Tab. 15.8 lists important definitions for the evaluation and treatment of nephrotic syndrome. When the use of steroids is ineffective or the side effects become intolerable, alternative pharmacologic therapy becomes necessary. ▶Tab. 15.9 lists the most frequently used nonsteroidal immunosuppressive agents available for the treatment of glomerular diseases. Only physicians familiar with the use of immunosuppressive medications should prescribe them.

During the second decade of life the prevalence of MCD decreases and nephrotic syndrome is increasingly associated with other forms of glomerular disease. Most frequent in the United States are focal segmental glomerulosclerosis (FSGS) and other forms of glomerular diastases, as listed in ▶Tab. 15.10. The concurrent findings of hypertension and hematuria in adolescents with new-onset nephrotic syndrome are unusual in MCD.

15.5.3 Focal segmental glomerulosclerosis

Focal segmental glomerulosclerosis (FSGS) is defined as a clinicopathologic syndrome characterized by proteinuria and a focal and segmental glomerulosclerosis pattern of injury by microscopic examination that is common to many different conditions (see ▶Tab. 15.10). A rigorous analysis of the characteristics and localization of the glomerular lesions and knowledge of clinical circumstances provides more specificity and clinically relevant information for the evaluation and treatment of patients. With advancement in knowledge of the structure and function of the filtering mechanism

Tab. 15.8: Useful definitions for management of the nephrotic syndrome.

Term	Adult	Adolescent/child
Relapse	Proteinuria ≥1 g day 1	Albustix 3+ or proteinuria >40 mg^2 per hour occurring on 3 days within 1 week
Frequently relapsing	2+ relapses within 6 months	2+ relapses within 6 months
Complete remission	Reduction of proteinuria ≤0.20 g/day and serum albumin >35 g/L	< 4 mg^2 per hour on at least 3 occasions within 7 days. Serum albumin >35 g/l-1
Partial remission	Reduction of proteinuria to 0.21g/day and serum albumin >35 g/L ± decrease in proteinuria of 50% from baseline	Disappearance of edema. Increase in serum albumin >35 g/l and persisting proteinuria >4 mg^2 per hour or >100 mg/m^{2}per day
Steroid-resistant	Persistence of proteinuria despite prednisone therapy 1mg per kg per day for 4 months	Persistence of proteinuria despite prednisone therapy of 60 mg/m^2 for 4 weeks and three methylprednisolone pulses
Steroid-dependent-nephrotic syndrome	Two consecutive relapses that occurring during therapy or within 14 days of completing steroid therapy	Two relapses of proteinuria 14 days after stopping or during alternated steroid therapy

in the glomerular basement membrane, many forms of genetically determined causes of FSGS have been identified. In addition, secondary causes of FSGS are also being more commonly encountered, including low birth weight, prematurity, obesity, and the use of anabolic steroids in adolescents and young adults (26).

Primary FSGS is of particular concern to the physician caring for adolescents. It is the most common cause of glomerular disease resulting in end-stage renal disease (ESRD) in this age group, particularly in African American adolescent males. It is now recognized that the prevalence of primary FSGS in nephrotic black patients is two to four times that of the Caucasian population. The incidence of FSGS in children and adults is increasing in all ethnic groups.

Treatment of primary focal segmental glomerulosclerosis

The response to treatment of primary FSGS is difficult to predict; however, based on the experience of the use of immunosuppression protocols, some patients do respond to medical management. Current treatment recommendations for primary FSGS include treatment of hypertension, use of antiproteinuric medications such as angiotensin converting enzyme inhibitors/angiotensin receptor blockers (ACEs/ARBs), treatment of hyperlipidemia, administration of immunosuppressive medications including steroids, and calcineurin inhibitors (cyclosporin, tacrolimus, and other medication as listed in ▶Tabs. 15.9 and 15.11). The recurrence of primary FSGS in the graft after transplantation is 23 to 40 percent; it is treated with plasmapheresis and intensification of immunosuppression. The response to plasmapheresis is well documented.

Tab. 15.9: Nonsteroidal immunosuppressive agents use in glomerular diseases.

Drug	Pediatric dose	Adult dose	Problem	Comment
Levamisol	2.5 mg/kg; limited experience ir the United States	Limited experience in adult patients in the United States.	No readily available in the United States.	Causes neutropenia.
Cyclophosphamide	2–3 mg/kg per day for 12 weeks	In refractory nephrotic syndrome, 2.5–3 mg/kg per day orally every day for 60 to 90 days. In proliferative lupus nephritis: 500 mg–1 g/m² IV every month for 6 months then quarterly for 2 years.	Need to monitor WCC.	Hemorrhagic cystitis, risk of sterility. particularly in adolescents boys more than in adolescent girls; premature ovarian failure in women. Repeated cycles not recommended.
MMF	600 mg/m² day in two doses (12.5 to18 mg/kg per dose twice a day)	0.5 to 3 g/day in two doses (lupus nephritis). Usual adult dose for other conditions 2 g/day.	Gastrointestinal distress.	Risk of immunosuppression, reactivation of latent viral infections, progressive multifocal leukoencephalopathy, lymphoproliferative disease.
Cyclosporin-A (Neoral)	6 mg/kg per day given every 12 hours; monitor trough levels to lower therapeutic range.	3–5 mg/kg per day in two doses; keep trough level low therapeutic range (150–225 µg/L.	Therapeutic leves are needed.	May cause interstitial renal fibrosis, hypertension (calcineurin nephrotoxicity), and decrease GFR.
Tacrolimus	0.075–0.2 mg/kg per day in two doses.		Therapeutic levels to be monitored.	May cause calcineurin nephrotoxicity, increased risk of diabetes mellitus in overweight patients.

(Continued)

Tab. 15.9: Nonsteroidal immunosuppressive agents use in glomerular diseases. (*Continued*)

Drug	Pediatric dose	Adult dose	Problem	Comment
Rituximab	375 mg/m² IV weekly in two to four doses.	375 mg/m² weekly in four doses.	U.S. boxed warning.	A CD20-depleting agent is primarily used to treat hematologic malignancies. Its use has been extended to immune-mediated diseases including renal diseases.
Eculizumab	Used for treatment of paroxysmal nocturnal hemoglobinuria; is an investigational drug for kidney diseases.	Has been use off label in some forms of atypical hemolytic uremic syndrome and kidney transplantation.	U.S. boxed warning; increases susceptibility to meningococcal disease.	Monoclonal humanized IgG antibody that binds to complement protein C5, preventing cleavage intoC5a and C5b and thus preventing the formation of membrane attack complex (MAC).

Tab. 15.10: Etiologic classification of focal segmental glomerulosclerosis.

Primary FSGS or idiopathic associated with vascular permeability factor.

Secondary forms of FSGS.
Familial/genetic.
Mutations in nephrin, podocin, α-actin-4, mutation in transient receptor potential cation 6 channel (TRPC6), mutations in WT1.

Viral infection associated with HIV, parvovirus 18.

Drug-induced (heroin, interferon, lithium, pamidronate, sirolimus).

Postadaptive response.
Reduced renal mass very low birth weight. Unilateral renal agenesis, renal dysplasia, reflux nephropathy, sequel to cortical necrosis, surgical renal ablation, any advance renal disease with reduction of functioning nephrons.
Initial normal renal mass hypertension, obesity, increased lean body mass, anabolic steroids, cyanotic congenital heart disease.

Tab. 15.11: Drugs commonly used to treat glomerular diseases.

Immunomodulatory agent	Proposed mechanism of action
Glucocorticoids	Steroids suppress B- and T-cell function inactivate NF-kBa, thereby decreasing cytokine generation.
Cyclophosphamide	An alkylating agent that covalently links DNA, RNA, and proteins leading to either cell death or protein function. Cyclophosphamide causes neutropenia and lymphopenia.
Mycophenolic acid	Inhibits T- and B-cell proliferation by blocking purine synthesis by inhibiting inosine monophosphate dehydrogenase.
Cyclosporine/tacrolimus	Inhibits the phosphatase calcineurin, preventing the translocation of nuclear factor of activated T cells (NFAT) and leading to reduced transcriptional activation of early cytokines genes. Cyclosporin may also stabilize the actin cytoskeleton of podocytes maintaining podocytes function.
Rituximab	Murine/human chimeric anti-CD20 monoclonal antibody that depletes B cells.
Azathioprine	Inhibits T- and B-cell proliferation by blocking purine synthesis.
Chlorambucil	An alkylating agent that cross links DNA; it reduces the number of both T and B cells.
Eculizumab	Monoclonal antibody to the complement protein C5. It blocks cleavage of C5, thereby preventing the formation of C5 and the membrane attack complex.
Plasma exchange	Removes high-molecular-weight substances such as antigen-antibody complexes, cryoglobulins, and myeloma light chains from the plasma.
Nonimmunomodulatory agents: ACE/ARBs	Decrease intraglomerular pressure; may also have antifibrotic properties.

An important form of familial FSGS nephrotic syndrome presenting in adolescents follows an autosomal dominant pattern of inheritance, and these patients are resistant to immunosuppression. Although no immunosuppressant medication is indicated, these individuals must have their hypertension and dyslipidemia treated. Many affected family members progress to end-stage renal disease (ESRD). Families with inherited forms of FSGS will benefit from genetic counseling. After renal transplantation, the disease does not recur in the renal graft. Patients with FSGS induced by obesity and the metabolic syndrome will respond to weight reduction, diet, exercise, and antihypertensive medication (27). There are reports of the beneficial effects of bariatric surgery for morbidly obese patients with nephrotic-range proteinuria (28).

Collapsing focal segmental glomerulosclerosis

The term *collapsing focal segmental glomerulosclerosis* was initially used in 1986 by Weiss et al. (17) to describe six African Americans who presented with febrile illness, severe nephrotic syndrome, and rapidly progressive renal failure leading to ESRD. Histopathologic findings included FSGS with glomerular capillaries membranes that were wrinkled and collapsed, with hyperplastic podocytes obliterating the urinary space.

Although the clinical and pathologic findings suggested HIV infection, only one patient in this group went on to develop AIDS. There are striking racial disparities in the predisposition of African American and European American populations for the development of FSGS and HIV infection. Research notes a genetic predisposition linking variants in the nonmuscle myosin heavy chain 9 gene (MYH9), which seems to play a major role in both FSGS and HIV–associated collapsing glomerulopathy (29). Although it is more common in patients with a history of HIV infection and intravenous heroin addiction, there is no history of high-risk behavior or serologic evidence of HIV infection in 20 percent of the affected patients.

Clinically this disorder is manifested by a severe nephrotic/nephritic syndrome associated with fever, general malaise, resistance to steroids, and rapid advancement to ESRD or death. There are a few reports indicating a response to immunosuppression with methylprednisolone and intravenous rituximab (30). In general the prognosis is poor. Genetic predisposition to the development of the disease has been linked to MYH9 gene variants, which may predispose African Americans to the disease.

Since the initial observations by Weiss et al, the disease has been increasing in frequency; it affects younger children and women and is becoming more recognized in other countries (including China and Pakistan) in association with a negative history of HIV infection or drug abuse. The disease has resulted from the use of certain medications, including pamidronate and interferon (IFN)-α, β, or γ and is typically accompanied by endothelial tubule reticular inclusions. Of interest is the observation that the condition improves following the discontinuation of the interferon treatment or the offending drug. The prognosis is in general poor for long- term renal function; however, there are occasional cases of successful treatment with immunosuppression including rituximab.

15.5.4 Membranoproliferative glomerulonephritis (MPGN)

MPGN, also known as mesangiocapillary glomerulonephritis, is characterized by histologic findings of diffuse proliferative lesions, thickening of the capillary wall, and splitting of the glomerular basement membrane by mesangial interposition, giving the aspect a of double contour. MPGN denotes a pattern of glomerular injury common to different diseases processes. By electron microscopic examination, three types of MPGN have described, labeled I, II, and III. The frequency of MPGN by type based on electron microscopy is listed in ▶Tab. 15.12.

Type I MPGN, the classic form of the disease and also the most common, is defined as the presence of immune complexes in the subendothelial space and in the mesangium; it is associated with activation of the classic pathway of complement activation. Type II MPGN is also known as dense deposit disease (DDD), which is the preferred nomenclature at present. It is considered to be a completely different clinical and pathologic entity from MPGN type I as well as type III.

In North America and Europe, types I and III are the most common forms of MPGN to cause nephrotic syndrome in children, adolescents, and adults. In the United States, 1.5 percent of the affected pediatric and adolescent patients reach ESRD. The incidence of MPGN type I varies significantly with geographic location and is more common in other countries. In Nigeria, for example, it represent up to 52 percent of cases of nephrotic syndrome in children and adolescents. The pathogenesis of MPGN types I and III seems to results from chronic antigen exposure in susceptible individuals. The disease is seen more often in adolescents as well as young adults; in the United States, it affects Caucasians more often than African Americans. There are three clinical presentations of MPGN types I and III: nephrotic syndrome, acute nephritis, and asymptomatic hematuria. The known causes of MPGN types I and III are listed in ▶Tab. 15.13.

Clinical observation indicates that the pathogenesis of type I MPGN is associated with chronic antigenemia with IgG antibodies, unknown antigen, and complement C3; there is also activation of the classic pathway. In patients with active hepatitis C infection, the development of cryoglobulinemia correlates better with the disease and is observed in older individuals. The pathogenesis of the disease in younger children is less clear.

The treatment of MPGN type 1 requires an investigation of the possible cause of the disease. This is especially important in adolescents and in young adults, in whom a secondary cause of the disease is more likely. Particular care must be taken to exclude the presence of active hepatitis C B infection. Treatment of the infection is necessary before immunosuppression is initiated. In children as a general rule, hepatitis B or C is of lesser concern.

MPGN type I is the most common form of this disease; it may be primary or secondary. The secondary forms of MPGN type I with immune deposits are associated with infections, autoimmune diseases, and dysproteinemias. In other cases, as in thrombotic microagiopathies and chronic liver diseases, immune deposits are absent. Of the MPGN type I associated with infections, those associated with hepatitis C and B are of particular relevance. Cryoglobulinemic glomerulonephritis type II has been linked with chronic hepatitis C; the clinical manifestations are those of systemic vasculitis with hypocomplementemia. IFN-α is the treatment of choice for patients with hepatitis

Tab. 15.12: The frequency of the various types of MPGN (18).

Totals	Type I (%)	Type II (%)	Type III (%)
412	213 (52%)	109 (26%)	90 (22%)

Tab. 15.13: Causes of MPGN.

MPGN I	Infectious
Primary/idiopathic	Hepatitis C
Familial	Hepatitis B
Secondary	*Schistosoma mansoni*
Malignancy	HIV
Lymphomas	malaria
Chronic Lymphocytic leukemia	Other
Non-Hodgkin's lymphoma	HIV
Immunologic	Malaria
Cryoglobulinemia	Other
Sjögren's syndrome	Heroin abuse
Complement deficiencies	Partial lipodystrophy
SLE	MPGN type III
	Primary/idiopathic
	Familial
	DDD/MPGN type II
	Primary
	Idiopathic/familial
	Complement deficiency

C–associated cryoglobulinemia. The immunosuppressive therapy for the vasculitis is with methylprednisolone and cyclophosphamide; this management is effective but poses the risk of activating hepatitis C and is reserved for those patients with multiple organ involvement.

A secondary form of MPGN type I is hepatitis C–associated glomerulonephritis in patients with positive serology for hepatitis C that may or not be associated with cryoglobulinemia. Hepatitis C–associated MPGN type I is currently recognized as one of the most important causes of infection-associated glomerulonephritis. The treatment is with long-term antiviral medications including IFN-α and ribavirin. No immunosuppression is indicated because of the risk of activating the hepatitis C infection.

Chronic hepatitis B infection has also been associated with MPGN type I. The pathogenesis involves deposition immune complexes in the glomeruli, and hepatitis B antigen can be demonstrated in the glomeruli. The condition is most common in children. Membranous nephropathy is the most common associated pattern of glomerular injury in hepatitis B. The serology is positive for hepatitis B surface antigen; the clinical manifestations include nephrotic syndrome and, less frequently, cryoglobulinemia with vasculitis. The cornerstone of treatment is antiviral therapy with IFN-α; however, immunosuppressive therapy increases the risk of activating the hepatitis B infection. Types I and III usually present in older children, adolescents, and young adults; it affects males and females with equal frequency and is responsible for 5 to 20 percent cases of the nephrotic syndrome in Europe and North America. The general impression is that the incidence of MPGN is declining in these parts of the world. The presence of persistent circulating immune complexes – as seen in chronic bacterial, viral, and parasitic diseases as well as immunologic diseases (autoimmune), neoplasia, and paraproteinemias – plays an important role in the development of MPGN type I.

The clinical presentation of MPGN may assume several forms that include nephrotic syndrome in about 30 percent of cases, persistent microscopic hematuria and proteinuria in 35 percent, chronic progressive glomerulonephritis in 20 percent, and rapidly progressive glomerulonephritis in 10 percent . Laboratory abnormalities include depletion of complement C3, total hemolytic complement (CH50), and in some cases C4. At least three mechanisms have been implicated as responsible for the hypocomplementemia in MPGN: circulating immune complexes activating the classic pathway, NF (an autoantibody directed against complement proteins), and excessive breakdown of C3 by C3 convertase of the alternative pathway.

The clinical course of MPGN is generally progressive and prognosis for renal survival is poor, particularly in adults with MPGN type II. The prognosis is better in younger individuals. Indicators of poor renal prognosis include hypertension, impaired renal function, nephrotic syndrome, more than 20 percent of crescents present, sclerosis, mesangial deposits, and tubulointerstitial disease. A less strong association is seen with being male and also having macroscopic hematuria; no correlation is seen with serum complement levels.

Treatment of primary MPGN type I

There is no specific therapy for primary MPGN. Children and adolescents with MPGN types I and III were treated by the Cincinnati group with steroids at 2 mg/kg per day, up to 80 mg every other day for up to 2 years; there was dose reduction according to clinical response and an improvement in renal survival was reported (31). A similar improvement was reported by the International Study of Kidney Disease in Children with alternate-day use of steroids (32). Long- term alternate-day prednisone treatment demonstrated stabilization and improvement in renal function and proteinuria with the administration of prednisone at a dose of 2 mg/kg to a maximal dose of 60 mg for 1 year (depending on the response), followed by 10 to 20 mg every other day for 2 to 5 years (31). The side effects of this regimen are considerable, including hypertension, growth retardation, obesity, and cataracts. Careful monitoring of the patients is necessary. With this regimen the renal survival rate has increased from 50 percent in previous decades to between 60 and 85 percent in the present decade. Nephrologists working with adults are using similar regimens for patients with active disease. Additional therapeutic measures include the use of anticoagulant agents such as dipyridamol, acetylsalicylic acid, and heparin. Other agents for immunosuppression that have been use include calcineurin inhibitor and mycophenolate mofetil.

Treatment of secondary forms of MPGN type I

The management of secondary forms of MPGN should be directed to the underlying cause, as, for example, IFN-α for hepatitis C and steroids as well as cyclophosphamide for lupus nephritis. Nonspecific treatment includes normalization of blood pressure with the use of ACE inhibitors or ARBs to decrease proteinuria.

The treatment of the secondary forms of MPGN type I is primarily directed to the cause of the disease. Particular consideration is given to those with MPGN type I induced by hepatitis C and B virus infections. In cryoglobulinemia type 2 vasculitis associated with chronic hepatitis C virus infection, the cornerstone of treatment is IFN-α and ribavirin. Immunosuppressive therapy with pulse methylprednisolone followed by oral prednisone and cyclophosphamide is effective in treating the vasculitis; however, the risk of reactivating the hepatitis C infection is high. Therefore, this regimen must be offered with caution only to patients with disseminated vasculitis involving several organ systems. For those with chronic hepatitis C–associated MPGN type I without cryoglobulinemia, the treatment is with antiviral agents IFN-α and ribavirin. The use of immunosuppressant agents poses a high risk of exacerbating the hepatitis C infection.

In secondary forms of MPGN type I associated with chronic hepatitis B infection, the treatment of choice is the administration of antiviral agents, IFN-α, and ribavirin; spontaneous resolution of the glomerulonephritis occurs or may follow the administration of antiviral agents. In general immunosuppression is contraindicated because of the risk of exacerbating the hepatitis B infection.

In the case of MPGN type I due to lupus (lupus nephritis class IV), the treatment is based in immunosuppression. The traditional management of these patients includes induction of remission with pulse methylprednisolone followed by oral prednisone with rapid tapering and cyclophosphamide; maintenance is with cyclophosphamide. Most recently mycophenolate mofetil has been used successfully with induction and maintenance therapy for patients with lupus class IV.

MPGN type II – dense deposit disease (DDD)

DDD is less common than MPGN type I, affecting mostly children and adolescents; but adults can also be affected. Its frequency of occurrence is two to three cases per 1 million of population. In DDD, the pattern of glomerular injury as noted by electronic microscopy is characterized by the presence of extremely osmophilic dense deposits in the capillary wall, giving a ribbon-like appearance of electron-dense material. The immunofluorescence staining is positive for C3, usually without immunoglobulins or C1q. Extrarenal manifestations may include partial lipodystrophy involving the face and upper body in some patients; there are also abnormalities of the retina (Drusen bodies), resulting in field and color defects and potential deterioration of the retina. Thus these youths will benefit from ophthalmologic evaluation.

DDD is due to dysregulation of the alternate pathway of complement activation. In 80 percent of cases there is an association with the presence of C3 nephritic factor (C3NeF), an antibody that stabilizes the enzyme C3 convertase (C3bBbp), resulting in continuous activation of the alternate complement pathway. Defects in other regulatory proteins of this pathway – such as factor H, factor I, complement membrane protein (CMP), and other factors – explain familial and acquired case of DDD (33).

With improved understanding of its various causes, the possibilities for the treatment of DDD have improved. A rational treatment of this condition requires careful evaluation of the alternate pathway of complement by specialized laboratories. Type III is considered to be a variant of type I and MPGN, in some cases with marked membrane thickening with double contours of the glomerular basement membrane (GBM), which is silver-negative. Abundant subendothelial ,and subepithelial deposits, as seen in membranous nephropathy, are present. In MPGN type III the complement activation profile involves both the activation of the alternate pathway with low C3, normal C4, and low C5-C9, implicating the presence of low-acting nephritic factor properdin-dependent stabilizing C5-convertase. Immunofluorescence is positive for IgG and

C3 plus or minus IgM, IgA, and C1 with electron-dense aggregates diffusely present in subendothelial and subepithelial areas of the membrane. The treatment of MPGN type III is similar to the treatment of MPGN type I.

Treatment of dense deposit disease

Current understanding of the causes of DDD has established a basis for a more rational therapeutic approach for the treatment of these rare and difficult conditions. In general the causes can be divided into three categories: deficiency of complement factor, functional abnormalities of complement factor, and autoantibodies against complement factor. For conditions associated with deficiency of complement factor, the treatment is replacement with plasma infusion or plasma exchange either in an acute form or in a chronic fashion, depending on the nature of the problem. Plasma exchange may be necessary to make room for the volume of plasma infused so as to avoid fluid overload concentrate. Concentrate of the deficient factor will avoid the need for plasma exchange. Patients with antibodies against complement factor C3 convertase, the most common cause of DDD, are treated by removal of the autoantibody via plasmapheresis, immunomodulation with intravenous immunoglobulins, and/or immunosuppression with steroids or rituximab.

Patients with DDD can also be treated with immunosuppression targeted to C5, the final step in the formation of the membrane attack complex (MAC). The IgG humanized monoclonal antibody eculizumab has been used with success in some patients with DDD. All patients with MPGN benefit from careful monitoring and treatment of hypertension, proteinuria, and renal function. These patients must be under the care of a physician familiar with these complexes disorders.

15.5.5 Membranous nephropathy

Membranous nephropathy is a chronic glomerular disease in which immune deposits of IgG and complement develop mainly in the subepithelial space of the glomerular capillary wall, inducing morphologic and functional changes. Morphologically, there is increasing thickening of the glomerular basement membrane; with silver methenamine staining, there are "spikes" surrounding the intramembranous deposits. Because inflammatory cell infiltration and hypercellularity are not characteristic finding of the disease, the term *membranous nephropathy* (MN) is preferred.

The incidence of MN in those from 1 to 12 years of age has been reported to be between 1 to 1.5 percent of nephrotic children; however, this increases to 22 percent in adolescents between 13 and 19 years of age (34,35). Most cases of MN develop in adults and older individuals. It is more frequent in Caucasian males, followed by those from Asia; it occurs less frequently in African American and Hispanic Americans. In the Caucasian adult population, it is responsible for 20 to 25 percent of cases of idiopathic nephrotic syndrome.

Based on histologic and ultrastructural features, four stages of the disease are described that give an approximation of the duration, severity, and progression of the disease. The clinical presentation is dominated by proteinuria and microscopic hematuria. The nephrotic syndrome is common but not specific. The diagnosis requires histologic examination of the renal tissue. Between 60 and 80 percent of cases are classified as idiopathic; the rest are secondary to a variety of causes including infections, autoimmune conditions, toxic agents, and malignancies (see ▶Tab. 15.14).

In the child or adolescent, the incidence of membranous nephropathy is not well established but is uncommon. In contrast to adults, in whom primary membranous nephropathy is more frequent, the secondary forms of the disease predominate in pediatric patients (35%). The nephrotic syndrome is the most common presentation of the disease, but in 7 percent nonnephrotic-range proteinuria and/or abnormal urinary sediment may be the presenting findings.

Etiology and pathogenesis of membranous nephropathy

The etiology of primary MN in humans is unknown; however, previous rat research has elucidated the in situ formation of immune complexes following the deposit of antibodies against locally induced or intrinsic antigens in the glomerular capillary wall membrane (17). The antibodies in rat studies are directed to megaline complex, a glycoprotein located in the sole of the foot processes. In humans that glycoprotein does not appear in this location. In recent years substantial advances in the understanding of MN in humans has occurred by the identification of two antigens responsible for the development of MN in humans. First, neutral endopeptidase (NEP) was identified as the antigen in membranous nephrotic syndrome in newborn infants resulting from fetomaternal alloimmunization in NEP-deficient mothers, who are able to transfer IgG antibodies to the fetus via the placenta and induce membranous nephropathy. The disease in the newborn resolves spontaneously within a few months with the disappearance of the circulating maternal antibodies.

Second, Salant and colleagues demonstrated the high proportion of patients with idiopathic membranous nephropathy having circulating antibodies to phospholipases

Tab. 15.14: Conditions associated with membranous nephropathy (18,20).

Autoimmune/collagen vascular disease	Medications
Autoantibodies against M-type phospholipase A-2 receptor (PLA2R) Autoantibodies against neutral endopeptidase (NEP) Lupus nephritis class V Rheumatoid arthritis Autoimmune thyroiditis Primary biliary cirrhosis Crohn's disease Sjögren's syndrome Ankylosis spondilitis Infectious and parasitic diseases Hepatitis B Hepatitis C Syphilis (congenital syphilis/latent syphilis) Malaria Schistosomiasis Filariasis	Penicillamine Gold salts Captopril Mercury Trimethadioine Neoplasms Carcinomas of colon, lungs, breast stomach, pancreas, kidney, prostate and cervix Melanoma Wilms' tumor Lymphocytic leukemia Hodgkin's disease Others: renal transplantation, sarcoidosis, sickle cell disease, Guillain-Barré syndrome

A2 receptor, a transmembrane protein located in podocytes; this group also noted that the anti–M type PLA2R-IgG4 subclass was the predominant antibody (36). These new developments will facilitate the diagnosis of patients that until now have been classified as having primary or idiopathic MN. The recurrence of MN after renal transplantation in association with high levels of anti-PLA2R antibodies – and remission of the disease with appropriate immunosuppression, correlating with a decline in the anti-PLA2R antibodies titer – is confirmatory evidence of the role of these antibodies in the formation of MN.

Diagnosis of membraneous nephropathy

There are no specific clinical or laboratory findings that permit the diagnosis of MN. However, some clinical features seem to be relevant. For example, there is a higher tendency for the development of thromboembolic disease (i.e., deep venous thrombosis, renal vein thrombosis, pulmonary embolism).

The diagnosis of MN requires renal biopsy and special histopathologic studies. Histopathologic diagnosis is established by renal biopsy, with special staining techniques (silver-methenamine, periodic acid–Schiff [PAS]), immunofluorescence, and electron microscopy. Plasma C3 is usually normal, whereas terminal complement component C5b-9 is reported to be elevated in urine. Because secondary forms of the disease are more common in the young, a report of the renal biopsy read as MN means that it becomes necessary to exclude secondary causes of the disease before starting the patient on potentially toxic immunosuppressive medication. This possibility is particularly relevant in the elderly.

All patients with MN and negative serology for lupus or SLE will require further evaluation before the disease is considered to be idiopathic. With the present level of understanding of the causes of MN, it is reasonable to look for the presence of M-type phospholipase A2 receptor antibodies (36). Complete evaluation for current or previous infection with hepatitis B (HBV) and C (HCV) is also necessary. Because serology studies may be negative in the presence of active infection, the most accurate test is DNA-polymerase chain reaction (PCR) for hepatitis B virus and RNA-PCR for hepatitis C virus infection.

Because of the serious risk of exacerbating the infection with immunosuppression, it is necessary to treat active hepatitis viral infections before starting immunosuppression; additionally, effective antiviral therapy alone may cause remission of the proteinuria in up to 60 percent of cases (37). The goal in treating HBV infection is to control replication, but the goal for HCV infection is to eradicate the virus. As a general rule the treatment of HCV infection is more difficult than the treatment of HBV infection. HBV infection can be treated with IFN-α or pegylated IFN-α. However, these agents cannot be used in advanced chronic kidney disease (CKD stage 3) with an estimated GFR (eGFR) below 30 mL/min; therefore nucleotide analogues to IFN-α (such as entecavir or adefovir) are commonly used. In addition, steroids or other immunosuppressive therapy or anti–B cell therapy may be indicated.

Accepted therapy for MN and MPGN due to HCV infection and the duration and the type of therapy are determined by the viral genotype and the GFR. For patients with eGFR greater than 30 mL/min and HCV genotype 1, pegylated IFN-α_{2a} with ribavirin is administered for 48 weeks. For HCV genotypes 2 and 3, the duration is 24 weeks. Steroids, immunosuppression, or anti–B cell therapy may also be indicated. For those with eGFR greater than 30 mL/min, pegylated IFN-α_{2a} is given as tolerated;steroids, immunosuppression, or anti–B cell therapy may also be indicated. In these patients monitoring of clinical condition, viral load, urinary protein/creatinine ratio, urinary sediment, eGFR, and cryocrit are necessary.

Treatment of membranous nephropathy

The decision to treat a patient with membranous nephropathy requires the consideration of many factors, including understanding the natural progression of the disease. Spontaneous remission of the disease is seen in up to 30 percent of cases, particularly in younger patients. There is also a correlation with male gender, older age, hypertension, severity of proteinuria at presentation, hypoalbuminemia, and elevated serum creatinine. In secondary forms of membranous nephropathy (i.e., Hashimoto's thyroiditis, membranous lupus nephritis), treatment consists in discontinuation of the offending agent and treatment of the viral infection or autoimmune disease. Nonimmune suppressive treatment includes control of blood pressure with antihypertensive and antiproteinuric medication such as ACE inhibitors or ARBs, lipid-lowering agents, prophylactic anticoagulation, and control of edema.

Immunosuppressive treatment of membranous nephropathy usually includes cytotoxic agents such as cyclophosphamide plus steroids, usually for several months (▶Tabs. 15.9 and 15.11). For those patients who do not respond traditional immunosuppressant therapy, other therapies are currently been evaluated, some of which have shown encouraging results (38,39,40) Autoantibodies to the M-type phospholipase A2 receptor are sensitive and specific for idiopathic membranous nephropathy. The anti–B cell monoclonal antibody rituximab is a promising new therapeutic agent for this condition; it is currently being evaluated. In a group of 25 patients with idiopathic membranous nephropathy whose M-type phospholipase A2 receptor antibody titers were known before treatment with rituximab (and the titers were repeated after treatment), the autoantibodies disappeared or declined within 12 months after the administration of this agent in 68 percent of those treated (41). The disappearance or decline of the autoantibodies predicted a positive response to treatment before changes in proteinuria were detected (41).

There is no specific treatment for membranous nephropathy. Additionally, spontaneous remission of membranous nephropathy may occur in up to 40 percent of children or adolescents with the nephrotic syndrome. A period of nonspecific treatment with ACE inhibitors, close supervision of renal function, and monitoring of severity of proteinuria is a reasonable approach for the adolescent with membranous nephropathy. Immunosuppression is indicated if there is deterioration of renal function or if the proteinuria is severe.

15.5.6 Management of nephrotic syndrome

General considerations

Current strategies for the treatment of nephrotic syndrome in these various disorders are continuously evolving and undergoing considerable reassessment. Most specific treatments require the use of high-dose corticosteroids and, frequently, systemic immunosuppressive agents. The potential short- and long-term side effects of these agents are considerable. Where eradication or medical control of the underlying disease is not possible, symptomatic treatment is often used. These treatments most often use a combination of modest dietary sodium restriction in conjunction with diuretics to control the degree of edema while taking care not to compromise the plasma volume. New strategies for the symptomatic medical control of nephrotic edema and the long-term management of intractable proteinuria are currently under investigation. Treatment of associated infections is always important (▶Tabs. 15.9 and 15.11).

15.6 Diabetic nephropathy

The incidence of childhood type 1 diabetes has dramatically increased, especially for children below 5 years of age. The development of vascular disease associated with diabetes represent a high risk for the long-term complications seen in this disease, resulting in significant decrease in the life expectancy of these individuals (42). Diabetic nephropathy, one of the serious complications of diabetes, affects up to 40 percent of patients with diabetes type 1 and is the principal cause of ESRD in developed and developing countries around the world. The development of microalbuminuria with type I diabetes occurs in pubertal and postpubertal patients and thus is an important concern for physicians caring for these populations. The natural evolution of diabetic nephropathy is summarized in ▶Tab. 15.15 (43).

Tab. 15.15: Stages of type 1 diabetic nephropathy: Structural and functional changes from reference.

	Main structural alterations	Albumin excretion	GFR	Blood pressure
Stage 1 at diagnosis of hyperfunction/ hypertrophy	Increased renal size	May be increased but normalizes after initiation of insulin treatment	Increased by 20%–50%	Normal
Stage 2 (after 2–5 years) normoalbuminuria, silent phase	Basement membrane thickening	Normal with increased; related to poor glycemic control or exercise	Normal or increased by 20%–50%	Normal
Stage 3 (after 6–15 years): incipient diabetic nephropathy/ microalbuminuria	Further basement membrane thickening and mesangial expansion	Increased: 20–200 µg/min or 30–300 mg/24 h	Normal/ increased	increasing
Stage 4 (after 15–25 years) overt diabetic nephropathy, macroalbuminuria	Marked renal abnormalities	Further increased: >200 µg/minor >300 mg/24 h	Decreased	Increased
Stage 5 (after 25–30 years)	Advanced glomerulopathy	Macroalbuminuria; often decreased owing to glomerular occlusion	Markedly decreased	Increased

There are several known risk factors for the progression of diabetes to diabetic nephropathy; some of these factors are amenable to modification and therefore prevention of progression. Other factors are not modifiable, such as duration of diabetes, genetic factors, and puberty. Because the initial morphologic and functional abnormalities develop at puberty and ESRD is seldom seen at this young age there is an opportunity for preventive measures to be implemented to control those factors (▶Tab. 15.16). It has been known for a long time that the renin angiotensin aldosterone system plays an important role in the progression of diabetic nephropathy. The most active component of the angiotensin II system, is a potent vasoconstrictor that induces hypertension, can induce cell proliferation, matrix expansion, and through the activation of transforming growth factor beta, induces fibrosis.

Current clinical data indicate that the development of nephropathy can be delayed with excellent glycemic control. Data also suggest that ACE inhibitors and ARBs are not indicated in diabetic patients without microalbuminuria or hypertension (44). Recommendations for patients with diabetes include vigorous glycemic control. After 5 years of the onset of diabetes, yearly screening for microalbuminuria is indicated. If microalbuminuria is detected, a repeat determination should occur 3 months later; if microalbuminuria is confirmed on three occasions, treatment with ACE inhibitors or ARBs is indicated. The dose is titrated to the therapeutic response. The simultaneous use of both classes of medications has been helpful in some cases.

15.7 Hematuria

15.7.1 Etiology

Gross or microscopic hematuria in an adolescent is a common occurrence. Evaluation of the possibility of RBC products in the urine requires both dipstick and microscopic analyses. Most dip-and-read urine stick products are very sensitive, with detection ranges as low as the equivalent of 2 to 5 RBCs per high-power field on microanalysis. Red or red-brown discolored urine or clear urine testing positive for blood on dipstick may indicate the the presence of hemoglobinuria or myoglobinuria rather than hematuria. The absence of RBCs on microanalysis should suggest either of the two former diagnoses, although the possibilities of RBC lysis in a very hypotonic urine (specific

Tab. 15.16: Strategies for prevention of diabetic nephropathy in children and adolescents (39).

Glycemic control, avoiding hypoglycemia.

Evaluation and treatment for microalbuminuria starting at 10 years of age if diabetes ≥5 years' duration.

Treatment of hypertension to bring blood pressure to normal levels using ACE inhibitors.

Monitoring and treatment of hyperlipidemia. There is no consensus in the use of statins in children and adolescents.

Prevention of obesity; avoid excess of protein intake.

Regular moderate exercise.

Avoidance of smoking.

gravity <1.007) or a false-positive result should also be considered. False-positives may occur in the presence of oxidizing contaminants, such as hypochlorite disinfecting solutions and high urinary bacterial contents with release of bacterial peroxidases. False-negative results occur in the presence of high concentrations of urinary ascorbic acid. Non-RBC products that may give the urine a reddish, smoky, or dark appearance should also be considered when the dipstick fails to be positive for blood. Urate crystals, berries, beets, and vegetable dyes as well as alcaptonuria, tyrosinosis, porphyrin compounds, and bile may all cause factitious hematuria.

The presence of 10 or more RBCs per high-power field on a spun urine specimen is considered abnormal in most laboratories. However, borderline RBC counts should be reaffirmed on at least two additional urinalyses, since as many as 80 percent of cases of microscopic hematuria detected on an initial urinalysis will be transient. Transient hematuria may be encountered in association with various conditions, as noted in ▶Tab. 15.17. Vigorous exercise or a period of strenuous training can also cause hematuria, which may be accompanied by proteinuria as well as casts; it typically clears within 24 hours.

15.7.2 Diagnosis

Persistent or recurrent hematuria warrants a thorough investigation for an underlying cause. The initial evaluation should include a carefully focused history, family history, and physical examination, all of which can contribute significantly to the diagnostic evaluation. ▶Tab. 15.18 describes general components of the initial clinical evaluation which often prove useful. The diagnostic studies appropriate to the adolescent with hematuria will largely depend upon the suspected site and etiology of the bleeding.

15.7.3 Laboratory studies

Localization of the site of urinary bleeding is often useful in the initial diagnostic evaluation. Hematuria originating in the kidney is often characterized by brown or cola-colored urine. The concomitant presence of greater than 2+ protein by dipstick, or RBC casts, WBC casts, deformed (dysmorphic) RBC, or renal tubular epithelial cells in urine sediment, increases the likelihood of bleeding from the renal parenchyma, especially from glomerular causes. Lower urinary tract bleeding is more often characterized by terminal hematuria, passage of blood clots, and/or normal RBC morphology on microanalysis.

If the cause of the hematuria is not evident from historical and physical findings, the initial empirical evaluation should begin with a urine microanalysis, from which it is

Tab. 15.17: Conditions associated with transient hematuria.

Ciprofloxacin: 250 mg twice daily for 3 days* (used off label for patients who are prepubescent)
Levofloxacin 250 mg once a day for 3 days
Nitrofurantoin: 50–100 mg four times daily for 7 days
Trimethoprim/sulfamethoxazole double strength (160 mg/800 mg) twice daily for 3 days
Trimethroprim: 100 mg twice daily for 3 days
Others: See text

---

*Used with permission from Torres AD, Greydanus DE: Genitourinary and renal disorders. In DE Greydanus, DR Patel, HD Pratt, eds. Essential Adolescent Medicine. New York: McGraw-Hill; 206:568.

Tab. 15.18: Common components of the clinical evaluation of hematuria.

History of	Suggests
Dysuria, fever	Upper or lower UTI
Headache, rash, arthralgias, others	Systemic infection, vasculitis, collagen vascular diseases, Henoch-Schönlein nephritis
Sinusitis, cough, headache, epistaxis	Wegener's granulomatosis
Flank pain	Renal calculus, acute urinary obstruction, subacute pyelonephritis, cystic diseases
Intermittent gross hematuria	IgA and IgG nephritis; urethritis, foreign body, hypercalciuria, neoplasm (rare)
Antecedent viral illness	Postinfectious nephritis, IgA nephropathy, other nephritis
Cola-colored urine, edema, hypertension	Glomerulonephritis
Bloody diarrhea	Hemolytic uremic syndrome (serotoxin-producing *E. coli* and others)
Family history of:	
Microhematuria	Thin basal membrane disease, hereditary nephritis, hypercalciuria
Hearing loss	Hereditary nephritis
Renal failure	Hereditary nephritis, cystic kidney disease
Anemia	Sickle cell disease or trait
Physical findings of:	
Hypertension	Acute or chronic glomerulonephritis
Edema, ascots	Glomerulonephritis, membranous nephropathy, focal sclerosis
Bruising	Coagulopathy, collagen vascular disease
Heart murmur, fever	Subacute bacterial endocarditis
Purpura	Systemic infection, Henoch-Schönlein nephritis
Flank mass	Polycystic kidney disease, obstructive uropathy, renal tumor, multicystic dysplastic kidney

Used with permission from Torres AD, Greydanus DE: Genitourinary and renal disorders. In DE Greydanus, DR Patel, HD Pratt, eds. Essential Adolescent Medicine. New York: McGraw-Hill; 206:568.

determined whether the bleeding is more likely glomerular or extraglomerular (i.e., nonparenchymal). As noted above, the presence of no RBCs and/or pigmented urine casts should raise the possibility of pigmenturia from hemoglobin or myoglobin. Others to consider in the appropriate setting include intravascular coagulation, mechanical RBC damage (e.g., artificial heart valves), hemolytic anemia (e.g., G6PD deficiency, mismatched blood transfusion), as well as muscle injuries (crush, electrical, posttraumatic compartment syndrome), myositis, and rhabdomyolysis.

A microanalysis showing a dysmorphic RBC subpopulation or RBC casts is indicative of glomerular or renal parenchymal bleeding. In this case, a serum C_3 is often useful to distinguish hypocomplementemic from normocomplementemic causes of renal parenchymal bleeding. In contrast, the absence of urinary casts and the presence of morphologically normal RBCs on microanalysis should suggest extraparenchymal bleeding.

Ultrasound of the kidneys and bladder is a useful and noninvasive tool in the initial evaluation of suspected renal structural abnormalities. Hypercalciuria also appears to be increasingly associated with hematuria and the subsequent risk of urolithiasis. A random daytime urine specimen, in which the ratio of the calcium concentration divided by the creatinine concentration (both expressed in the same units) is greater than 0.21, suggests the presence of hypercalciuria. In the setting of a history or family history suggestive of renal parenchymal disease, or the identification of physical or laboratory findings compatible with underlying glomerulonephritis or renal dysfunction, the decision as to the most appropriate subsequent evaluation (including the possible need for renal biopsy) and/or treatment should be made in conjunction with a specialist in nephrology.

15.8 Glomerulonephritis (GN)

15.8.1 General

Infection-related glomerulonephritis (▶Tab. 15.19) is declining, particularly in developed countries; specifically, acute poststreptococcal glomerulonephritis is in decline

Tab. 15.19: Causes and important characteristics of postinfectious GN (45).

Name	Site of infection	Organism	Comment
Acute poststreptococcal GN	URI, pharyngitis tonsillitis, cellulitis	*Streptococcus* group A (*Streptococcus pyogenes*) especially those with specific M types or C (*Stertococcus zooepidemicus*)	Onset of GN is between 7 and 21 days after onset of the infection; GN can be severe; recovery is the rule especially in children.
Acute flare of IgA nephritis	URI, pharyngitis, tonsillitis, gastroenteritis, cystitis, vaginitis	Bacterial or viral pathogens	Onset of the GN is usually 1–3 days after onset of the infection; usually the GN is mild, although gross hematuria may be present
Other acute infection	Pneumonia, gastroenteritis	*Streptococcus pneumoniae, Klebsiella, Mycoplasma, Salmonella,* enterohemorrhagic *E. coli*	The GN appears during the acute infection; the GN is usually mild, manifested by hematuria, but not always, it may be severe in some cases.

URI, upper respiratory infection; GN, glomerulonephritis.

owing to the successful treatment of streptococcal infections. However, because of the emergence of antibiotic-resistant staphylococcal strains such as methicillin-resistant *S. aureus* (MRSA), the acute form of glomerulonephritis with active infection is on the rise. These conditions must be considered as separated entities, diagnosed, and treated accordingly (45)

In postinfectious GN the patient has had an infection that resolves naturally or with the help of antibiotics. After 2 to 22 days of the initiation of the infection, the first manifestations of GN appear with gross hematuria, hypertension, and proteinuria; usually by this time the infection has resolved. However, the postinfectious GN is just beginning and the clinical manifestations may be mild or severe. The use of antimicrobial therapy will not modify the disease process at this point.

In the case of GN of active infection (▶Tab. 15.20), the patient develops an infection that does not resolve naturally. If the infection is considered superficial, local antibiotics may be applied and the seriousness of the infection may be missed. The renal involvement will become manifest weeks later with hematuria, proteinuria, hypertension, decreased complement C3 levels, decreased total complement, and elevated serum creatinine. Contrary to what is seen in postinfectious GN, in active infection-related GN, antimicrobial agents are necessary to treat and resolve the GN. If the infection is not treated, the GN may progress to chronic GN.

15.8.2 Poststreptococcal glomerulonephritis

General

Acute poststreptococcal glomerulonephritis (PSGN) is the most commonly encountered form of postinfectious nephritis in children and younger adolescents. This inflammatory renal disorder results from immune complex formation and localization within the

Tab. 15.20: Causes and important characteristics of active infection–related GN (45).

Name	Site of infection	Organism	Comment
Staphylococcal-related GN	Ischemic limb, cellulitis, endocarditis, osteomyelitis, shunts, pneumonia, CVC, unknown	Coagulase-positive *Staphylococcus*, often MRSA.	Likely the most common cause of GN from chronic bacterial infection.
Other bacterial-related GN	Deep-seated visceral abscess (thoracic, abdominal) osteomyelitis, endocarditis, shunts, CVC infection	Gram-positive or gram-negative organisms.	Severe acute kidney injury is common.
Viral infections	HBV. HCV, HIV, CMV, parvovirus	The GN can be mitigated by antimicrobial therapy.	
Nonbacterial, nonviral infections	Visceral organs are the usual sites	Parasites, spirochetes, fungi, others.	These are rare in North America and western Europe.

CVC, central venous catheter; CMV, cytomegalovirus.

glomerulus associated with specific M-serotype nephritogenic group A as well as group C streptococcal infections. Most commonly the sites of infection are the upper respiratory tract (pharyngitis, otitis, sinusitis) and the skin. The appearance of respiratory tract–associated PSGN is typically 7 to 14 days after onset of the infection, whereas onset of pyoderma-associated nephritis may take as long as 3 weeks. Late treatment (more than 36 hours after the onset of infection) or treatment at the time of appearance of the nephritis does not appear to modify the course of the renal disease. The typical clinical findings of PSGN include the triad of sudden onset of gross hematuria, volume overload (often manifesting as edema or cardiopulmonary congestion), and hypertension. However, many patients may be discovered to have asymptomatic disease, especially during periods of epidemic streptococcal disease.

PSGN: Laboratory studies

The diagnosis of PSGN relies upon the demonstration of the causative organism, although prior empiric therapy may preclude this option. Serologic tests for evidence of a preceding streptococcal infection are often useful; however, both chronic asymptomatic streptococcal carriage as well as elevated streptococcal-associated antibody levels are frequently present in unaffected individuals.

Most patients with suspected PSGN are screened with the streptozyme test, which screens for antibodies to several streptococcal antigens. A positive test should be confirmed with specific titers. Approximately 70 percent of patients with pharyngitis-associated PSGN will have increased titers of antistreptolysin-O (ASO), although the rise of the ASO titer in pyoderma-associated PSGN is less common. The combination of ASO, antihyaluronidase, and antideoxyribonuclease B (anti–DNAase B) titers should provide evidence of a recent streptococcal infection in almost all patients. Renal biopsy is not routinely indicated; however, it may be required when the presentation is atypical, as in rapidly progressive renal insufficiency, severe nephrotic syndrome, or persistent hypocomplementemia lasting for more than 8 weeks, suggesting other renal disease. Renal biopsy shows a diffuse mesangioproliferative pattern of injury. In severe cases crescentic lesions may be observed.

Decreased serum C3 levels are detected in approximately 90 percent of the cases. Therefore adolescents with acute glomerulonephritis who have normal C3 values at the time of onset should have consideration for other forms of nephritis. In addition, the serum C3 levels almost invariably return to normal within 6 to 8 weeks of onset of the nephritis. Thus serial complement measurements are necessary to document the diagnosis. Since other forms of chronic glomerulonephritis may become clinically exacerbated in association with an acute viral illness, variation from the typical clinical presentation and course should prompt a more thorough evaluation. Also, other acute bacterial and viral illnesses may be associated with a similar clinical presentation of acute nephritis.

Management

Culture, early diagnosis, and prompt treatment of any residual streptococcal infection may prevent the development of the disease. The antibiotic of choice is penicillin by injection or oral administration. Other suitable antibiotic may be used if penicillin cannot be administered. Preventive use of antibiotics may be indicated in siblings.

The management of acute nephritis requires evaluation and treatment of the associated hypertension. Long-acting calcium channel blockers may be the better antihypertensive medications, particularly in the presence of decreased renal function and/or hyperkalemia. In hypertensive encephalopathy we prefer nicardipine because is easy to administer. ACE inhibitors can be used if renal function is not compromised and hyperkalemia is not an issue. A low-sodium diet and fluid restriction may be necessary. The use of loop diuretics is indicated to treat edema and hypertension when there is intravascular congestion. Renal replacement therapy by peritoneal dialysis or hemodialysis is less frequently needed in the child or adolescent than in the adult. In rapidly progressive deterioration of renal function, a renal biopsy may demonstrate crescentic glomerulonephritis; the use of pulse methylprednisolone is then indicated (46).

Prognosis

Current data indicate that the vast majority of patients with PSGN can fully recover if morbidity associated with the clinical presentation (e.g., hypertensive encephalopathy, congestive heart failure, mineral imbalance associated with acute renal failure, and serious infection) can be avoided. This favorable prognosis excludes the very small percentage of patients who have PSGN manifesting as the clinical syndrome of acute oliguric renal failure associated with crescentic glomerulonephritis and individuals in the older population.

15.9 Henoch-Schönlein purpura (HSP) nephritis

The European League against Rheumatism/Pediatric Rheumatology European Society (EULAR/PReS) endorsed criteria for childhood vasculitis criteria for HSP that include the presence of palpable purpura as a mandatory criterion and any one of the following: diffuse abdominal pain, any biopsy showing IgA deposition arthritis or arthralgias, renal involvement, and any hematuria and/or proteinuria (47). HSP is the most common vasculitis in childhood, with an annual incidence of 14 cases in 100,000 children; however, the incidence varies with the geographic area studied. The purpura/petechiae and palpable rash primarily involve the lower extremities, buttocks, and distal upper extremities. It can also involve the scrotum and mimic torsion of the testicle.

Factors triggering HSP is frequently preceded by an infection in up to 50 percent of the cases; however, no specific antigen has been identified causing the disease. Bacterial as well as viral infections have been linked to the disease, including *Streptococcus* β, *Yersenia,Mycoplasma*, *Toxoplasma*, varicella, measles, rubella, adenovirus, and HIV. The HSP clinical manifestations are generally mild, and therapy is basically supportive, with treatment of symptoms. The arthralgias/arthritis can be treated with the appropriated NSAIDs; the abdominal pain usually responds to small dose of steroids, with rapid resolution. Recurrent severe abdominal pain and necrotizing skin lesions have been treated by the infusion of immunoglobulin. Early steroidal treatment of HSP has been reported to prevent the development of HSP nephritis (48). Renal manifestations of HSP include isolated gross or microscopic hematuria, proteinuria, and occasionally the nephrotic syndrome.

There is a selection bias related to the severity of the renal manifestations of the disease between those patients seen in a general practice as compared with those seen by the pediatric or adult nephrologist. Glomerulonephritis occurs in 20 to 30 percent of the patients, although severe nephritis (nephrotic-range proteinuria, hypertension, and azotemia) occurs less than 10 percent of the time; progression to ESRD occurs in severe cases of HSP affecting adults and children.

Renal biopsy is indicated in patients with deteriorating renal function, persistent proteinuria, and hypertension. The predominant renal lesion is that of a mesangioproliferative disease; characteristically, immunofluorence reveals predominant deposition of immunoglobulin A and codominance of C3 in some cases. There is a good correlation between the severity of the histologic lesions and the clinical severity of the disease. Patients with active disease may respond to treatment with corticosteroids and azathioprine (49). Adolescents with rapidly progressive glomerulonephritis and crescents on renal biopsy benefit from aggressive therapy including pulse methylprednisolone, cyclophosphamide, and plasmapheresis (▶Tabs. 15.9 and 15.11). Up to 15 percent of patient with severe HSP nephritis (histology IV–VI) will advance to ESRD. The disease has the tendency to recur in the transplanted kidney.

15.10 IgA nephropathy

Since the initial description by Jean Berger in 1968, IgA nephropathy is now recognized as the most common pattern of glomerulonephritis around the world, including in those countries that regularly perform renal biopsies in patients with hematuria and proteinuria. It is known as an important cause of chronic kidney disease and ESRD. The triggering mechanisms for the development of IgA nephropathy are not well known. In the case of HSP, infections have been considered important in some cases and the association with systemic diseases is well established, including chronic inflammatory bowel disease, dermatitis, malignancies, and chronic liver disease. A particularly severe disease is seen with *S. aureus* infection.

There is a wide range of clinical manifestations of IgA nephropathy, including recurrent macroscopic hematuria as well as asymptomatic urinary abnormalities (microhematuria and mild proteinuria), nephrotic syndrome, and chronic kidney disease. The renal biopsy most often reveals mesangial proliferation with dominance of immunoglobulin IgA deposition. The severity of the histologic manifestations also correlates with the clinical manifestations. From the histopathologic viewpoint, the lesions seen in IgA nephropathy are very similar to those observe in HSP nephritis.

The transformation of IgA nephropathy to HSP has been documented. In IgA nephropathy it is known that abnormal glycosylation of the IgA1 molecule occurs. It seems that the relationship between HSP and IgA nephropathy is more fundamental than superficial. IgA nephropathy becomes a chronic kidney disease in up to 40 percent of adults and leads to ESRD 15 years after renal biopsy.

The treatment of IgA nephropathy includes normalization of blood pressure, reduction of proteinuria, and decreased IgA formation. Recurrence of IgA nephropathy after transplantation of a related-donor graft is higher than in patients who received a deceased-donor renal graft (51).

15.11 Hemolytic-uremic syndrome

15.11.1 General

Hemolytic-uremic syndrome (HUS) is not truly a glomerulonephritis. Rather, it is a thrombotic microangiopathy affecting the kidney whose causes are multiple and include infections, genetic conditions, and acquired disorders of the alternate pathway of complement activation; other genetic and acquired disorders include von Willebrand proteinase deficiency (ADAMS13), defects in cobalamin metabolism, cancer chemotherapy, ionizing radiation, calcineurin inhibitors, pregnancy, sclerodermas crisis, and unclassified causes.

The most common cause of HUS in the United States is infection by Shiga toxin–producing organisms, in particular enterohemorrhagic *E. coli* (EHEC), especially 0157-H7. Other Shiga toxin–producing bacteria include *Shigella dysenteriae* type-1, *Citrobacter freundii*, and others. In outbreaks of EHEC HUS, 1 in 10 infected individuals develops diarrhea; between 5 and 15 percent of individuals who experience hematochezia will develop HUS. Some 12.9 percent of children below 5 years of age with bloody diarrhea develop HUS, whereas 6 to 8 percent of children 5 years old or older with EHEC will develop HUS.

Shiga toxin–associated HUS is one of the common causes of acute kidney injury (AKI) in the United States and in the world. It is commonly designated as diarrhea-positive HUS (D+HUS), and/or typical HUS. AKI in children has an average age of onset at 3 years (2–6 years), although it can also affect younger and older individuals. In the United States it often follows a diarrheal illness due to exotoxin (Shiga toxin)-producing *E. coli* (especially 0157-H7) and other infectious agents, including *Salmonella typhi*, *Shigella*, and *Campylobacter*.

Atypical forms of HUS are usually diarrhea-negative or D-HUS and have been associated with such infectious disease agents as *S. pneumoniae* as well as HIV; other associations include cancer chemotherapy, immunosuppressant drugs (e.g., cyclosporine), pregnancy (including preeclampsia and during the postpartum period), malignant hypertension, and scleroderma. D-HUS has also been reported in families with an autosomal recessive or dominant pattern of inheritance usually related to abnormal regulation of the alternate pathway of complement activation, the most common of which is abnormalities of factor H (53).

15.11.2 Diagnosis

The clinical manifestation include a prodromal diarrhea illness with cramping abdominal pain and blood in the stool; when the diarrhea subsides the child appears pale; petechiae may be observed as well as gross hematuria and decreased urinary output. The triad of microangiopathic hemolytic anemia (with schistocytes and helmet cells), thrombocytopenia, and AKI establishes the clinical diagnosis of HUS. These conditions may frequently be associated with hypertension, seizures, and/or encephalopathy. With the application of the pediatric criteria for the severity of AKI – including risk, injury, failure, loss, and ESRD (pRIFLE), the clinician will be able to assess the severity of renal injury and the need for renal support therapy.

The treatment of EHEC Shiga toxin–induced HUS is basically supportive and the use of antibiotic is controversial, particularly in case of HEEC infection. Treatment of anemia with packed RBCs when needed, control of hypertension, restoration of fluid electrolyte and acid-base homeostasis, and careful attention to nutritional needs are the corner-stones of treatment. The use of platelet transfusion is seldom indicated. Renal support should be initiated early rather than late. Adolescents presenting with features of HUS in whom CNS and hemorrhagic findings predominate should also be considered to have thrombotic thrombocytopenic purpura (TTP); TTP is a distinct entity from HUS.

15.11.3 Prognosis

With aggressive and early treatment of fluid and electrolyte imbalances (especially po-tassium imbalance), control of elevated blood pressure, and institution of early dialysis when required, the prognosis associated with the epidemic (D+HUS) form is good; with excellent management, the mortality is less than 5 percent in young children. Currently the mortality rate for patients with D+HUS in the United States is less than 5 percent. However, these individuals compared with controls with negative history of D+HUS more often have microalbuminuria as well as hypertension, have decreased glomerular filtration rates, and in general manifest a higher prevalence of chronic kidney disease and the need for long-term follow-up (50).

Other infectious causes of HUS (such as those associated with *S. pneumoniae* sepsis) require specific therapeutic approaches, particularly in relation to the administration of blood products. There is currently no consensus among nephrologists regarding the use of washed blood products in patients with this disease. However, some still use them caution.

The severity of the HUS is worse in the atypical cases (D-HUS). Important new developments have recently occurred in understanding the diagnosis and therapeutic in-terventions in atypical cases of hemolytic uremic syndrome (D-HUS) associated with complement dysregulation, which occurs in less than 10 percent of cases of HUS in the United States (51). In D-HUS, particularly in the familial and recurrent forms of the disease, and in patients with TTP, management includes plasma exchange and plasmapheresis therapy. The short- and long-term prognosis in these patients is less favorable, and they should be managed in collaboration with a nephrologist.

15.12 Lupus nephritis

Systemic lupus erythematosus (SLE) is an autoimmune chronic inflammatory disease with protean clinical manifestations. In SLE, multiple autoantibodies in the serum react to multiple cell components, mainly those of nucleosome origin (54). It is now known that genetic factors play a significant role in the development of the disease. The prevalence of the disease is about 40 in 100,000 of the Caucasian population in Europe and in North America. Populations from Asia have a greater incidence than African Americans, followed by Hispanics. Females are more frequently affected than males in all populations; the female-to-male ratio is 2:1 in the prepubertal age group, 4.5:1 among adolescents, and 8:1 among adults. Twenty percent of SLE cases develop in childhood.

The most frequent clinical manifestations in patients with lupus include fever and weight loss, which affect all patients. Musculoskeletal findings include arthralgias, synovitis, and arthritis. Serosal involvement include pleuritis, pericarditis, and oral ulcers. Skin manifestations consist of butterfly facial rash, photodermatosis, and alopecia. Hematologic manifestations are anemia, leukopenia, thrombocytopenia, and thrombosis associated with antiphospholipid antibodies.

Lupus glomerulonephritis is a common and serious feature of SLE . The term *lupus glomerulonephritis* denotes the spectrum of immune complex–mediated renal diseases secondary to SLE. The renal manifestations are extremely heterogeneous and may affect the glomeruli, tubules, interstitium, and blood vessels. Proteinuria is present in 100 percent of cases with nephrotic-range proteinuria occurring in between 45 percent and 65 percent. Clinical or morphologic involvement of the kidneys occurs in 50 to 80 percent of lupus patients at any time during the course of their disease. Moreover, renal alterations are found in 90 percent of patients at autopsy. The lowest 5-year survival has been reported in patients with CNS and renal involvement. Abnormal urinary sediment includes granular casts and red cell casts. Microscopic hematuria is seen in up to 80 percent of cases, and gross hematuria in 1 to 2 percent. Reduced renal function at presentation is present in 40 to 80 percent of cases. Rapid progressive glomerulonephritis occurs in up to 30 percent of patients. Acute renal injury with failure occurs at presentation in 1 to 2 percent of cases. Hypertension is common, affecting up to 50 percent of cases. Hyperkalemia is reported in 15 percent of patients. Tubular abnormalities (distal renal tubular acidosis type IV), are usually asymptomatic and are described in about 60 percent of patients.

15.12.1 Serology

Anti-dsDNA is noted in 40 to 90 percent of patients with a high specificity and with an association with disease activity. Anti-SSA/Ro is noted in 35 percent with a low specificity and no disease activity association. Anti-SSB/La is seen in 15 percent with no disease activity association and low specificity. Anti-Sm is noted in 5 to 30 percent with high specificity and no disease activity association. Finally, Anti-C1q has a frequency of 80 to 100 percent; it has high specificity and is associated with disease activity.

15.12.2 Classification

There have been several pathologic classifications of lupus nephritis. The current classification, according to the in the International Society of Nephrology/Renal Pathology Society (ISN/PRS) 2004 is depicted in ▶Tab. 15.21.

15.12.3 Treatment of lupus nephritis

Treatment of lupus nephritis depends on the classification of the severity of the disease in the individual patient. Treatment of classes I and II is supportive in nature. The treatment of classes III, IV, and V requires, in addition to supportive measures (i.e., treatment of hypertension, pain, hyperlipidemia, and avoidance of sun exposure), immunosuppression. It is useful to divide the treatment of lupus nephritis of classes III, IV, and V into two phases: induction therapy and maintenance therapy.

Tab. 15.21: Lupus neprhitis.

Class I
Minimal mesangial lupus nephritis – normal by light microscopy but mesangial deposition by immunofluorescence.

Class II
Mesangial proliferative lupus nephritis – mesangial hypercellularity and mesangial deposits by immunofluorescence.

Class III
Focal lupus nephritis –
IIIA – Purely active lesions – focal proliferative lupus nephritis
IIIA/C – Active and chronic lesions – focal proliferative and sclerosing lupus nephritis
IIIC – Chronic inactive lesions with glomerular scars – focal sclerosing lupus nephritis

Class IV
Diffuse lupus nephritis –
IVA – purely active lesions – diffuse proliferative lupus nephritis
IVA/C – active and chronic lesions – diffuse segmental or global proliferative and sclerosisng lupus nephritis
IVC – inactive with glomerular scars

Class V
Membranous lupus nephritis

Class VI
Advanced sclerosing lupus nephritis – 90 percent of glomeruli globally sclerosed without residual activity

---

The induction phase of treatment consists of high-dose intravenous pulse methyl-prednisolone 600 to 1,000 mg/m^2 (maximum 1 g) daily for 3 days. This is followed by oral prednisolone 1 to 2 mg/kg per day (maximum 60–80 mg/day) with a rapid taper. Concomitantly intravenous pulse cyclophosphamide is given monthly for 6 months, 500 to 1,000 mg/m^2. In very severe cases or when the patient does not respond to this therapy, plasma exchange daily for 5 to 10 days has been used, or rituximab may be used in more severe cases following a protocol.

Side effects of immunosuppressive therapy for lupus nephritis with methylpredniso-lone and cyclophosphamide include amenorrhea, cervical dysplasia, avascular necrosis, herpes zoster, infections, and death. These side effects are more common with cyclophosphamide given intravenously for 6 months except for vascular necrosis, which is more common with the use of intravenous methylprednisolone.

Owing to the severe toxicity of the drugs in the above protocol, the Euro-Lupus Nephritis Trial (ELNT) was developed (55). In this trial, 90 patients with diffuse proliferative or focal proliferative nephritis or membranous nephritis were randomized to receive the 6-month pulse cyclophosphamide followed by either infusion of cyclophosphamide every third month or a shorter treatment course consisting of 500 mg of cyclophosphamide given intravenously every 2 weeks for six total doses and then switched to azothiophrine maintenance therapy for 30 months. Both treatments were equally effective in several renal and extrarenal parameters, with fewer infections in the shorter-treatment group (55). Because this trial was largely performed in a Caucasian population, it is unknown if it will be equally effective in other populations.

Sequence therapies for lupus nephritis using pulse methylprednisolone 500 to 1,000 mg daily for three doses are followed by oral prednisone in a rapid taper plus a standard dose of intraveous cyclophosphamide. Maintenance therapy with mycophenolate mofetil was developed in a study involving more than 100 patients; this protocol was proven to be as effective as the previously used protocol (57).

Currently mycophenolate mofetil (MMF) and methylprednisolone have been successfully used for induction therapy, followed by MMF for maintenance therapy, without the use of cyclophosphamide. Four randomized controlled studies involving 268 patients showed a significant reduction in the risk of treatment failure in the MMF group as compared with the cyclophosphamide group (58). The risk of death or ESRD may be lower with MMF compared with cyclophosphamide, which is an important clinical finding not previously demonstrated. There was no increase in adverse events associated with MMF (58). The MMF pediatric dosage is based on body surface area (BSA). Patients with a BSA of $1.25/m^2$ to $1.5/m^2$ should receive 750 mg twice a day. Patients with a BSA greater than $1.5/m^2$ should receive 1 g twice a day. Alternatively, a dosage of 12.5 to 18 mg/kg twice a day to a daily maximum of 2 g/day for 1 to 2 years can be used.

15.13 Conclusion

The renal system is a critically important and complex organ system needed for normal growth and health in the adolescent. This chapter reviews paramount issues in this regard including urinary tract infections, proteinuria, hematuria, and glomerulonephritis. Concepts of diagnosis and management are presented. Consultation with colleagues in nephrology is recommended for adolescents with complex and refractory renal conditions.

References

1. Litza JA, Brill JR. Urinary tract infections. Prim Care 2010;37(3):491–507.
2. Dielubanza EJ, Schaeffer AJ. Urinary tract infectins in women. Med Clin North Am 2011; 95 (1): 27–41.
3. Bonny AE, Brouhard BH. Urinary tract infections among adolescents. Adolesc Med 2005; 16:149–61.
4. Meier S, Weber R, Zbinden R. Extended-spectrum β-lactamase-producing Gram-negative pathogens in community-acquired urinary tract infections: an increasing challenge for antimicrobial therapy. Infection 2011 Jun 25. [Epub ahead of print]
5. Bader MS, Hawboldt J, Brooks A. Management of complicated urinary tract infections in the era of antimicrobial resistance. Postgrad Med 2010;122 (6):7–15.
6. Saadeh SA, Mattoo TK. Managing urinary tract infections. Pediatr Nephrol 2011 Mar 16. [EPub ahead of print]
7. Neuman I, Moore P. Pyelonephritis (acute) in non-pregnant women. Clin Evid (Online) 2011 Jan 13. [EPub ahead of print]
8. Shields J, Maxwell AP. Acute pyelonephritis can have serious complications. Practitioner 2010;254:19–24.
9. Vazquez JC, Abalos E. Treatments for symptomatic urinary tract infections during pregnancy. Cochrane Database Syst Rev 2011;19(1):CD002256

10. Williams G, Craig JC. Long-term antibiotics for preventing urinary tract infection in children. Cochrane Database Sys Rev 2011;16(3):CD001534.
11. Ejernaes K. Bacterial characteristics of importance for recurrent urinary tract infections caused by Escherichia coli. Dan Med Bull 2011;58(4):B4187.
12. Epp A, Larochelle A, Lovatsis D, et al. Recurrent urinary tract infection. J Obstet Gynaecol Can 2010;32(11):1082–101.
13. Kodner CM, Thomas-Gupton EK. Recurrent urinary tract infections in women: diagnosis and management. Am Fam Physician 2010;82(6):638–43.
14. Damiano R, Quarto G, Bava I. Prevention of recurrent urinary tract infections by intravesical administration of hyaluronic acid and chondroitin sulphate: a placebo-controlled randomized trial. Eur Urol 2011;59(4):645–51.
15. Barbosa-Cesnik C, Brown MB, Buxton M, et al. Cranberry juice fails to prevent recurrent urinary tract infection: results from a randomized placebo-controlled trial. Clin Infect Dis 2011;52(1):23–30.
16. Schnarr J, Smaill F. Asymptomatic bacteriuria and symptomatic urinary tract infections in pregnancy. Eur J Clin Invest 2008;38(Suppl 2):50–57.
17. Torres AD, Greydanus DE. Orthostatic proteinuria genitourinary and renal disorders. In: Greydanus DE, Patel DR, Pratt HD, eds. Essential adolescent medicine. New York: McGraw-Hill;2006:335–36.
18. Fogo A. Renal pathology. In: Avner ED, Harmon WE, Niaudet P, Norishige Y, eds. Pediatric nephrology, 6th edition. Berlin: Springer, 2009:555.
19. Peter J Lavin PJ, Winn MP. TORcin up the importance of calcium signaling. J Am Soc Nephrol 2011;22:1391–93.
20. Hildebrandt F, Herringa SF. Specific podocin mutations determine the age of onset of nephrotic syndrome all the way into adult life. Kidney Int 2009;75:669–71.
21. Peter F. Hoyer PF. Minimal change nephrotic syndrome. In: Floege J, Johnson RJ, Feehally J, eds. Clinical nephrology, 4th ed. St Louis, MO: Elsevier Saunders, 2010:222–45.
22. Garin EH, Diaz LN, Mu W. Urinary CD80 excretion increases in idiopathic minimal-change disease. J Am Soc Nephrol 2009;20:260–66.
23. Becker DJ. Minimal change disease. Nephrol Rounds 2008;34:111–34.
24. Hodson EM, Night JF, Willis NS, Craig JC. Corticosteroid therapy for nephrotic syndrome in children. Cochrane database Syst Rev 2005;1:CD001533.
25. Hiraoka M, Tsutkahara H, Matsubara K, et al. West Japan Cooperative study Group of Kidney Disease in Children. Am J Kidney Dis 2003;41(6):1155.
26. Herlitz LC. Markowitz AB. Farris JA. Development of focal segmental glomerulosclerosis after anabolic steroid Abuse. Jam Soc Nephrolo. 2010;21:163–72.
27. Kambham N, Markowits GS, Valeri AM, et al. Obesity related glomerulopaty: An emerging epidemic. Kidney Int 2001;59(4):1498–509.
28. Ritz E, Kolgeganova T, Piecha G. Is there an obesity- metabolic syndrome related glomerulopaty? Curr Opin Hypertens 2010;45:222–31.
29. Winkler CA, Nelson G, Oleski TK, et al. Genetics of focal segmental glomerulosclerosis and human immunodeficiency virus – associated collapsing glomerulopaty: the role of the MYH9 genetic variation Sem Nephrol 2010;30(2):111–25.
30. Kaito H, Kamel K, Kikuchi E. Successful treatment of collapsing focal segmental glomerulosclerosis with a combination of rituximab, steroids and ciclosporin. Pediatr Nephrol, 2010;25(5):957–59.
31. McEnery PT, McAdams AJ, West CD. Treatment of mesangiocapillary glomerulonephritis: improved survival with alternated day prednisone therapy. Clin Nephrol 1980;13:117–24.
32. Tarshis P. Treatment of mesangiocapillary glomerulonephritis with alternate day prednisolone: a report from the international study of kidney diseases in children. Pediatr Nephrol 1992;6:123–30.

33. Smith RJ. Dense deposit disease focus group, new approaches to the treatment of dense deposit disease. J Am Soc Nephrol 2007;18:2447–56.
34. International Study of kidney diseases in Children. Nephrotic syndrome in children: Prediction of histopathology from clinical and laboratory characteristic at time of diagnosis. A report of the International study of International Study of Kidney Diseases in Children. Kidney Int 1978;13:159–65.
35. Moxey-Mims MM, Stapleton FB, Feld LG. Applying decision analysis to management to adolescents with idiopathic nephrotic syndrome. Pediatr Nephrol 1994; 8:660–64.
36. Beck LH Jr., Bonegio RG, Lambeau G. M-type phospholipases A2 receptor as target antigen in idiopathic membranous nephropathy. N Engl J Med 2009;361(1):11–21.
37. Duffield JS, Qamar A Advances in the etiology and management of immune-mediated glomerulonephritides Nephrol Rounds 2008;6(10):111–18.
38. Remuzzi G, Chiurchiu C, Abbate M. Rituximab for idiopathic membranous nephropathy. Lancet 2002;360:923–24.
39. Flavio V, Cohen SD, Appel G. Novel B cell therapeutic targets in transplantation and immune -mediated glomerular diseases. Clin J Am Soc Nephrol 2010;5:142–51.
40. Fernando C. Fervenza, Roshini S. Rituximab therapy in idiopathic membranous nephropathy: A 2-year study. Clin J Am Soc Nephrol 2010;5:2188–98.
41. Beck LH Jr., Fervenza FC, Beck DM et al. Salant Rituximab-induced depletion of anti-PLA2R autoantibodies predicts response in membranous nephropathy J Am Soc Nephrol 2011;22:1543–50.
42. Narayan KM, Boyle JP, Thompson TJ. Life time risk for diabetes mellitus in the Unites States. JAMA 2003;29:184–89.
43. Marcovecchio ML, Chiarelli F. Diabetic nephropathy. In: Avner ED, Harmon WE, Niaudet P, Yoshikawa N, eds. Pediatric nephrology, 6th ed. Berlin: Springer, 2009:324–40.
44. Bilous R, Chatuverdi N, Sjolie AK, et al. Effect of candesartan on microalbuminuria and albumin excretion rate in diabetes: Three randomized trials. Ann Intern Med 2009; 151 (1):11–20.
45. Nadasdy T, Herbert LA. Infection related glomerulonephritis: understanding mechanisms. Sem Nephrol 2011;31:369–75.
46. Rodriguez-Iturbe B, Burdmann EA, Barsoum RS. Glomerular diseases associated with Infection. In: Floege J, Johnson RJ, Feehally J, eds. Clinical nephrology, 4th edition. St Louis, MO: Elsevier Saunders, 2010:662–67.
47. Ozen S. Ruperto N Dillon MJ, et al. EULAR/PReS endorsed consensus criteria for the classification of child hood vasculitis. Ann Rheum Dis 2006;65:936–41.
48. Weiss PF, Feinstein JA, Luan X, et al. Effects of corticosteroids on Henoch-Schoenlein purpura: A systemic review. Pediatrics 2007;120:1079–87.
49. Shin JI, Park JM, Shin YH. Can Azathioprine and steroids alter the progression of Henoch-Schoenlein purpura nephritis? Pediatr Nephrol 2005;20:1087–92.
50. Sharma AP, Filler G, Dwight P, Clark WF. Chronic renal disease is more prevalent in patients with hemolytic Uremic Syndrome who had a positive history of diarrhea.Kidney Int 2010;78:598–604.
51. Waters AM, Licht C. aHUS caused by complement dysregulation: New therapies on the Horizon.Pediatr Nephrol 2011:26:41–57.
52. Koyama A, Sharmin S, Sakurai H. Staphylococcus aureus cell envelope antigen is a new candidate for the induction of IgA nephropathy, Kidney Int 2004;66:121.
53. Johnson S, Taylor CM. Hemolytic uremic Syndrome. In: Avner ED, Harmon WE, Niaudet P, Yoshikawa N, eds. Pediatric nephrology, 6th ed. Berlin: Springer, 2009:1156–58.
54. Van der Vlag J, Berden JHM. Lupus nephritis role of antinucleosome autoantibodies. Sem Nephrol 2011;31:386–89.

55. Houssiau FA, Vasconcelos C, D'Cruz D. Immunosuppressive therapy in lupus nephritis: the Euro-Lupus Trial, a randomized trial of low-dose versus high-dose intravenous cyclophosphamide. Arthritis Rheum 2002;46(8):2121–31.
56. Contreras G, Pardo V, Leclercq B. Sequential therapies for proliferative lupus nephritis. N Engl J Med 2004;350(10):971–76.
57. Appel GB, Contreras G, Dooley MA. Lupus Management Study Group. J Am Soc Nephrol 2009;20(5):1103.
58. Walsh M,. Mycophenolate mofetil for induction therapy of lupus nephritis: A systemic review and meta-analysis. Clin J Am Soc Nephrol 2007;2:968–75.

Acknowledgments

16 About the editors

Donald E. Greydanus, MD, Dr. HC (ATHENS), FAAP, FSAM (Emeritus), FIAP (HON) is Professor of Pediatrics and Human Development at Michigan State University College of Human Medicine (East Lansing, Michigan) and Director of the Pediatrics Residency Program at Michigan State University/Kalamazoo Center for Medical Studies (Kalamazoo, Michigan). Received the 1995 American Academy of Pediatrics' Adele D. Hofmann Award for "Distinguished Contributions in Adolescent Health," the 2000 Mayo Clinic Pediatrics Honored Alumnus Award for "National Contributions to the field of Pediatrics," and the 2003 William B Weil, Jr., MD Endowed Distinguished Pediatric Faculty Award from Michigan State University College of Medicine for "National and international recognition as well as exemplary scholarship in pediatrics." Received the 2004 Charles R Drew School of Medicine (Los Angeles) Stellar Award for contributions to pediatric resident education and awarded an honorary membership in the Indian Academy of Pediatrics – an honor granted to only a few pediatricians outside of India. Was the 2007–2010 Visiting Professor of Pediatrics at Athens University, Athens, Greece and received the Michigan State University College of Human Medicine Outstanding Community Faculty Award in 2008. In 2010 he received the title of Doctor Honoris Causa from the University of Athens (Greece) as a "distinguished scientist who through outstanding work has bestowed praise and credit on the field of adolescent medicine (Ephebiatrics)." In 2010 he received the Outstanding Achievement in Adolescent Medicine Award from the Society for Adolescent Medicine "as a leading force in the field of adolescent medicine and health." Past Chair of the National Conference and Exhibition Planning Group (Committee on Scientific Meetings) of the American Academy of Pediatrics and member of the Pediatric Academic Societies' (SPR/PAS) Planning Committee (1998 to present). Member of the Appeals Committee for the Pediatrics' Residency Review Committee (RRC) of the Accreditation Council for Graduate Medical Education (Chicago) in both adolescent medicine and general pediatrics. Numerous publications in adolescent health and lectureships in many countries on adolescent health. E-mail: Greydanus@kcms.msu.edu

Dilip R Patel, MD, FAAP, FSAM, FAACPDM, FACSM, is professor in the Department of Pediatrics and Human Development at the Michigan State University College of Human Medicine, East Lansing, Michigan. He is a full time teaching faculty member in the Pediatric Residency Program at the Michigan State University Kalamazoo Center for Medical Studies, Kalamazoo, Michigan. Dr Patel has subspecialty training and interests in neurodevelopmental disabilities, developmental-behavioral pediatrics, adolescent medicine and sports medicine. He has published numerous papers on wide ranging topics in these areas and has edited several special symposia and books. E-mail: patel@kcms.msu.edu

Cynthia L Feucht, PharmD, BCPS is adjunct professor in the Department of Pharmacy Practice at Ferris State University in Big Rapids, Michigan. She completed a specialized pharmacy residency in ambulatory care and obtained recognition as a Board Certified Pharmacotherapy Specialist. Dr. Feucht has practiced in a variety of settings including hospital, ambulatory care, academics and currently practices in ambulatory care and has interests in the areas of pediatrics and geriatrics. Dr. Feucht has taught pharmacology for different institutions and continues to teach for the School of Pharmacy at Ferris State University. She has published several papers and chapters and has also served as coeditor. E-mail: Cynthia.feucht@gmail.com

Hatim A Omar, MD, FAAP, Professor of Pediatrics and Obstetrics and Gynecology and Director of the Section of Adolescent Medicine, Department of Pediatrics, University of Kentucky, Lexington. Dr. Omar has completed residency training in obstetrics and gynecology as well as pediatrics. He has also completed fellowships in vascular physiology and adolescent medicine. He is the recipient of the Commonwealth of Kentucky Governor's Award for Community Service and Volunteerism He is the recipient of the Commonwealth of Kentucky Governer's Award for community service and volunteerism in 2000, KY teen Pregnancy Coalition Award for outstanding service 2002, Awards for suicide prevention from the Ohio Valley Society for Adolescent Medicine and Kentucky Pediatric Society in 2005 and 2007, Sexual Abuse Awareness Month Award for his work with sexual abuse victims from the KY association of sexual assault professionals in 2007, Special Achievement Award from the American Academy of Pediatrics 2007 and the Founders of Adolescent Medicine Award from the AAP in 2007. He is well known internationally with numerous publications in child health, pediatrics, adolescent medicine, pediatric and adolescent gynecology. E-mail: haomar2@uky.edu

Joav Merrick, MD, MMedSci, DMSc, is professor of pediatrics, child health and human development affiliated with Kentucky Children's Hospital, University of Kentucky, Lexington, United States and the Division of Pediatrics, Hadassah Hebrew University Medical Centers, Mt. Scopus Campus, Jerusalem, Israel, the medical director of the Health Services, Division for Intellectual and Developmental Disabilities, Ministry of Social Affairs and Social Services, Jerusalem, the founder and director of the National Institute of Child Health and Human Development in Israel. Numerous publications in the field of pediatrics, child health and human development, rehabilitation, intellectual disability, disability, health, welfare, abuse, advocacy, quality of life and prevention. Received the Peter Sabroe Child Award for outstanding work on behalf of Danish Children in 1985 and the International LEGO-Prize ("The Children's Nobel Prize") for an extraordinary contribution towards improvement in child welfare and well-being in 1987. E-mail: jmerrick@zahav.net.il

17 About the Department of Pediatrics and Human Development, Michigan State University College of Human Medicine, MSU/Kalamazoo Center for Medical Studies, Kalamazoo, Michigan, United States

The Department of Pediatrics and Human Development (PHD) at Michigan State University College of Human Medicine (MSUCHM) was developed in 1968 with the formation of the College of Human Medicine (CHM) at Michigan State University (MSU) in East Lansing, Michigan. It is a nationally recognized Department of PHD that involves four Michigan State University (MSU) campuses including East Lansing and Kalamazoo, Michigan. Michigan State University/Kalamazoo Center for Medical Studies (MSU/KCMS) is a nationally recognized university/community based residency program with over 170 residents in over 12 disciplines including pediatrics that is located in Kalamazoo, Michigan.

Mission and service

The MSUCHM PHD has a unique balance between behavioral science, basic biological research, and clinical pediatrics. The department has a commitment to a comprehensive approach to the health and development of the child, adolescent, and the family. PHD has a unique blend of community integrated medical training centers with a unified educational mission that serves medical students, pediatric residents, and four communities in Michigan.

The mission is to "advance the healthy development and well-being of children and adolescents through innovative medical education, research, clinical care, and advocacy, emphasizing community-based partnerships." To this end, the department offers a broad range of clinical and laboratory services to the children and adolescents of Michigan. PHD draws on the talents of over 100 faculty members and over 500 volunteer teaching faculty members. The mission of the Kalamazoo program (MSU/KCMS Pediatrics Program) is to train both medical students in their third and fourth years as well as many residents in the field of pediatrics. MSU/KCMS pediatrics is a fully accredited 3-year program preparing physicians for board-certification in pediatrics.

Values of MSU/KCMS include compassionate service, leadership training, commitment to lifelong learning, emphasis on teamwork, and commitment to excellence in health care. Trainees at MSU/KCMS become skilled at providing patient care that is compassionate, appropriate, and effective for the treatment of health problems and the promotion of health. They learn to demonstrate interpersonal and communication skills that result in the effective exchange of information and collaboration with patients, their families, and health professionals. They are taught to develop a commitment to carrying out professional responsibilities and an adherence to ethical principles throughout their training with a goal of these values becoming a lifelong habit that reveals professional compassion, integrity, and respect for others. Kalamazoo is the home of the Kalamazoo Promise, a truly unique program that guarantees college education for students who graduate from the Kalamazoo public schools.

Research activities

MSU/KCMS has a variety of research projects in adolescent medicine, neurobehavioral pediatrics, adolescent gynecology, pediatric diabetes mellitus, asthma, cystic fibrosis, and pediatric oncology. MSU/KCMS Pediatrics is involved with a number of studies with the Children's Oncology Group in the United States.

MSU/KCMS Pediatrics has recently published a number of medical textbooks, including Essential Adolescent Medicine (McGraw-Hill Medical Publishers), The Pediatric Diagnostic Examination (McGraw-Hill), Pediatric and Adolescent Psychopharmacology (Cambridge University Press), Behavioral Pediatrics, 2nd ed. (iUniverse Publishers in New York and Lincoln, Nebraska), Behavioral Pediatrics, 3rd ed. (New York: Nova Biomedical Books). Pediatric Practice: Sports Medicine (McGraw-Hill), Handbook of Clinical Pediatrics (Singapore: World Scientific), and Neurodevelopmental Disabilities: Clinical Care for Children and Young Adults (Dordrecht: Springer).

MSU/KCMS Pediatrics has edited a number of journal issues published by Elsevier Publishers covering pulmonology (State of the Art Reviews: Adolescent Medicine – AM:STARS), genetic disorders in adolescents (AM:STARS), neurologic/neurodevelopmental disorders (AM:STARS), behavioral pediatrics (Pediatric Clinics of North America), pediatric psychopharmacology in the 21st century (Pediatric Clinic of North America), nephrologic disorders in adolescents (AM:STARS), college health (Pediatric Clinics of North America), adolescent medicine (Primary Care: Clinics in Office Practice), behavioral pediatrics in children and adolescents (Primary Care: Clinics in Office Practice), adolescents and sports (Pediatric Clinics of North America), and developmental disabilities (Pediatric Clinics of North America). The department has also edited a journal issue on musculoskeletal disorders in children and adolescents for the American Academy of Pediatrics' AM:STARS.

The department has developed academic ties with a variety of international medical centers and organizations, including the Queen Elizabeth Hospital in Hong Kong, National Taiwan University Hospital (Taipei, Taiwan), Indian Academy of Pediatrics (New Delhi, India), the University of Athens Children's Hospital (First and Second Departments of Paediatrics) in Athens, Greece, and the National Institute of Child Health and Human Development in Jerusalem, Israel.

Contact

Professor Donald E Greydanus, MD and Professor Dilip R. Patel, MD
Pediatrics and Human Development
Michigan State University College of Human Medicine PHD Department
Michigan State University/Kalamazoo Center for Medical Studies
1000 Oakland Drive, Kalamazoo, MI 49008–1284 United States
E-mail: Greydanus@kcms.msu.edu and Patel@kcms.msu.edu
Website: http://www.kcms.msu.edu/ and http://phd.msu.edu/

18 About the Division of Adolescent Medicine at the University of Kentucky, Lexington, Kentucky

The Division of adolescent medicine was founded in 1998 to provide state-of-the-art care for adolescent patients from all areas of the commonwealth of Kentucky, to serve as a statewide resource for education and training for local providers on adolescent issues, to study specific factors on the local level affecting youth in the state, to help teach medical students and residents and to provide community service to help improve the future of teens in the commonwealth.

The division provides comprehensive, holistic team approach to adolescents, where teens receive all aspects for care from mental health to routine care from a team of professionals including physicians, mental health providers, social workers, nutritionists and nursing staff. One unique program within the division is the Young Parent Program, where pregnant teens are cared for throughout pregnancy; then they and their babies are cared for together in the program.

The division is active in research with several peer-reviewed articles published each year as well as books and special journal editions.

In the community, the program has founded several grass route programs to help prevent youth suicide, teen pregnancy, accidental death, and substance abuse among adolescents in Kentucky.

The division has provides lectures, workshops, media events and teaching for community providers, parents, teachers and school counselors. It also provides advocacy work on behalf of teens with active work at the state legislative and executive government as well as local governments to help improve the lives of teens.

Collaborations

The division collaborates locally with school boards, youth service centers, state and local governments, other universities and child advocacy centers as well as with regional adolescent medicine programs.

Internationally there are collabotations with the Institute for Child Health and Human Development in Israel, the Division of Adolescent Medicine at Santa Casa University, Brazil, Quality of Life Research Center, and Nordic School of Holistic Health, Copenhagen, Denmark, and the Department of Applied Social Sciences, Hong Kong Polytechnic University, Hong Kong.

The vision

The vision of the Division of Adolescent Medicine is to improve the health and long-term well-being of Kentucky Youth to grow into productive adults. We also envision global work to help positive youth development worldwide.

Target areas of interests

The interest areas of the division are all aspects of youth development and adolescent health with focus on prevention and community involvement in colloboration on the local, national and global level with programs having the same goal.

Contact

Hatim A. Omar, MD, FAAP
Professor, Pediatrics and Obstetrics/Gynecology
Children's Miracle Network Chair
Chief, Division of Adolescent Medicine and Young Parents Program (J422)
Kentucky Children's Hospital
UK Healthcare, Department of Pediatrics
University of Kentucky College of Medicine
Lexington, KY 40536 United States
Email: haomar2@uky.edu

19 About the National Institute of Child Health and Human Development in Israel

The National Institute of Child Health and Human Development (NICHD) in Israel was established in 1998 as a virtual institute under the auspices of the Medical Director, Ministry of Social Affairs and Social Services, in order to function as the research arm for the Office of the Medical Director. In 1998 the National Council for Child Health and Pediatrics, Ministry of Health, and in 1999 the Director General and Deputy Director General of the Ministry of Health endorsed the establishment of the NICHD. In 2011 the NICHD became affiliated with the Division of Pediatrics, Hadassah Hebrew University Medical Centers, Mt. Scopus Campus, Jerusalem.

Mission

The mission of the National Institute for Child Health and Human Development in Israel is to provide an academic focal point for the scholarly interdisciplinary study of child life, health, public health, welfare, disability, rehabilitation, intellectual disability, and related aspects of human development. This mission includes research, teaching, clinical work, information, and public service activities in the field of child health and human development.

Service and academic activities

Over the years many activities became focused in the south of Israel due to collaboration with various professionals at the Faculty of Health Sciences (FOHS) at the Ben Gurion University of the Negev (BGU). Since 2000 an affiliation with the Zusman Child Development Center at the Pediatric Division of Soroka University Medical Center has resulted in collaboration around the establishment of the Down Syndrome Clinic at that center. In 2002 a full course on "disability" was established at the Recanati School for Allied Professions in the Community, FOHS, BGU and in 2005 collaboration was started with the Primary Care Unit of the faculty and disability became part of the master of public health course on "children and society." In the academic year 2005–2006 a one-semester course on aging with disability was started as part of the master of science program in gerontology in our collaboration with the Center for Multidisciplinary Research in Aging. In 2010 began collaborations with the Division of Pediatrics, Hadassah Medical Centers, Hebrew University, Jerusalem, Israel.

Research activities

The affiliated staff have over the years published work from projects and research activities in this national and international collaboration. In the year 2000 the International Journal of Adolescent Medicine and Health and in 2005 the International Journal on Disability and Human development of De Gruyter Publishing House (Berlin and New York), in the year 2003 the TSW-Child Health and Human Development and in 2006 the TSW-Holistic Health and Medicine of the Scientific World Journal (New York and Kirkkonummi, Finland), all peer-reviewed international journals were affiliated with the National Institute of Child Health and Human Development. From 2008 also the International Journal of Child Health and Human Development (Nova Science, New York), the International Journal of Child and Adolescent Health (Nova Science) and the Journal of Pain Management (Nova Science) affiliated and from 2009 the International Public Health Journal (Nova Science) and Journal of Alternative Medicine Research (Nova Science).

National collaborations

Nationally the NICHD works in collaboration with the Faculty of Health Sciences, Ben Gurion University of the Negev; Department of Physical Therapy, Sackler School of Medicine, Tel Aviv University; Autism Center, Assaf HaRofeh Medical Center; National Rett and PKU Centers at Chaim Sheba Medical Center, Tel HaShomer; Department of Physiotherapy, Haifa University; Department of Education, Bar Ilan University, Ramat Gan, Faculty of Social Sciences and Health Sciences; College of Judea and Samaria in Ariel and in 2011 affiliation with Center for Pediatric Chronic Diseases and Center for Down Syndrome, Department of Pediatrics, Hadassah-Hebrew University Medical Center, Mount Scopus Campus, Jerusalem.

International collaborations

Internationally with the Department of Disability and Human Development, College of Applied Health Sciences, University of Illinois at Chicago; Strong Center for Developmental Disabilities, Golisano Children's Hospital at Strong, University of Rochester School of Medicine and Dentistry, New York; Centre on Intellectual Disabilities, University of Albany, New York; Centre for Chronic Disease Prevention and Control, Health Canada, Ottawa; Chandler Medical Center and Children's Hospital, Kentucky Children's Hospital, Section of Adolescent Medicine, University of Kentucky, Lexington; Chronic Disease Prevention and Control Research Center, Baylor College of Medicine, Houston, Texas; Division of Neuroscience, Department of Psychiatry, Columbia University, New York; Institute for the Study of Disadvantage and Disability, Atlanta; Center for Autism and Related Disorders, Department Psychiatry, Children's Hospital Boston, Boston; Department of Paediatrics, Child Health and Adolescent Medicine, Children's Hospital at Westmead, Westmead, Australia; International Centre for the Study of Occupational and Mental Health, Düsseldorf, Germany; Centre for Advanced

Studies in Nursing, Department of General Practice and Primary Care, University of Aberdeen, Aberdeen, United Kingdom; Quality of Life Research Center, Copenhagen, Denmark; Nordic School of Public Health, Gottenburg, Sweden, Scandinavian Institute of Quality of Working Life, Oslo, Norway; Centre for Quality of Life of the Hong Kong Institute of Asia-Pacific Studies and School of Social Work, Chinese University, Hong Kong.

Targets

Our focus is on research, international collaborations, clinical work, teaching and policy in health, disability and human development and to establish the NICHD as a permanent institute at one of the residential care centers for persons with intellectual disability in Israel in order to conduct model research and together with the four university schools of public health/medicine in Israel establish a national master and doctoral program in disability and human development at the institute to secure the next generation of professionals working in this often nonprestigious/low-status field of work.

Contact

Joav Merrick, MD, DMSc
Professor of Pediatrics, Child Health and Human Development
Medical Director, Health Services, Division for Intellectual and Developmental Disabilities, Ministry of Social Affairs and Social Services, POB 1260, IL-91012 Jerusalem, Israel.
E-mail: jmerrick@inter.net.il

Index